DR. PERRICONE'S

7 *Secrets to Beauty, Health, and Longevity*

The Miracle of Cellular Rejuvenation

BALLANTINE BOOKS • NEW YORK

DR. PERRICONE'S

7 *Secrets to Beauty, Health, and Longevity*

NICHOLAS PERRICONE, M.D.

No book can replace the diagnostic expertise and medical advice of a trusted physician. Please be certain to consult with your doctor before making any decisions that affect your health, particularly if you suffer from any medical condition or have any symptom that may require treatment.

ISBN-10 0-345-49245-5
ISBN-13 978-0-345-49245-6

Printed in the United States of America on acid-free paper

www.ballantinebooks.com

9 8 7 6 5 4 3 2 1

First Edition

Book design by Mary A. Wirth

Acknowledgments

Anne Sellaro again deserves star billing in these acknowledgments. Anne's untiring enthusiasm, hard work, creativity, and vision as friend, agent, producer, and collaborator continue to help me share my message and mission with millions of people worldwide.

I would also like to extend a warm thank-you to the great many friends and colleagues who have generously assisted me, including

Caroline Sutton, Gina Centrello, Libby McGuire, Tom Perry, Kim Hovey, Brian McClendon, Rachel Bernstein, Cindy Murray, Lisa Barnes, Christina Duffy, and the entire team at Ballantine, including the outstanding sales force

David Vigliano and the team at Vigliano Associates

Tony Tiano, Lennlee Keep, Eli Brown, and the team at Sante Fe Productions

The Public Broadcasting Service (PBS-TV)

Harry G. Preuss, M.D., M.A.C.N., C.N.S.

Stephen Sinatra, M.D., F.A.C.N., F.A.C.C.

Michigan State University College of Human Medicine

Department of Dermatology, Henry Ford Hospital

Fuji Health Sciences, Inc.

Dr. Cass Ingram

Chris Kilham

Ehud Sperling and the team at Inner Traditions/Healing Arts
    Press

The team at the N.V. Perricone M.D., Ltd. Flagship Store

The team at N.V. Perricone M.D., Ltd.

Edward Magnotti

Terence Sellaro

Craig Weatherby

Sharyn Kolberg

Chim Potini

Lori Bush

Dr. Peter Pugliese

Steven Pugliese

Mahnaz Badamchian

Randy Hartnell and the team at Vital Choice

Our retail partners, Sephora, Nordstrom, Neiman Marcus,
    Bloomingdale's, Saks Fifth Avenue, Henri Bendel, Parisian, and
    Belk

My parents

My children, Jeffrey, Nicholas, and Caitie

My brother and sisters, Jimmy, Laura, Barbara, and June

Contents

Introduction

Tremendous strides have been made in the field of anti-aging medicine since the publication of my first book, *The Wrinkle Cure*, in 2000. It was there that I first introduced my inflammation–aging theory, which firmly places chronic, low-grade invisible inflammation at the center of aging, age-related diseases, and a host of degenerative conditions.

This theory was often dismissed with either ridicule or skepticism—however, science has now recognized its validity, and inflammation has been overwhelmingly recognized as a serious threat to health and longevity.

As you will learn in this book, we do not need elaborate, expensive, and possibly dangerous pharmaceuticals to halt the inflammatory response and its resultant negative effects. *Dr. Perricone's 7 Secrets to Beauty, Health, and Longevity* will give you all of the tools you need, starting with the single most important—the food we eat.

Every day multiple studies are published linking diet to disease. A recent study reported that diets high in saturated fats increase our risk for Alzheimer's disease, which is an inflammatory disease. Conversely, the anti-inflammatory diet reduces our risk for this debilitating and growing epidemic. Just as important as choosing the right foods is choosing how they are grown and raised. A new study has clearly linked exposure to pesticides with Parkinson's disease. As I have always emphasized, buy organic and protect yourself and your loved ones from exposure to proven toxic substances.

But it goes even further than the anti-inflammatory foods. We have also made great technological strides in the development of novel nutritional supplements to complement foods and provide the missing links in health and wellness. For the first time, as outlined in this book, we have proven methodologies to revitalize our tired, worn-out bodies *at the cellular level* and recharge them with increased energy, improved mood, a greater sense of well-being, and renewed purpose.

These targeted supplements are worlds beyond the original vitamins of past generations. Today we can target the key parts of the cells, such as the mitochondria, to restore energy to the cell. As we age, energy levels decline in the cells—in fact, they eventually lose their ability to repair themselves altogether. With the use of a newly discovered class of mitochondrial rejuvenators, we can recharge the cells in all of our organ systems, including the skin, for total body rejuvenation. Being a dermatologist, I find this particularly exciting. Learning how to restore bone structure and muscle mass to the aging face is one of our greatest strategies in maintaining a youthful face.

However, the good news doesn't stop there. Science has recently learned that brain cells can also be rejuvenated. It was long and widely believed that we were born with a genetically determined brain of fixed size and potential, for better or worse. This is far from the truth. We now know that the brain is a growing and changing organ. As we will learn in this book, we have many strategies to optimize this growth, including the *essential fatty acid phosphatidylserine, which is a powerful prevention for memory loss, Alzheimer's, and dementia.* Other fatty acids, such as the omega-3s and fish oils, dramatically improve brain health, mood, attention span, and more.

We will also learn about forms of exercise that will not only deliver powerful anti-aging benefits to the body but will also increase our powers of focus and concentration while restoring physical and mental equilibrium.

As you will learn in *Dr. Perricone's 7 Secrets to Beauty, Health, and Longevity,* our bodies, minds, and spirits have the potential for tremendous growth, rebirth, and regeneration, given the proper tools. Thank you for accompanying me on this exciting journey.

NICHOLAS PERRICONE, M.D.
Madison, Connecticut
July 2006

DR. PERRICONE'S

7 *Secrets to Beauty, Health, and Longevity*

Cellular Rejuvenation

This book is the culmination of a lifetime of work and research into why and how we age. In my previous books, I laid the blame on chronic, subclinical inflammation for everything from wrinkles and obesity to chronic degenerative diseases such as heart disease, Alzheimer's, certain cancers, arthritis, and more. Although the concept was not universally accepted by physicians and scientists—in fact, it was often ridiculed—inflammation has now made it into the accepted list of causative factors in aging and disease. A quick look at the National Library of Medicine website reveals hundreds of studies verifying this, including a recent study reported by the University of Texas Department of Physiology stating that "the activation of inflammatory genes acts as a bridge linking normal aging to pathological processes." Another recent study, this one out of Columbia University, found that "with most age-associated diseases, individuals manifest an underlying chronic inflammatory state. . . ."

In each of my books I have set forth strategies to combat this inflammation. As inflammation and its destructive effects have become widely recognized and accepted, many leading scientists are making it the focus of their research.

Now my goal, in addition to learning how to prevent and reverse inflammation in our daily lives, is to build on my previous work and go even deeper than I have before. Exciting new scientific developments are showing us that there is even more we can do—we can actually *rebuild* our bodies on a cellular level. Brain, bone, muscle, and skin can all benefit in a process known as *cellular rejuvenation*.

Once the realm of salesmen of questionable supplements and potions, the field of anti-aging has now taken its place at the forefront of legitimate scientific research. Each day new reports on studies are published, studies showing that science is on the brink of learning how to trigger the cellular self-repair mechanisms that appear to be a driving force in life extension.

In this book we will explore multiple disciplines, all of which are accessible to everyone. We will learn how cellular rejuvenation works; it is a new and exciting science that will restore mental and physical health to all areas of the body, both inside and outside. For the first time we have the means and the methods to stop the age-related decline of all organ systems. Some of our tools are thousands of years old, long forgotten and ready to be reintroduced in this book, while others are current discoveries. Together they provide us with up-to-the-minute strategies to both delay and reverse the negative effects of aging.

In researching and writing this book, I have found numerous approaches that greatly enhance our ability to delay (and prevent) the onset of the undesirable effects of aging. There are proven foods, botanicals, and nutritional supplements that offer genuine physical and mental restorative benefits. And while we cannot turn back the clock, we can learn to slow it down—to the inestimable benefit of ourselves, our loved ones, our community, and our planet. A sick and aging populace is the greatest threat we have in terms of destabilizing our future. The seven anti-aging secrets you will find here are your tools to circumvent such a disaster and ensure healthy, happy, active years for decades to come.

Which brings us to *secret 1: Jump-start your cellular metabolism.*

The Mighty Mitochondria

There's a reason I'm starting this book with the mitochondria. They're the part of the cell that creates energy, the very foundation of cellular rejuvenation. A young cell is characterized by optimal energy production. Slow down that production, and you begin the aging process. The goal, therefore, is to rev up your cellular metabolism—the chemical and physiological processes by which the body builds and maintains itself and by which it breaks down food and nutrients to produce energy.

To understand the concepts of cellular metabolism and rejuvenation, we need to understand the inner workings of the cell—in particular, the mitochondria, sometimes called the "cellular power plants" because they metabolize food-derived chemicals to produce energy. Mitochondria are responsible for converting nutrients and oxygen into the energy-yielding molecule adenosine triphosphate (ATP) to fuel the cell's activities. Without energy, the cell can no longer repair itself, resulting in cellular breakdown.

One of the things that makes the mitochondria unique is that they have their own set of DNA (deoxyribonucleic acid) molecules. We are all familiar with DNA, which is the material inside the nucleus of cells that carries genetic information. But what many people are not aware of is that the mitochondria also contain DNA, above and beyond the DNA found in the nucleus of the cell. Unfortunately, the primary site of damage to the cell is in the DNA found in the mitochondria. The DNA in the mitochondria is at exceptional risk because of the free radicals produced in this tiny furnace during energy production. The cell automatically fixes much of the damage done to nuclear DNA; however, the DNA in the mitochondria cannot be as readily fixed. Therefore, extensive DNA damage accumulates over time and shuts down the mitochondria, causing the cells to die and the organism to age.

There have been many theories of aging; one of the most significant is the free-radical theory proposed by Denham Harman, M.D., Ph.D. A free radical is a molecule that is missing an electron in its outer orbit. Dr. Harman first suggested that free radicals alter the molecular structure of the cell, causing damage to the cell. They do this by stealing their missing electron from other molecules to complete their outer orbit. In other words, free radicals are molecules that want to join with other molecules, and by doing so they cause cellular damage.

As is often the case with pioneering work in the scientific worlds, Dr. Harman's theories were essentially ignored for decades. However, scientists now recognize and acknowledge the importance of free radicals in the aging process. It is also well established that free radicals play an active role in very diverse, age-related diseases. In my first book, *The Wrinkle Cure*, I introduced Dr. Harman's free-radical theory of aging and proposed that free radicals initiate the inflammatory process that is ultimately responsible for aging and age-related disease.

The Inflammation Theory of Aging

The majority of the free radicals are derived from oxygen. Thus, the damage being done by these free radicals is known as *oxidative damage*. When a cell has a high level of free radicals present, we call this *oxidative stress*, and oxidative stress leads to the production of chemicals that create inflammation within the cell. This process is a vicious cycle, as free radicals can initiate inflammation and inflammation can initiate the production of free radicals.

The scientists who argue in favor of the free-radical theory of aging must now go beyond this premise if we are to stop and help reverse cellular degeneration. Free radicals exist only for a nanosecond and therefore do very little *direct* damage to cellular molecules. However, what they do accomplish, in their very brief life, is the initiation of an *inflammatory cascade*, which can continue for hours or even days. The long life of the inflammatory cascade results in most of the cellular damage that leads to aging and age-related diseases.

Fortunately for us, our bodies already contain certain defenses against free radicals and inflammation. Our bodies can actually make a variety of enzyme antioxidants that suppress or alter free radicals. (An enzyme is a protein that accelerates the rate of chemical reactions.) They are referred to as *endogenous* antioxidants because they are made internally by the body. Another way of obtaining antioxidants is through our diet or by taking nutritional supplements. We call these *exogenous* antioxidants because they come from outside of the body. We are all familiar with many of these antioxidants, such as vitamins C and E, as well as the multitude of phytonutrients that are available in fresh fruits and vegetables.

Antioxidants are critical in anti-aging medicine because they act as natural anti-inflammatories, giving us protection against the inflammation initiated by free radicals that causes cellular damage. When this damage occurs internally to our vital organs, such as the brain, it results in problems such as Parkinson's disease, Alzheimer's, and dementia. It can also damage the lungs, resulting in decreased respiratory function, as well as the heart and the kidneys.

And it is not just our internal organs that suffer. Free-radical damage and inflammation is apparent in our appearance with each passing year. It manifests in very visible damage to skin, resulting in the thinning of the skin, deep lines, wrinkles, sagging, and loss of tone, texture, and radiance. Negative changes in our muscle mass, known as sarcopenia, along with the loss of critical bone mass (osteopenia and osteoporosis), also occur. Each of these changes, whether external or internal, is the initial result of damage on a molecular and cellular level.

Recharging the Mitochondrial Batteries

Now that we know what causes cells to age, we can concentrate on what we need to (1) protect them from inflammatory damage and (2) recharge the mitochondrial "batteries" to keep them up and running with energy to spare. There are two ways to do this: through diet and through nutritional supplements. We'll begin with diet.

The foods we eat are of critical importance because they either create or prevent the free radicals and inflammation implicated in aging and disease, meaning our diet can be either pro-inflammatory or anti-inflammatory. It is very exciting that scientific breakthroughs and discoveries now allow us to actually rejuvenate and revitalize our bodies on a cellular level—but if our diet is pro-inflammatory, we will undermine the effects of even the most powerful remedies. So the first step in cellular rejuvenation is to establish a firm base, beginning with the foods we eat, thus ensuring the success of mitochondrial and other cellular rejuvenators.

As it turns out, the dietary advice I have given in my previous books has been right on the money—not only for preventing inflammation but also in terms of enabling our bodies' cells to repair themselves. The following six categories of foods, familiar to my loyal readers, each have important and particular properties for maintaining and improving cellular metabolism.

CATEGORY 1: PROTEIN (FOR CELLULAR REJUVENATION)

Protein plays a very important role in a successful health, beauty, and anti-aging program. It is the basic material of life. In fact, the word *protein* comes from an ancient Greek root meaning "of first importance." The body could not grow or function without it.

As protein is digested, it breaks down into amino acids, which are then used by the cells to repair themselves. Since the human body can manufacture only 11 of the 20 amino acids that are essential for life, the remaining 9 must be provided through the intake of dietary protein.

Without adequate protein, our bodies enter into an accelerated aging mode. Our muscles, organs, bones, cartilage, skin, and the antibodies that protect us from disease are all made of protein. Even the enzymes that facilitate essential chemical reactions in the body—from digestion to building cells—are made of protein. If your cells do not have complete access to all the essential amino acids, cellular repair will be incomplete and also much slower.

It's important to note that protein cannot be stored in our bodies; therefore, we need to have a good source of quality protein at each meal for optimum health and cellular repair.

As to where protein rates on the "inflammatory scale," we will find that protein, on the whole, is neutral. However, some sources of protein, such as wild salmon, provide powerful anti-inflammatory benefits because they are high in anti-inflammatory omega-3 essential fatty acids (EFAs) and astaxanthin, a superpowerful carotenoid antioxidant with potent anti-inflammatory properties.

Conversely, forms of protein that are high in saturated fats can have a pro-inflammatory effect in the body. Limit your intake of red meats, choose the leaner cuts, and substitute leaner choices such as chicken breast without the skin, light turkey meat, and even bison and ostrich. Increase your intake of all forms of seafood except those known to have high mercury or pesticide levels (www.vitalchoice.com offers lists of recommended fish with excellent safety profiles).

Category 2: Carbohydrates (for Cellular Energy)

Carbohydrates are sugars and starches, which are the most efficient source of food energy. They are stored in the muscle and liver as glycogen and in the blood as glucose. However, to make the most efficient use of this stored energy, sugar needs to be consumed in the form of complex carbohydrates like those found in whole fruits

ASTAXANTHIN, THE MULTIFUNCTIONAL ANTIOXIDANT

Astaxanthin is a unique and multitalented antioxidant. It is also one of the reasons for wild salmon's status as a leading superstar in the realm of anti-aging foods. However, it is also important to take astaxanthin as a nutritional supplement to ensure optimum benefits.

Astaxanthin has the ability to protect the cell membrane from free radicals also known as reactive oxygen species, or ROS, including the most damaging of all, the singlet oxygen. *Carotenoids* in general, and astaxanthin in particular, effectively absorb energy from free radicals and the singlet oxygen.

Astaxanthin provides powerful protection to the lipid bi-layer that surrounds our cells as well as the mitochondria and the nucleus within the cells. This dual function of protection is unique to astaxanthin and one of the reasons it plays such an important role in the protection of cells. Because astaxanthin can penetrate different portions of the cell, it protects all organs and systems throughout the body. This broad-based protection is the foundation for the multifunctional benefits that have become associated with astaxanthin and its anti-aging properties. The health areas that have been studied include

- *Cardiovascular:* Recent studies have indicated the tendency of astaxanthin to reduce blood pressure. The antihypertensive mechanism may in part be explained by the tendency of astaxanthin to increase blood flow. It is hypothesized by the researchers that this results from blood vessel relaxation and dilation. Also, in one of the studies, a 50% drop in the incidence of stroke was noted in the astaxanthin-treated group.
- *Type 2 diabetes:* A preliminary study indicates that astaxanthin supplementation may improve control of type 2 diabetes and inhibit progressive kidney

damage. This study also supports the findings of an earlier study that indicates that astaxanthin may preserve pancreatic function as well as insulin sensitivity.

Other benefits include

- Improved skin elasticity and reduced appearance of fine lines
- Eye fatigue (asthenopia) reduction
- Improved muscle endurance and recovery following vigorous exercise
- Reduced gastric inflammation and dyspepsia

It is important to note that all of these studies were performed using the AstaREAL brand of natural astaxanthin, which is produced from the microalgae *Haematococcus pluvialis*, a natural carotenoid pigment and biological antioxidant believed to be the world's richest source of astaxanthin, in fully enclosed and protected biosystems either in Sweden or on the island of Maui in Hawaii. As with so many nutritional supplements, it is critical to know that you are getting the highest-quality, most vigorously tested—for both safety and efficacy—formula possible. AstaREAL is a trademark of Fuji Chemical Industry.

(preferably organic so we can eat the skin, which contains high levels of nutrients and fiber); starches need to be eaten in the form of beans, legumes, and some whole grains, which break down slowly and won't cause spikes in blood sugar and insulin. If the carbohydrate choices we make are fruits, vegetables, beans, and legumes, along with whole grains such as old-fashioned oatmeal, we will reap great anti-aging benefits—from wrinkle protection to weight reduction.

In addition to choosing anti-inflammatory carbs, we must also learn how to avoid pro-inflammatory carbs, which degrade cellular

NATURE-MADE

A simple rule to remember is this: If the food was made by nature and you are eating it in its unadulterated form, it is a good choice, with the possible exception of the potato. Juice, for example, doesn't exist in nature but must be extracted from the fruit by physical means, making it a less desirable form of carbohydrate. If the food is processed in some way (other than cooked), it is more than likely not a good choice.

function. Pro-inflammatory carbohydrates are the "simple" sugars and starches, as opposed to the "complex" carbohydrates described above.

Just about everyone knows by now that sugar and all forms of sweeteners, flour, processed foods, sodas, juices, energy drinks, baked goods, pasta, and snack foods (chips, pretzels, etc.) are categorized as "high-glycemic" carbohydrates and come under the "Not a Good Choice" heading. This simply means that they rapidly convert to sugar when eaten, creating inflammation on a cellular level throughout the body. These foods cause the pancreas to release insulin in an effort to control the level of blood sugar in the body. Eventually, this leads to obesity, even though caloric intake may not necessarily be excessive. These foods also cause wrinkles and sagging in the face. There is no upside, other than the momentary rise in the "feel good" neurotransmitter, serotonin. Unfortunately, serotonin levels quickly drop, setting our bodies up for a roller-coaster ride of food cravings, mood swings, wrinkled skin, fatigue, and weight gain. Additionally, it is now almost universally accepted by anti-aging researchers worldwide that controlling blood sugar levels may be the greatest anti-aging tool we have—bar none.

CATEGORY 3: OMEGA-3 ESSENTIAL FATTY ACIDS (FOR CELLULAR STABILIZATION)

Our diets also need to include anti-inflammatory fat sources. This is a topic that I have covered extensively over the years. In fact, because they cause increased inflammation in the brain, I hold extreme low fat and fat-free diets culpable in the epidemic of depression that has swept the United States since the 1980s. Ideally our diets will be free from excess saturated fats and all trans-fatty acids—another reason to avoid all processed and prepared foods.

The EFAs found in fish (such as salmon, anchovies, sardines, sablefish, trout, etc.), nuts and seeds, and avocados are anti-inflammatory. They also have the unique ability to stabilize the cell plasma membrane, the outer portion of the cell. When we stabilize the cell plasma membrane, we decrease our risk of oxidative stress and its resultant production of the cascade of inflammatory chemicals that causes damage throughout the cell, especially the mitochondria.

The result of following the anti-inflammatory diet will be the prevention of inflammation produced by free radicals. There will be a great improvement in our physical appearance, decreased wrinkling and sagging of the skin, increased energy levels, elevated mood, better brain function, decreased body fat, greater muscle mass, stronger bones, and a powerful immune system.

CATEGORY 4: CAROTENOIDS (FOR CELLULAR GROWTH AND REPAIR)

Carotenoids are fat-soluble pigments that give a red-orange-yellow color to fruits, vegetables, egg yolks, wild salmon, steelhead trout, shellfish (e.g., shrimp and lobsters), and the feathers of birds, notably brilliant pink flamingos. Fish and fowl alike get their red-orange-yellow hues from eating large quantities of carotenoid-rich aquatic plants, such as algae and plankton.

The deep, vibrant colors, such as those found in fruits, vegetables, beans, legumes, nuts, extra virgin olive oil (EVOO), and seafood such as wild salmon, signify the presence of antioxidants, making these foods an essential part of this program. The carotenoid family of antioxidants offers very special and targeted properties for cellular rejuvenation—in fact, as you will see, they play a significant role in cellular growth and repair.

Dark, leafy greens such as spinach, kale, chard, and collards are also rich in carotenoids, but their red-orange-yellow colors are masked by green-hued chlorophyll, which is a more dominant pigment.

Because they are fat-soluble, carotenoids can enter both the cell plasma membrane and the mitochondria, where they protect these parts of the cell from oxidative stress, free-radical damage, and pro-inflammatory chemicals. This is very important for protecting our immune systems, because it is well known that immune cells are particularly sensitive to oxidative stress.

The vivid hues of foods colored by these natural antioxidant pigments impart more than just eye appeal (and serious eye protection and regeneration). Here are some of the key benefits you may enjoy from eating carotenoid-rich foods:

- The body converts the carotenoids in spinach to vitamin A (retinol) as needed.
- Carotenoids may reduce the risk of cardiovascular disease, in part because of their antioxidant, anti-inflammatory properties. (*Note:* Unlike food sources, supplemental carotenoids such as alpha- and beta-carotene do not produce consistently positive results against cardiovascular disease.)
- Carotenoids neutralize the free radicals responsible for general oxidative stress, which damages the cell and is the primary force behind the symptom-free "subclinical" inflammation that accelerates the internal aging process and manifests externally as wrinkles.
- Carotenoids may reduce the risk of cancer, especially cancers of the lung, bladder, breast, esophagus, and stomach.

- Carotenoids help block sunlight-induced inflammation in the skin, which leads to wrinkles and can cause skin cancer.
- The lutein and zeaxanthin abundant in spinach, kale, and collard greens exert protective antioxidant effects in the retina, and, accordingly, they appear to help prevent cataracts and macular degeneration. They also help protect against prostatic changes.

In fact, calorie for calorie, spinach and other dark-green leafy vegetables offer extraordinary amounts of more preventive-health nutrients and anti-aging antioxidants than most other foods. Together with their potent antioxidant, anti-aging pigments, these metabolic basics make them a preventive-health powerhouse. They

- Are excellent sources of vitamins C and K, which are essential to bone health
- Are excellent sources of magnesium, which can help lower high blood pressure and protect against heart disease
- Are good sources of calcium but are also high in oxalic acid, which blocks its absorption. For this reason, spinach is not as good a source as its calcium content suggests. Add calcium-rich foods such as cottage cheese and yogurt to meals to compensate for this effect
- Are an excellent source of folate, a B-complex vitamin essential for cell growth, reproduction, and proper fetal development. (Cooked, spinach contains 146 micrograms of folate per 3.5-ounce serving, or about 37% of the recommended daily allowance, or RDA.) Folate also allows the body to neutralize a blood chemical called homocysteine that can lead to heart attack or stroke. And low folate intake has been linked to increased risk of a number of cancers. The combination of high folate and carotenoids in these vegetables increases their cancer-protective properties

Researchers at Tufts University report that men who consumed foods high in folate (such as spinach) for 3 years displayed sharper cognitive skills at the end of the study period. Two mental capacities that typically decline with age were tested: verbal skills and the ability to copy complex figures. Tufts nutritional epidemiologist Katherine Tucker described the challenges copying a figure presents to the brain: "You have to visualize it spatially, locate it in your brain, and then tell your hand to draw it."

Another study, this one involving young women, found that those who consumed at least 1,000 micrograms of folate a day were 46% less likely to develop high blood pressure than those who consumed less than 200 micrograms. Since high blood pressure is a major cardiovascular risk factor, this is a very exciting finding. Experts recommend that all adults consume at least 400 micrograms a day, which is the amount considered essential for women to take to prevent birth defects. (*Note:* A high-folate diet can cause seizures in those taking anticonvulsion medications.).

It's not just the carotenoids found in plant foods that protect and rejuvenate the cells. Astaxanthin is the type of carotenoid found in wild salmon and gives salmon its deep pink or red hue. Astaxanthin is often referred to as "red gold from the sea," because it is the antioxidant leader of all carotenoids: 10 times more potent than beta-carotene and 100 times stronger than vitamin E. Rainbow trout, shrimp, lobster, crawfish, crabs, and red caviar also owe their rich coloring to the astaxanthin in their diets. Wild Alaskan sockeye salmon delivers a remarkable 4.5 milligrams per 4-ounce serving. In terms of antioxidant capacity, 4.5 milligrams of astaxanthin is equivalent to 450 milligrams of vitamin E—the amount widely recommended for optimal health.

As if all that weren't enough, researchers at the University of Hawaii have produced additional evidence to show how carotenoids work to increase cellular health, encourage cell-to-cell communication, and prevent cancer.

Researcher Dr. John Bertram reported that dietary carotenoids increased the activity of a molecule called connexin 43. This molecule forms small channels between cells, and by doing so, connects virtually all cells in the body. Through these channels, cells exchange nutri-

Eat Broccoli, Prevent Cancer

Food plays a critical role, for both good and bad. New research continues to unlock the secrets of how foods (and nutritional supplements) influence every aspect of our physical and mental well-being or lack thereof. A quick example is the following: We have all been told that broccoli and the cruciferous vegetables help prevent cancer. But until now, we didn't know how or why.

In an outstanding example of cellular rejuvenation, a study conducted at Georgetown University and reported in the *British Journal of Cancer* found that indole-3-carbinol, a chemical in vegetables such as broccoli, cauliflower, and cabbage, actually boosts DNA repair in cells and may stop them from becoming cancerous. This is a critical finding because DNA is the material inside the nucleus of cells that carries genetic information. If we are genetically predisposed to cancer, could this mean that we can repair our cells and thus prevent cancer simply by eating broccoli? It is certainly a fascinating premise, and scientists are ardently pursuing this line of study.

According to Professor Eliot Rosen, who led the research, "it is now clear that the function of crucial cancer genes can be influenced by compounds in the things we eat: Studies that monitor people's diets and their health have found links between certain types of food and cancer risk. Our findings suggest a clear molecular process that would explain the connection between diet and cancer prevention." As we've learned, carotenoids also show powerful chemoprotective properties. Do try to always buy organically grown vegetables—the pesticides and chemical fertilizers used on nonorganically grown vegetables may counteract the positive effects of these foods.

Hollywood's Newest Star . . .
the Goji Berry

Hollywood has at last made a true discovery. Apparently, many superstars have heard about this ancient Tibetan berry that is one of the most nutritionally dense foods on Earth and has a sweet mild cherry–cranberry flavor.

Goji berries contain more than 500 times more vitamin C by weight than oranges do and are the most abundant source of carotenoids on Earth. (They have more beta-carotene than carrots do.) They contain 18 amino acids and more iron than spinach does and are loaded with many other vitamins and minerals, including calcium, magnesium, zinc, selenium, and vitamins B_1, B_2, B_6, and E.

This tiny berry (available as either dried berries or a juice) is a powerful antioxidant, rating 18,500 on the Oxygen Radical Absorbance Capacity (ORAC) scale, a standardized measurement by the U.S. Department of Agriculture of the antioxidant potency of foods. (In comparison, blueberries have 2,400 ORAC units and strawberries have 1,540.) Fortunately, the goji berry ranks low on the glycemic scale, which means it will not cause an age-accelerating spike in blood sugar and insulin.

Here are just a few of the major benefits of eating goji berries:

- They stimulate the pituitary gland to release human growth hormone (HGH), which aids in reduction of body fat, helps you sleep, improves memory, and gives you a more youthful appearance.
- They help keep coronary arteries open and functioning smoothly and maintain their strength and integrity. Goji berries also increase the levels of an important blood enzyme that fights against the sticky lipid peroxides that can lead to cardiovascular disease, heart attack, atherosclerosis, and stroke.

- They can increase the level of testosterone in the blood, thereby increasing libido in both men and women. According to an old Chinese proverb, "He who travels one thousand kilometers from home should not eat goji!"
- They heighten immune system responses. Research has shown that goji berries' polysaccharides help enhance and balance the activity of immune cells, including T-cells, cytotoxic T-cells, and the immunoglobulins IgG and IgA.

ents and many vital signals that ensure normal cellular growth. When we understand that the word *cancer* is a general term for about 100 diseases characterized by uncontrolled, abnormal growth of cells, we realize how important normal cellular growth is in its prevention.

It is believed that restoring communication between cells may stop tumor growth and also prevent cancer from developing in the first place. Studies have shown that up to 70% of human cancer is preventable, and 40% of this can be attributed to diet. This is of critical importance when we consider that aging itself is a potent carcinogen. According to the American Cancer Society, nearly 80% of cancers are diagnosed in people older than 55. After reaching late middle age, men face a 50% chance of developing cancer, and women have a 35% chance. No one knows why cancer typically surfaces later in life, although a multitude of scientific theories abound. It may well be due to years of following a pro-inflammatory lifestyle and eating pro-inflammatory foods that cause serious damage to our cells. Fortunately we can stop a lot of this damage by simply changing the way we eat and adding targeted nutritional supplements.

CATEGORY 5: FLAVONOIDS (FOR PROTECTING THE CELL MEMBRANE)

Another important source of cell protection is the flavonoid. If an antioxidant found in a fruit or vegetable is not a carotenoid, chances are it's a flavonoid. Scientists have so far classified more than 5,000 naturally occurring flavonoids.

Flavonoids are a category of polyphenols, a large group of phytochemicals that are found in many plants and give some flowers, fruits, and vegetables their color. Research conducted since the 1990s has provided ample evidence that the water-soluble polyphenol antioxidants in some foods and herbs can also provide substantial protection against free-radical damage to cell membranes (the outer boundaries of the cells). This is highly significant, because any reduction in the number of free radicals in the cell membrane will inevitably result in a reduction in the number of free radicals available to damage the membrane surrounding our mitochondria.

However, the ability of polyphenols in food to protect the cell membrane is highly variable and depends on the chemical structure of each compound. One of the most abundant—and one of the most protective—flavonol-class polyphenols is quercetin, because it has the right chemical structure for scavenging free radicals.

The available research results indicate that most of the polyphenols found in fruits and vegetables offer some protection for cell membranes and therefore strengthen the body's first line of defense against free-radical damage to the mitochondria in our cells.

The following are the major classes of dietary polyphenols (that is, flavonoids), along with their chief food sources:

- *Flavonols (quercetin, myricetin, rutin)*: Onions, apples, apple peels, berries, tea, red wine, fruits, vegetables, herbs, buckwheat
- *Flavanones (hesperetin, naringenin, fisetin)*: Citrus fruits (especially the white pith), vegetables, fruits, red wine

- *Flavanols/flavan-3-ols (epigallocatechin gallate, epicatechin, (+)-catechin, epicatechin gallate)*: Tea, cocoa, berries
- *Anthocyanins:* Grapes, berries
- *Procyanidins:* Cocoa, berries, grapes, red apples, eggplant, red cabbage, red wine, cranberries
- *Proanthocyanidins:* Grapes, red wine, grape seed extract
- *Curcuminoids:* Whole turmeric spice, curcumin supplements

THE COLOR OF CURRY

Curcumin, the antioxidant, anticancer, anti-inflammatory polyphenol pigment that makes turmeric yellow and gives the characteristic color to curry dishes, protects the mitochondria in two ways:

- It appears to protect against oxidation of membrane lipids on the exterior and interior of cells.
- It appears to protect against mitochondrial dysfunction, probably because it is a potent inhibitor of the inflammatory compound in our cells called nuclear factor kappa B (NFkB).

I should note that certain of the dietary antioxidants from plant foods—including many carotenoids and polyphenols—do not pass through the intestinal lining easily and are therefore active primarily in the gastrointestinal tract. Their localized antioxidant action in the gut may nevertheless be important because the intestine is particularly exposed to oxidizing agents and affected by inflammation and numerous diseases such as cancer. Together with a few carotenoid compounds, polyphenols constitute the only dietary antioxidants present in the colon, because vitamins C and E are absorbed in the upper segments of the intestine.

CATEGORY 6: GREEN FOODS
(UNSURPASSED CELLULAR REJUVENATORS)

Green foods is a popular term used to describe young cereal grasses such as barley, wheat, rye, and oats before the grass is converted into grain. These cereal grasses have long been cultivated for their energy-dense grain; however, the nutrient profiles of green cereal plants change quickly as they grow. As the plant grows, the chlorophyll, protein, and vitamin content of cereal grasses declines sharply and the level of cellulose (indigestible fiber) increases. Over a period of several months, the green leafy cereal grasses become amber waves of grain bearing the kernels we harvest to make into flour—an unhealthy, pro-inflammatory food.

But this doesn't mean that we should eliminate these foods from our diet. The most nutritious part of these plants resides in their young green blades of grass, which offer great health and anti-aging benefits. However, these delicate grasses are highly perishable and prior to modern processing techniques were not widely available. Fortunately, we can now capture and protect the abundant nutrients in freshly harvested young green cereal grasses, making their everyday use practical and beneficial for everyone.

Of the green cereal grasses, wheatgrass and barley grass have been found to contain the most balanced nutrient profile, with barley grass being especially rich in the micronutrients so critical to cellular rejuvenation. Here are some of its most important benefits:

- *Enhanced metabolism:* Efficient metabolism of fats and carbohydrates inhibits the accumulation of fat and cholesterol in our tissues, a condition believed to contribute to the risk of both heart disease and diabetes. Dr. Kazuhiko Kubota at the Science

University of Tokyo found that barley grass juice reduces serum cholesterol in rats fed a high-cholesterol diet. Enhanced cellular metabolism through increased activity may also help control the amount of body fat. Dr. Kubota found that mice fed a diet containing barley grass juice were 150% more active than mice fed a control diet. (For more information on barley grass and weight loss, see Chapter Two, "Lean for Life.")

• *Anti-inflammatory action:* Barley grass juice contains important anti-inflammatory substances, including superoxide dismutase (SOD) and chlorophyll, so it is not surprising that Dr. Kubota and other researchers have found that it reduces inflammation in both animals and humans. Along with SOD and chlorophyll, Dr. Kubota has isolated two other potent anti-inflammatory glyco-proteins in barley grass juice.

• *Antioxidant protection:* Barley grass juice contains a synergistic blend of antioxidants, such as the all-important carotenoids, vitamin C, vitamin E, SOD, catalase, chlorophyll, and 2"-*O*-glycosyli-sovitexin (2"-*O*-GIV), a potent antioxidant recently isolated and studied by Dr. Takayuki Shibamoto, Dr. Yoshihide Hagiwara, and colleagues at the University of California, Davis. They found 2"-*O*-GIV was effective in preventing oxidation of blood lipids by free radicals and the formation of two toxic by-products of oxidation, acetaldehyde and malonaldehyde.

Beer drinkers may be particularly interested in Dr. Shibamoto's latest research on the antioxidative properties of 2"-*O*-GIV from barley grass. Recently, Dr. Shibamoto and colleagues have found that 2"-*O*-GIV prevents the oxidation of beer and inhibits the formation of acetaldehyde, a compound that may be responsible for the damaging effects of alcohol on the liver—as well as that unpleasant feeling called a hangover that we get in the morning after drinking the night before.

• *Effective detoxification:* Health-conscious consumers today are looking for more than wholesome, nutritious food to maintain good health; they also want to protect themselves from the ever-increasing number of toxins in our environment. While periodic use of internal cleansing and detoxification programs helps eliminate the body's toxic overload, a more effective method would be to gently detoxify our bodies every day through our diet. Therefore, optimal nutrition should include foods that not only supply us with all the nutrients necessary for cellular metabolism but also help remove toxins.

- *Longevity and immunity enhancement:* When we are exposed to excessive ultraviolet (UV) light, it can result in the oxidation of fats, which plays a key role in damaging tissue. This oxidation is known as "lipid peroxidation." It creates free radicals, which are responsible for extensive damage to the tissue. This process can occur in foods before they are eaten; when this occurs in nuts, for example, which are rich in unsaturated fats, they are said to be rancid. Rancid fats are responsible for increased rates of heart disease and atherosclerosis and are also carcinogenic (cancer causing), so we want to avoid them at all costs.

  This process can also take place inside of the body. When squalene, an important lipid found in skin, is associated with peroxidation, it results in skin aging and may also be responsible for mutations in the DNA that can lead to cancer.

  Flavonoids in barley grass may help prevent these mutations and protect the body from cancer, including skin cancer, as well as the premature aging conditions associated with free radicals.

  Adding barley grass juice powder to your diet is a convenient and effective way to ensure that you reap the benefits of nature's green bounty, which provides those phytonutrients and phytochemicals necessary for maintaining optimal health.

- *Cardiovascular benefits:* Good cardiovascular function and proper blood flow are absolute prerequisites for good health. Restrictions in the ability of the heart and blood vessels to deliver nutrients to the body's cells obviously weaken the body and its ability to stave off disease. People suffering from chronic health problems, especially those associated with aging, often have arteriosclerosis, or "clogged arteries," that affects blood flow, increases heart rate, and leads to high blood pressure as a result of narrower arteries. Oxidation of blood lipids, particularly that of the so-called bad low-density lipoprotein cholesterol (LDL-C), is known to play a role in the development of arteriosclerosis. While dietary, lifestyle, and genetic factors all play a role in cardiovascular function, relatively simple dietary changes, including the use of dietary supplements, offer a convenient way to kick-start a program for promoting a healthy heart.

- *Cholesterol reduction and prevention of LDL oxidation in type 2 diabetes:* People with type 2 diabetes have an elevated risk for atherosclerosis. Dr. Ya-Mei Yu and colleagues found that supplementation with barley grass reduced the levels of both cholesterol and oxygen free radicals in the blood of type 2 diabetics. Additionally, they showed that barley grass supplementation acted synergistically with vitamins C and E in reducing LDL oxidation. The researchers concluded that barley grass "acts as a free radical scavenger and may help protect type 2 diabetic patients from vascular diseases."

- *Cellular regeneration:* Cellular repair and regeneration depend on the adequate intake of nutrients, reduction of the inflammatory response, and protection against noxious stimuli. Each of these actions depends on the delivery of an adequate supply of nutrients, anti-inflammatory substances, and antioxidants by a healthy cardiovascular system. As research has shown, barley grass not only helps support cardiovascular activity but also contains a variety of essential nutrients, antioxidants, and anti-inflammatory substances (chlorophyll, SOD, the glycoproteins P4-D1 and D1-G1) that significantly support cellular repair and rejuvenation. The demonstrated ability of Green Magma brand barley grass (the form of barley grass used in these studies) to restore cellular function is related to its anti-aging properties in fighting free-radical activity, reducing inflammation, and supporting healthy blood flow, as well as in its possible ability to prevent and reverse damage to genetic material.

SARAH'S STORY

Feeling Tired and Run Down

Sarah was one of those rare talents. As a singer-songwriter she had successfully bridged multiple musical genres. Her albums consistently topped both the country and the popular charts. However, as much as her fans loved her—and they did—perhaps her greatest claim to fame was the near reverence accorded to her by her fellow musicians. Sarah was in continual demand to record and appear in concert with the world's biggest stars—an accolade her many Grammys proved was well deserved.

As might be expected, Sarah's schedule was both grueling and hectic. She needed to keep herself in top shape to meet the ongoing demands on her time and energy. But with a new tour on the horizon, Sarah admitted to me that for the first time, she was dreading being on the road. "Dr. Perricone," Sarah said, "I don't know if I have chronic fatigue or what, but I feel tired and run down. I can't seem to build up enthusiasm for this tour, and there is no way I can back out at this late date." Sarah's physician had recently given her a complete physical, which she had passed with flying colors, so I knew there was no underlying disease causing her fatigue. My first job was to secure Sarah's nutritional profile, because diet is often the primary culprit behind many mental and physical symptoms.

"I love salad," Sarah confessed. "Because I keep a close watch on my weight, I always use a nonfat salad dressing." While eating salads is always recommended, using nonfat dressing is not. Unless we add a good form of fat, such as EVOO, our bodies can't absorb all the important nutrients in the salad. I also learned, much to my dismay, that Sarah relied heavily on so-called power drinks for her energy. These popular beverages are very high in caffeine and sugar; this combination can leave you exhausted and dehydrated—a dangerous combination. Sarah also admitted trouble sleeping, another side effect of consuming excess caffeine.

Equally alarming was Sarah's ongoing lack of protein. Without adequate protein, our bodies enter into an accelerated aging mode. Our muscles, organs, bones, cartilage, skin, and the antibodies that protect us from disease are all made of protein. Even the enzymes that facilitate essential chemical reactions in the body—from digestion to building cells—are made of protein. If our cells do not have complete availability of all the essential amino acids, cellular repair will be not only incomplete but also much slower than it should be.

Since the body can't store protein for future use, we need to have a good source of quality protein at each meal. Ideally, we should eat three meals and two snacks per day, evenly spaced, to provide a steady flow of nutrients, fats, protein, and carbohydrates for optimum performance and to avoid physical and mental fatigue.

Getting Sarah on the Road to Cellular Repair

I instructed Sarah to fill her tour bus refrigerator with plain yogurt, hard-boiled eggs, raw and unsalted nuts, olives, gallons of spring water, and lots of fresh fruits and vegetables. My favorite yogurt is made from a goat or sheep's milk in the Greek style. This is a much richer yogurt because the Greek method removes the watery whey from the finished product. Also, goat and sheep's milk have much smaller molecules than cow's milk, making them much more digestible and also ideal for those who are lactose-intolerant. (See the "Resources" section for sources of this excellent product.) I also advised her to stock her shelves with individual cans of salmon. These simple basic foods would provide her with the nutrient structure she needed to regain her energy and diminish any signs of aging in her face (directly attributable to protein deficiency). Because these foods are also rich in anti-inflammatory antioxidants, Sarah would soon begin to see major changes in her skin, including the radiant, healthy glow that is one of the hallmarks of a young face.

I also had Sarah begin a supplement regimen. In addition to a good multivitamin, we added carnitine and acetyl-L-carnitine, both important because they enhance cellular energy production. Also recommended was alpha lipoic acid, the only antioxidant that can boost cellular levels of glutathione, the tripeptide antioxidant critical to health and longevity, which decline with age, and Co-Q$_{10}$. Coenzyme Q$_{10}$ works synergistically with alpha lipoic acid and acetyl-L-carnitine to assist with many metabolic processes and helps elevate levels of other antioxidants, such as vitamins C and E.

Sarah was also eager to try topical anti-inflammatoriess.

About eight weeks later I received two tickets to Sarah's sold-out concert at a major venue in the New York metro area. After the opening acts of two legendary and world-famous bands, the lights went down and a hush fell over the crowd. As the lights came back up, the crowd went wild as Sarah began to sing one of her famous Grammy award–winning songs. I could see a new bounce to Sarah's step. She radiated a healthy, natural energy. Her skin glowed—in fact, she was positively radiant—a fact not lost on the huge numbers of young male fans in the audience who were cheering wildly.

All in all, it was a thrilling evening—the perfect kickoff to her world tour. Fortunately few of us have the kinds of physical demands for stamina that a performer such as Sarah has. However, with each passing decade we all lose a little bit more of the spark of youth. Luckily, with a little knowledge and lifestyle modification, we really can do something about it.

Boosting Cellular Rejuvenation with Nutritional Supplements

Another important strategy for reducing inflammation and protecting the mitochondria is the use of targeted nutritional supplements. Although this is still somewhat controversial among many mainstream physicians, I firmly believe in the anti-aging, health, and beauty benefits of nutritional supplements. I also believe that this anti-supplement bias is harmful, as it deprives people of safe and effective methodologies proven to reduce inflammation and thereby lessen their risk for age-related diseases.

Fortunately, there are several very powerful antioxidant, anti-inflammatory compounds that provide the mitochondria with significant protection from free-radical damage. As stated earlier, the cell plasma membrane, which is made up of lipids, is the most vulnerable portion of the cell in terms of the production of free radicals and resultant inflammation.

Like cells, the mitochondria are also enveloped by a lipid membrane. Accordingly, the antioxidants that confer the greatest protection are *lipid (fat) soluble*, a chemical characteristic that enables them to concentrate in the lipid membranes that enfold the cell as well as in its mitochondria and nucleus.

THE NEW NEWS ABOUT ALPHA LIPOIC ACID

The first line of defense belongs to a compound in the body called alpha lipoic acid (ALA). Readers of my previous books already know the importance I place on this multitasking, multiprotective supplement. But recent studies have shown that it is even more powerful than previously thought.

ALA is a very powerful antioxidant, anti-inflammatory agent, but additional amounts can be obtained only from supplements, because it is almost nonexistent in foods. ALA is unique among antioxidants because it is soluble in both fat and water.

It is also unique in having the ability to penetrate the lipid-soluble portions of the cell. Because ALA can protect both the fat- and the water-soluble parts of the cell, scientists have named it the "universal antioxidant." Because ALA is found as part of an enzyme complex in the mitochondria that converts food to energy, it is also known as the "metabolic antioxidant." Here are some of the highlights of the amazing properties of ALA:

- ALA is the only antioxidant that can boost cellular levels of glutathione, an antioxidant of tremendous importance in overall health and longevity and essential for the functioning of the immune system. People with chronic illnesses such as acquired immunodeficiency syndrome (AIDS), cancer, and autoimmune diseases generally have very low levels of glutathione. White blood cells are particularly sensitive to changes in glutathione levels, and even subtle changes may have profound effects on the immune response.
- ALA helps regulate glucose metabolism. Sugar can be extremely damaging to our cells if it is not well controlled, as it can react with molecules within the cell in a permanent bond called glycation. Once these bonds between sugar and protein are formed, they become mini factories for the generation of free radicals that can attack our cells and their mitochondria and produce inflammation. ALA helps prevent damaging glycation while also increasing the cell's ability to use glucose. When taken orally as a supplement, ALA can concentrate in both the cell and mitochondrial lipid membranes, where it protects both from free-radical damage, thus preventing the commencement of an inflammatory cascade.
- ALA is especially protective to the mitochondria in nerve cells and can therefore help prevent degeneration of the brain seen with aging and age-related diseases of the central nervous sys-

tem. In addition, ALA has been used successfully to treat patients with diabetic neuropathy (nerve damage).

- ALA works synergistically with other antioxidants in the skin to reduce the damaging inflammatory effects of UV radiation. ALA's capacity to regulate production of nitric oxide, which controls blood flow to the skin when applied topically, helps to transform the complexion from dull, pasty, and pale to vibrant and glowing. Topical ALA will also reduce puffiness in the face and eye area and decrease wrinkles and pore size.

DIVIDE AND CONQUER: THE NEWEST RESEARCH ON ALPHA LIPOIC ACID

ALA is found naturally in our cells, locked up in the mitochondria in an enzyme complex responsible for the conversion of food to energy. Only recently were scientists able to reveal the structure of ALA and produce it for use as a supplement.

It is interesting to note that when lipoic acid is taken into the cell, it forms dihydrolipoic acid (DHLA), which confers additional benefits over ALA. The body best uses a form of lipoic acid called R-lipoic acid (RLA), and RLA automatically converts to R-dihydrolipoic acid (R-DHLA). ALA is fat soluble, while DHLA is water soluble. It is because of this automatic conversion that lipoic acid confers protection throughout the cell, both the fat- and water-soluble compartments. RLA and DHLA make up what is known as a "redox couple." Redox reactions primarily involve the transfer of electrons between two chemical compounds. The compound that loses an electron is said to be *oxidized*, and the one that gains an electron is said to be *reduced*. In a somewhat complicated process, RLA and R-DHLA are constantly swapping electrons. RLA donates an electron to R-DHLA (and is therefore oxidized); when that happens, the R-DHLA obtains the electron and is therefore reduced. When RLA obtains an extra electron, it is reduced into R-DHLA, and when R-DHLA donates an electron, it is oxidized into RLA. These reactions occur constantly to meet the body's metabolic and free-radical defense needs. This is why the health benefits of ALA are associated with both forms: RLA and R-DHLA.

When we take ALA it is converted automatically to R-DHLA. Here are the likely benefits of taking ALA:

- R-DHLA regenerates the antioxidants vitamin C, thioredoxin (a small protein that has multiple enzymatic and regulatory roles in the cell), and glutathione, which in turn can recycle vitamin E.
- R-DHLA scavenges hypochlorous acid, peroxyl radicals, and hydroxyl radicals.
- R-DHLA is believed to prevent lipid peroxidation by reducing oxidized glutathione, thus altering in a beneficial way the glutathione-to-glutathione disulphide (GSH:GSSG) ratio, which decreases steadily in our bodies after 45 years of age.
- While both forms—R-DHLA and RLA—possess the ability to chelate (bind to) toxic metals and scavenge free radicals, only R-DHLA can regenerate the body's internal antioxidants and repair oxidative damage.
- Only R-DHLA blocks the formation of cells (osteoclasts) that break down bone in inflammatory conditions.
- R-DHLA inhibits the activity of a key pro-inflammatory enzyme called cyclo-oxygenase-2 (COX-2).
- R-DHLA is the most effective of all the sulfur-dependent antioxidants. Sulfur is a key constituent of amino acids and enzymes found in our cells.
- R-DHLA enhances the transport of glucose into cells via the insulin-signaling pathway.
- R-DHLA—but not RLA—can prevent oxygen-starvation damage in heart tissues resulting from the blocking of an artery.

This wonderful redox combo, which is obtained through taking ALA, accomplishes the following:

- Studies suggest that RLA and R-DHLA cross the blood–brain barrier to protect brain cells. The brain is particularly vulnerable because it contains high concentrations of easily oxidized polyunsaturated fatty acids, uses oxygen at a high rate, and has a relatively weak antioxidant defense system.
- RLA plus R-DHLA helps control blood sugar, increases ATP (mitochondrial energy) levels, detoxifies heavy metals, and can reverse oxidative damage to enzymes and DNA.
- RLA plus R-DHLA acts as an antioxidant both directly and indirectly, by recycling of other antioxidants and by increasing cellular levels of glutathione.
- R-DHLA may increase absorption, blood levels, and bioavailability of RLA.
- Studies have shown that the combination of RLA and R-DHLA prevents either from becoming a dangerous pro-oxidant if high concentrations are reached or transition metals are present, and maintains the redox status of blood, which may be one of the most effective means of controlling age-related increases in oxidative stress.

ACETYL-L-CARNITINE (FOR CELLULAR STABILIZATION)

Acetyl-L-carnitine (ALC) is a derivative of carnitine and is responsible for the transport of fatty acids into a cell's mitochondria. ALC also improves energy production within brain cells, increases cellular respiration, and is considered a neuroprotective agent because of its antioxidant and membrane-stabilizing effects. Carnitine and ALC are important because they enhance energy production—the hallmark of a young, healthy cell. ALC is synthesized from carnitine; therefore, it cannot be found in food and must be taken as a nutritional supplement. Acetylated carnitine is far superior to normal L-carnitine in terms of bioavailability because it is absorbed by the gastrointestinal tract, enters cells, and crosses the blood–brain barrier more readily than unacetylated carnitine does. ALC can pass through the mitochondrial membrane, where it functions as a natural anti-inflammatory antioxidant. ALC is an indispensable mitochondrial rejuvenator because it can help repair the mitochondria, while working synergistically with other powerful anti-inflammatory antioxidants, such as ALA, coenzyme Q_{10}, and glutathione.

In animal studies, ALA administered in conjunction with ALC actually rejuvenated the mitochondria of aging mice and improved memory and energy levels. Many researchers, including me, believe that ALC has significant potential for improving the quality of life and perhaps even extending the average life span of humans. Like many nutrients, ALC functions best in the presence of the omega-3 EFAs.

In a nutshell, the main benefits of ALC include

- Improved energy in brain cells
- Increased cellular respiration
- Reduced inflammation
- Assistance in repairing the mitochondria

COENZYME Q_{10} (FOR CELLULAR REPAIR)

Since cellular energy production declines as we age, substances such as coenzyme Q_{10} (Co-Q_{10}), also known as ubiquinone, are critical in maintaining enough energy in the cell so that it can repair itself. This antioxidant is found in the mitochondrial portion of the cell, where it performs two essential functions: It transports electrons in energy production and protects cells against the free radicals formed during normal metabolism. Co-Q_{10} interrupts the chemical chain reaction that transforms EFAs into destructive free radicals; thus, it protects against the high level of free radical activity found in our cells' mitochondria and is vital for maintaining cells' ability to generate energy.

Studies also indicate that Co-Q_{10} decreases the depletion of nucleotides (involved in making and storing energy and carrying DNA) and calcium, which suggests that it may be able to protect us against the age-related mutations in mitochondrial DNA characteristic of advancing age.

Co-Q_{10} is fat soluble, which enables it to protect the lipid-rich membranes of the cell and the mitochondria, and works synergistically with ALA and ACL to assist with many metabolic processes. It also helps elevate levels of other antioxidants, such as vitamins C and E. Co-Q_{10} also reduces the amount of lipid peroxides in the blood, which are the key markers of overall oxidative stress in the body.

Co-Q_{10} is probably one of the best researched of the antioxidant, anti-inflammatory vitamins; extensive studies show that it provides protection to all organs of the body, especially the heart, brain, and kidneys. It is these vital organs that appear most affected by age-related declines in Co-Q_{10} levels. Because Co-Q_{10} is such a powerful anti-inflammatory, it is extremely protective against cardiovascular disease by keeping the heart muscle healthy while preventing inflammation of the arteries that leads to arterial sclerosis.

For optimal absorption into the bloodstream, Co-Q_{10} should be taken with foods that contain healthy fats, such as nuts and seeds, a salad dressed with extra virgin olive oil, a piece of grilled salmon, and avocado slices. And while Co-Q_{10} can be found in fish such as salmon, it is important to supplement this key nutrient for the purposes of mitochondrial protection, rejuvenation, repair, and anti-aging.

In general, Co-Q_{10}

- Protects against free-radical activity in the mitochondria
- Decreases age-related mutations of mitochondrial DNA
- Assists with metabolic processes
- Protects against cardiovascular disease

NIACIN-BOUND CHROMIUM (FOR LIFE EXTENSION)

My colleague at Georgetown University's School of Medicine, Dr. Harry Preuss, recently alerted me to very new and exciting findings. Animal studies found that niacin-bound chromium (NBC) increased the average life span by 20% compared with a placebo. The NBC helps to lower the levels of circulating glucose (sugar) in the body. One of the reasons I advocate eliminating (as much as possible) sugar and simple starches from your diet is because high levels of circulating glucose in the body increase the presence of free radicals, which are the primary cause of metabolic disorders that can lead to diabetes. Scientists have repeatedly demonstrated that diabetes represents a premature form of aging, because of the damage caused by the excessively perturbed glucose–insulin system. This is really exciting news and one of the first strategies (other than caloric deprivation) shown to positively impact life span. (For additional benefits of this remarkable nutrient, see Chapter Two, "Lean for Life.")

Chromium is a very important trace mineral that promotes normal insulin function and is essential for proper protein, fat, and carbohydrate metabolism. As any anti-aging scientist well knows, elevated levels of insulin and blood sugar significantly accelerate cellular aging. Research now shows that the type of chromium known as NBC has a superior anti-aging and safety profile.

Extensive clinical and basic research using a unique form of *oxygen-coordinated* NBC—generally known as chromium nicotinate or polynicotinate (generic name for ChromeMate) has shown that the niacin-bound form of chromium is the superior form. (Some forms have a worrisome profile; therefore, I recommend using the ChromeMate brand for both safety and efficacy.) This form of NBC provides significant health benefits to those with diabetes and with metabolic syndrome and is indeed the optimal form of chromium available as a dietary supplement.

The main benefits of NBC include

- Promotion of proper insulin function and normal blood sugar levels
- Promotion of healthy blood cholesterol levels, normal blood pressure, and cardiovascular health
- Promotion of healthy body weight and lean body mass

Lean for Life

As we age, life can have many surprises in store for us. Some of them are positive and life affirming, such as an increase in wisdom and a greater appreciation for all of the simple pleasures. However, there are also a few unpleasant surprises in store—and one of them is a slow, creeping weight gain that sneaks up on us when we aren't looking. In fact, we may discover that by the time we are 40, we weigh a solid 10 or 20 pounds more than we did in our twenties. And it gets worse. Statistics show that we gain an average of 10 pounds of body fat while losing 5 pounds of muscle mass with each decade.

One of my strongest motivations in writing this book has been to offer exciting, cutting-edge information that will enable us to halt or reverse the undesirable signs of aging. However, like the search for a cure for the common cold, successful, safe, and long-term interventions for weight loss have eluded us. In fact, as we all hear on a daily basis, the world is getting fatter. We are in the midst of a worldwide obesity—or, as some term it, "globesity"—epidemic affecting all age groups, including young children.

Beyond following the mantra "eat less, exercise more," there have been no proven strategies or safe pharmacological interventions that work for the long term when it comes to losing weight. And even "eat less, exercise more" is not a surefire guarantee of weight loss. This is because a number of so-called healthy or low-calorie foods can sabotage our best intentions. These include foods that interfere with our ability to burn fat and foods that stimulate the appetite, making it almost impossible to eat less.

In this chapter I will not only teach you simple ways to avoid these common pitfalls but also let you in on *secret 2: We don't need to fanatically count grams of fat, carbs, or calories to maintain an ideal weight and/or to lose excess weight. All we have to do is learn how to control our blood sugar.* If you take away just one discovery from this book, let it be that. We can experience cellular rejuvenation in the body by helping to "reprogram" our genetic code to stop the storage of excess fat and the loss of youthful muscle mass. As I will demonstrate, we can even turn on the genes that suppress appetite and turn off the genetic switch that tells the body to store fat.

If we can prevent wild swings in blood sugar, we can avoid an inflammatory response and thereby prevent our insulin levels from going too high or too low. If they are too low, we cannot nourish our muscles and they begin to break down. If insulin levels are too high, we put a lock on the body's ability to burn fat for energy, and the body will store the fat instead. We can learn to avoid overeating or craving junk food by taking two simple steps: (1) avoid the insulin highs and lows by spacing meals and snacks evenly throughout the day and (2) cut out sugars and starchy foods that stimulate appetite and substitute proteins, good fats, fruits, and vegetables.

Obesity: The Cellular Rejuvenation Inhibitor

In *The Perricone Weight-Loss Diet*, I introduced new strategies to control three critical factors—blood sugar, insulin, and inflammation—the formula that ensures that we will be lean for life. To quickly recap the inflammation–obesity connection: When we eat foods that cause a sharp spike in blood sugar, it results in elevated levels of the hormone *insulin*, causing an inflammatory response. This results in a number of negative effects, one of which is blocking the body's ability to burn fat for energy, resulting in the storage of unwanted body fat (and beginning the aging process that comes with loss of energy). When blood sugar drops and insulin levels go down, the result is the eventual breakdown of muscle mass.

This one-two punch has important ramifications because it brings home the following point: It is not scale weight that is of primary importance. We can and will actually weigh more if our bodies are well muscled, because muscle weighs more than fat. However, our appearance will be leaner-looking, trim, and more compact, because muscle is denser and more compressed than fat. We will look much more attractive with good muscle mass. A quick look at any of the men and women on the pro tennis circuit will verify this. Yes, they may weigh more than the current batch of skeletal supermodels and actresses, but who can deny their physical strength, health, and beauty? Muscle also burns calories, even when we are sleeping or resting, making it much easier to stay lean. Controlling inflammation by *carefully controlling our blood sugar and insulin levels* through the foods we eat is critical (and also easy) if we want to lose body fat and preserve muscle.

IT'S IN THE GENES

Several weeks after the publication of *The Perricone Weight-Loss Diet* in October 2005, a team of international researchers discovered that a specific gene on chromosome 15 regulates inflammation. As I have taught and written for the past several decades, inflammation is implicated in a wide range of disorders, including cancer, cardiovascular disease, diabetes, infections, arthritis, Alzheimer's, and obesity.

According to John Blangero, Ph.D., a scientist at the Southwest Foundation for Biomedical Research (SFBR) in San Antonio, Texas, and the senior author of the research article on the discovery, "Practically every common disease involves an inflammatory component, so the discovery of a new player in the inflammation pathway opens up many potential avenues for intervention on a broad range of health issues."

This discovery has great significance for anyone interested in disease prevention, anti-aging, and weight loss. Perhaps most exciting for me personally is mainstream scientific validation of my teachings, which places inflammation at the root of many health problems—a concept that unfortunately was not always well received. In fact, on more than one occasion, it has been met with great skepticism!

Even more unfortunate is that not all physicians, scientists, and other experts keep current with the plethora of scientific studies prior to passing judgments. The latest peer-reviewed studies are published daily on the National Library of Medicine's website: http://www.ncbi.nlm.nih.gov/entrez/query.fcgi. It is free to all, scientist and layperson alike, and an outstanding resource for the best and brightest peer-reviewed studies from international university research. These studies and others in the same vein firmly identify inflammation as the culprit in many of the aforementioned degenerative conditions. A great many studies also verify the role of vitamins and antioxidants in the form of nutritional supplements in the prevention and reversal of many signs of aging—contrary to the media health gurus who imply otherwise.

Scientists are now eager to find a pharmaceutical to counter this inflammatory gene. But why wait for a drug that might be a decade in the making when the answer may be no farther away than your next meal? It is my belief that these findings underscore the importance of adopting a lifestyle whose cornerstone is the anti-inflammatory diet

HIGH-FRUCTOSE CORN SYRUP—
UPSETTING THE APPETITE APPLECART

The introduction of highly glycemic high-fructose corn syrup (HFCS) in the 1970s has, in my opinion, a direct corollary in the rise in obesity in both children and adults. Prior to the 1970s, popular soft drinks such as Coke and Pepsi were made with pure cane sugar. The average bottle of soda was 6 ounces. In the ensuing decades as we and our meals have become super-sized, an average can or bottle of soda holds 12 ounces and a large soda can contain 32 ounces or more.

The April 2004 issue of the *American Journal of Clinical Nutrition* reported that the consumption of HFCS increased 1,000% between 1970 and 1990, far exceeding the changes in intake of any other food or food group. HFCS now represents 40% of caloric sweeteners added to foods and beverages and is the sole caloric sweetener in soft drinks in the United States. Sweetened beverages (and they are ubiquitous—even in the health food store) set us up for calorie overconsumption.

According to the *Alternative Medicine Review* December 2005 issue, fructose promotes the formation of toxic advanced glycation end-products (this is the glycation I often write about that degrades the collagen in our skin, resulting in deep wrinkles, and that is implicated in the complications of diabetes and in the development of atherosclerosis). In addition, excessive fructose consumption may be responsible in part for the increasing prevalence of obesity, diabetes mellitus, and nonalcoholic fatty liver disease.

When we consume simple sugars such as HFCS, we are causing an immediate pro-inflammatory spike in our blood sugar. Unlike glucose, however, fructose *does not* stimulate insulin secretion or enhance leptin production—key hormones that regulate the appetite. Because insulin and leptin act as signals to the brain for the regulation of food intake and body weight, the ability of fructose to bypass these mechanisms may contribute to overeating. In short, the body's natural checks and balances are thrown out of balance. Fructose bypasses the natural mechanisms that prevent overeating and actually makes the body think it is still hungry—even after eating a large meal.

This is because the digestive and absorptive processes for glucose and fructose are different. Also, when we consume large amounts of fructose, which is basically an unregulated source of fuel for the liver, it is converted to both fat and cholesterol. Fructose also significantly raises triglyceride levels. As Perricone readers know, I am no advocate of sugar—in fact *sugar is toxic*. But the effects of fructose, particularly in the form of HFCS, are an even more significant cause for alarm. (I am not talking about the naturally occurring fructose found in fresh fruit.)

Thus, the increase in consumption of HFCS is directly related to the epidemic of obesity: As the consumption of HFCS has increased around the world, so has the incidence of obesity. However, that is not the only negative effect of HFCS and corn syrup. According to Michael Pollen, writing in the *New York Times* (June 4, 2006), 70 percent of America's corn fields are treated with the powerful herbicide atrazine. He states that traces of the chemical routinely turn up in American streams and wells and even in the rain; the U.S. Food and Drug Administration also finds residues of atrazine in our food. This herbicide was recently banned by the European Union and is a suspected carcinogen and endocrine disruptor in humans. Use of these types of toxins pose a potentially devastating threat to the environment and everything in it—including humans.

and targeted nutritional supplements, the foundation for my entire body of work, to optimize cellular rejuvenation.

In "The Anti-Aging Kitchen," you will find a list of *pro-inflammatory foods*, which are mainly simple sugars, starches (including breads, pasta, desserts, juices, soda, French fries, and snack foods, such as rice and corn cakes, potato chips, and pretzels), and the wrong type of fats (margarine, shortening, products containing trans-fatty acids, and most vegetable oils). The simple sugars and starches quickly convert to sugar in the bloodstream with the resulting negative effects described above. The *anti-inflammatory foods,* also listed in Appendix A, are those rich in antioxidants, EFAs, fiber, and phytonutrients. These include fresh fruits and vegetables, cold-water fish such as wild salmon, beans and lentils, healthy fats such as EVOO, and so on. Food in its most natural, least processed form is always the best choice.

Food for Thought

Every day a new study hits the newswire demonstrating the health benefits of anti-inflammatory foods. Recently, for instance, scientists at University College London have discovered that beans, lentils, and nuts contain inositol pentakisphosphate, a potent natural anticancer compound that blocks a key enzyme involved in tumor growth. Beans and lentils also stabilize blood sugar and help offset the inflammatory effects from other foods. In fact, a meal with legumes raises blood sugar very slowly and moderately, and even moderates the blood sugar response to the next meal you eat, whether this next meal includes beans or not.

Simply put, if we avoid foods that cause a rise in blood sugar and insulin, we will avoid an inflammatory response and thus be able to burn fat as opposed to storing it. We will also be able to effectively stop out-of-control appetites and we will prevent our muscle mass from breaking down.

APPETITE SUPPRESSANTS

As we saw in Chapter One ("Cellular Rejuvenation"), we can protect our bodies from an incredible array of diseases—including cancer— via the foods we eat. Can we also influence our ability to lose weight and prevent unwanted weight gain with food? The answer is yes, and there are several very good ways to accomplish this.

The first, and probably the most obvious, way to lose weight is to eat less. And the best way to do that is to find a way to suppress the appetite. A good way to start is to eat protein.

It appears that a protein-rich diet can work on a cellular level to decrease appetite. An interesting animal study from INSERM, the French national medical research institute, and the Université Lyon has uncovered new evidence that explains how protein-rich diets stunt the appetite, according to a report in the journal *Cell Metabolism*. The findings suggest a novel link that connects macronutrients in the diet to hunger. (Macronutrients are proteins, fats, and carbs that generate hormonal responses and provide the body with building blocks to function properly and to repair damaged cell tissue.)

"It is well known that protein feeding decreases hunger sensation and subsequent food intake in animals and humans," said study author Gilles Mithieux. However, the mechanism of how protein affects appetite remains unclear. Earlier studies have shown that eating dietary protein has little effect on the major hormones that regulate hunger. What this new study found was surprising: Protein-rich diets spark the production of glucose in the small intestine. That rise in glucose, sensed in the liver and relayed to the brain, led the animals to eat less.

Without getting overly technical, the upshot of the study is this: In addition to protein's ability to diminish appetite, the intestinal synthesis of glucose activates the part of the brain involved in the control of appetite, causing a subsequent decline in food consumption. That's why I always recommend eating your protein first at the start of each meal and snack.

However, protein isn't the only macronutrient that helps suppress appetite. A meal of fish (for protein) and fresh vegetables (for low-glycemic carbs), for example, will provide satiety without encouraging the body to overeat. This is in direct opposition to the high-glycemic

Keep *on* the Grass

Part of the rise in obesity can be attributed to the changes in the way we raise beef and other animals. According to Jo Robinson, the author of an excellent book, *Pasture Perfect,* "grass-fed beef is healthier than grain-fed beef, and may even be healthier than chicken."

Grass-fed beef is up to three times leaner than grain-fed beef and can have up to 15 fewer calories per ounce than grain-fed beef. Grass-fed meat also provides more balanced omega-3s and omega-6 fatty acids, which help guard against a variety of ailments.

Like wild salmon, grass-fed beef is an excellent source of high-quality omega-3 EFA, as well as conjugated linoleic acid (CLA; see pages 51–52). Researchers have also compared key antioxidants in meat from pasture-fed and grain-fed cattle. The grass-fed meat was higher in vitamin C, vitamin E, and folic acid. It was also 10 times higher in beta-carotene. These health benefits decline significantly after just 3 months of grain feeding, even if the grain is organic.

"What's not in grass-fed beef that is in grain-fed beef is important, too," Robinson wrote in an article published in the magazine *Mother Earth News.*

For instance, mad cow disease has never been found in grass-fed beef, which is also far less likely to contain dangerous *Escherichia coli* (*E. coli*) bacteria. Grass-fed beef has "no extra hormones and no traces of antibiotics and is both cleaner and more wholesome than ordinary beef by far. Feedlot cattle may eat . . . all kinds of products in addition to grain, including chicken manure, chicken feathers, newsprint, cardboard and municipal garbage waste."

Expansion of the grass-fed beef market in the United States still faces hurdles, owing to the fact that most livestock expertise has centered on grain-fed animals for many years, and the feeding, slaughter, and handling of grass-fed animals is very different. Robinson says, "Everything has to be right for it to be an excellent product, and there isn't a school or an extension agent to teach you the ropes." She hopes that the U.S. Department of Agriculture will start supporting the research and extension offices needed to bring better-quality beef to more American consumers. For more information on grass-fed beef, visit www.deliciousorganics.com.

carbohydrates we frequently consume. In fact, these foods and beverages create a vicious cycle of overeating—the more you eat, the more you want. The ubiquitous bread basket placed before diners as soon as they sit down in a restaurant is a prime example—just one slice will immediately begin to stimulate the appetite and encourage overeating. Next time you're dining out, pass up that predinner roll and opt instead for smoked salmon or shrimp cocktail.

CARALLUMA FIMBRIATA—SUPERSTAR OF THE WEIGHT-LOSS FIRMAMENT

So far in this chapter we have learned how to avoid the common dietary pitfalls that cause us to overeat and gain unwanted weight. Now I would like to introduce a revolutionary, new (to Americans) plant-based remedy, *Caralluma fimbriata*, an outstanding weapon against overeating, the accumulation of body fat, and the loss of muscle mass.

As for so many miracle healing plants, the *Caralluma* story begins in India, where thousands of medicinal plants and vegetables have been used for millennia. Although you may not find them documented in medical textbooks, these botanicals are an important part of the daily lives of the native populations and are highly valued for their many proven, curative properties.

Edible, succulent cacti grow wild all over India and are part of the daily diets of several native populations. *Caralluma fimbriata* is the most prevalent of these species, and it flourishes in large parts of interior India. It grows wild in urban centers as well and is planted as a roadside shrub and as a boundary marker in gardens.

Caralluma is eaten in several forms. It is cooked as a regular vegetable, with spices and salt, used in preserves such as chutneys and pickles, and is even eaten raw. Indian tribals chew chunks of *Caralluma* to suppress hunger when on a day's hunt.

Caralluma has been used for centuries in India. Its benefits include increased energy, increased lean muscle mass, and significant, measurable decrease in arm and waist circumference, along with fat loss. *Caralluma* not only inhibits fat synthesis but also increases the burning of fat, which makes more energy available to the body for cellular repair. In ad-

SAFETY PROFILE

To see testimonials from botanical experts, noted Ayurvedic practitioners, university professors, and botanists across India about the safety and complete lack of toxicity of *Caralluma fimbriata*, see the "References" for this chapter. These testimonials also attest to its use in the daily diets of local populations in the regions of India in which *Caralluma* grows. The tribal community treats *Caralluma fimbriata* as a food item for daily consumption. They believe that *Caralluma* is a unique herb that cures common health problems apart from its excellent ability to suppress appetite and thirst. They eat a handful of *Caralluma* chunks during their hunting trips, which may last many days at a stretch. A bag full of *Caralluma* chunks is enough to cater to the needs of the entire tribal group when hunting, eliminating the necessity of carrying food.

dition to historical and anecdotal data, *Caralluma* has also been clinically demonstrated to suppress appetite and stop hunger pangs. In fact, the U.S. Food and Drug Administration (FDA) has published excellent and comprehensive information regarding *Caralluma* and its many benefits.

How *CARALLUMA* Works

Caralluma works by

- *Blocking fat formation.* During a complicated chemical process called the Krebs cycle, glucose is broken down into a compound called *pyruvic acid*, which enters the mitochondria. Pyruvic acid in turn is broken down to acetic acid and is ultimately converted to *acetyl coenzyme A* and citric acid. During this cycle, *ATP* is formed, which in turn generates the energy the body needs for its day-to-day activities. What happens when too much energy is generated? It is stored by the body in the form of fat. The basic building block of fatty acids is acetyl coenzyme A. However, the formation of acetyl coenzyme A requires a vital enzyme called *citrate lyase*. If this enzyme is blocked, then the body cannot make fat. This is where *Caralluma fimbriata* comes in—it contains pregnane glycosides, plant substances that are believed to block the activity of citrate lyase. By blocking this enzyme, *Caralluma fimbriata* blocks the formation of fat by the body.

  Caralluma fimbriata also blocks another enzyme called *malonyl coenzyme A*. By blocking this enzyme and the subsequent fat formation, the body is forced to burn its fat reserves, accelerating the rate of fat loss by the body.
- *Suppressing appetite.* Controlled clinical trials with *Caralluma fimbriata* extract clearly demonstrate its ability to suppress appetite, probably due to its activity on the appetite-control mechanism of the brain. When we eat, nerves from the stomach send a signal to the hypothalamus, the part of the brain that controls appetite. When the stomach is full, the hypothalamus signals the brain to

stop eating. When a person is hungry, the hypothalamus sends a signal to the brain that food is needed.

By interfering with this signal, or by creating a signal on its own, *Caralluma fimbriata* seems to fool the brain into thinking that the stomach is full, even when the person has not eaten. It is believed that the pregnane glycosides in *Caralluma fimbriata* inhibit the hunger sensory mechanism of the hypothalamus.

This is very exciting because the search for substances that can effectively suppress excessive hunger has long been on the scientific radar screen as a potentially important approach to weight management. However, conventional drugs that can work as appetite suppressants carry with them serious risks, including cardiac disturbances, elevated blood pressure, anxiety, insomnia, and hypersensitivity. Another downside is that our appetite comes back with a vengeance when the drug wears off—thus potentially causing us to overeat and undo the drug's effects. None of this is true with *Caralluma*—when it wears off, your appetite returns to normal.

• *Generating lean muscle mass.* The main reason most weight-loss programs fail is that we always feel dull and tired after losing weight. This makes us revert to old eating habits and results in rebound weight gain. However, the opposite occurs when we take *Caralluma*. People report that they feel more energetic and that they have lost body fat and strengthened lean muscle mass.

The reason for this is that *Caralluma* not only *inhibits fat synthesis* as mentioned above but also *increases the burning of fat*. It is a well-known fact that fat cells tend to store calories, while muscle cells burn calories. Therefore, when more energy is available to the body, muscle cells burn energy faster. This results in the shrinking of fat cells, while muscle becomes stronger. And while muscle cells are heavier than fat cells, they are also denser—more compact—than fat cells. Consequently they occupy less space and our bodies appear trim and compact.

Rarely have I come across a botanical that has personally impressed me as much as *Caralluma fimbriata.* Here in the West, extract of *Caralluma* is used as a supplement. If you're taking it in powder form, mix ⅛ teaspoon with water one hour before meals. If you're taking capsules, follow the directions on the label. (See the "Resources" section for sources of *Caralluma fimbriata.*)

I have often joked during lectures and TV appearances that I carry a photo of the nutrient ALA in my wallet—right next to photos of my beloved children. While this is a slight exaggeration, I freely confess to holding ALA in the highest esteem for its many inimitable anti-aging

GO FOR PISTACHIOS

Contrary to popular belief, nuts will not sabotage your ability to lose weight. In fact, they are a great addition to your daily diet. Almonds, filberts, walnuts, pine nuts, pecans, macadamia nuts, and other varieties of tree nuts are recommended—as is the pistachio, which has a delicious buttery flavor. Similar to almonds, the pistachio has a high nutritious value, being very rich in proteins and vitamins. Pistachios are also high in healthy monounsaturated fats, making them a highly satisfying food or snack.

Pistachios are gaining fame as one of the healthiest nuts available because of their high levels of phytosterol, a plant compound known to reduce cholesterol levels and improve heart health. According to an article published in December 2005 by the American Chemical Society's *Journal of Agricultural and Food Chemistry,* pistachios have the highest levels of phytosterols among snack nuts most commonly consumed in the United States. The unique green color of this delightful nut is due to its high level of chlorophyll, a plant pigment that makes leaves green. Avoid the dyed red shells and select the natural tan shelled variety.

properties. My experiences thus far with *Caralluma* have convinced me that this amazing plant deserves an equally elevated status.

Nutrients That Help Control Blood Sugar

There are many supplements, including some that we discussed in Chapter One ("Cellular Rejuvenation") for mitochondrial rejuvenation, that will also assist in weight management and cellular repair. Here are a few of the best:

CONJUGATED LINOLEIC ACID—THE MISSING LINK IN OBESITY AND WEIGHT GAIN

Conjugated linoleic acid (CLA) is a fatty acid that is found in many of the foods we eat. However, with the dietary change from grass to grain, levels of CLA dramatically decreased in meat and dairy products. When CLA is present, it is found in the fatty portion of milk. Drinking skim milk prevents us from receiving the benefits of CLA. However, since CLA levels are now so low in animal products, skim versus full-fat milk is a moot consideration. Unless you are eating meat and dairy from grass-fed animals, avoid full-fat dairy products and choose only the leanest cuts of meats—or better yet, avoid grain-fed beef and opt for organic, free-range poultry and wild fish.

When taken in effective doses, CLA decreases body fat, especially in the abdominal area. There are several mechanisms of CLA's activity that accomplish these feats:

- CLA actually concentrates in the cell membrane, stabilizing it and thus preventing the breakdown of arachidonic acid into a pro-inflammatory prostaglandin. It helps the insulin receptors remain intact, thus increasing insulin sensitivity, which will then decrease blood sugar and circulating insulin levels.
- Remarkably, studies show that CLA also helps block the absorption of fat and sugar into fat cells (adipocytes). It even induces a

reduction in the actual size of the fat cells. (One reason people gain weight as they age is that their fat cells literally become fatter.)

- Although one article published in the *Journal of Nutrition* reported that CLA supplementation for 1 year does not prevent weight or body fat regain, another relatively recent and large-scale study published in the same journal showed that taking 3.4 grams of CLA a day for 2 years led to a small but significant decrease in body fat in overweight people. Interestingly, CLA appears to have no effect on the body fat of people who are not overweight. It appears to have the most effect on women with a body mass index of 25 to 30 kilograms per square meter. To learn how to calculate your BMI visit www.americanheart.org.

Many studies show that in addition to having antioxidant, anti-inflammatory, and insulin-sensitizing actions, CLA helps prevent muscle loss and weakness associated with aging and disease. This is one of the reasons CLA has long been a favorite supplement of athletes and body builders. What could be more exciting or encouraging than a supplement that shrinks body fat while increasing and preserving lean muscle mass? (*Note:* Do not take CLA if you are pregnant, nursing, or have diabetes or any other health problem. Always consult with your primary care physician before taking it.)

Dosage information: Take one 500-milligram capsule in the morning and one 500-milligram capsule in the evening.

NIACIN-BOUND CHROMIUM

It isn't just CLA that helps us to preserve lean muscle mass. There are several key nutrients that help control blood sugar, including chromium polynicotinate, also known as NBC. My friend and colleague Dr. Harry Preuss (whom I mentioned in Chapter One, "Cellular Rejuvenation") is currently researching the use of dietary supplements and nutraceuticals to favorably influence or even prevent a variety of conditions, especially those related to obesity, insulin resistance, loss of lean muscle mass, and cardiovascular perturbations. Dr. Preuss recently examined a number of chromium compounds and found NBC to be among the most efficacious. Nutrition experts report that generally, Americans have a chromium deficiency—and low levels of chromium are associated with type 2 diabetes and cardiovascular disease.

Articles on studies have also been published noting that increased consumption of sugar depletes our body stores of chromium, placing us at further risk for hyperglycemia and hyperinsulinemia (too much blood sugar and too much insulin). In a placebo-controlled crossover study, Dr. Preuss and a team of researchers at Georgetown University Medical Center showed that overweight African-American women consuming 600 micrograms of chromium as NBC (the ChromeMate brand) for 8 weeks had a significant loss of body fat and sparing of muscle (lean body mass) compared with a prior placebo period of the same duration. Increased fat loss was also observed among women who were randomized to consume chromium first, followed by placebo, suggesting a carryover effect of the supplementation on fat loss. No adverse effects were observed.

Dosage information: Take one 200-microgram ChromeMate capsule daily, preferably with a meal.

OMEGA-3 FATTY ACIDS

Head for the seafood counter or stock up on fish oil capsules if you want to lose weight. One key strategy that will stop your waistline from spreading and help you to lose existing body fat is to favor certain dietary fats: namely, the long-chain "marine" omega-3 fatty acids abundant only in fatty cold-water fish and high-quality supplemental fish oil.

Marine-source omega-3s cause the body to burn calories for immediate energy needs, before they are turned into hard-to-lose, inflammation-inducing abdominal fat. This metabolic magic trick means that we will end up carrying less weight. No one ever got fat from eating fish—as long as it's not batter-dipped and fried in inflammatory omega-6 vegetable fats. Unfortunately we cannot say the same about sirloin steaks or cheeseburgers made from grain-fed beef rich in saturated fat. Cold-water fish and omega-3 fish oil capsules stabilize blood sugar and lower insulin levels—key factors in preventing weight gain and achieving successful weight loss.

Dosage information: As a dietary supplement, take one 1,000-milligram wild sockeye salmon oil softgel with or after a meal up to three times daily. To maximize benefits, higher doses should be approved by your health care professional.

No Weight-Loss Benefit from Farmed Salmon

The results of several recent studies show that eating farmed salmon—whose plant-based feed makes them high in inflammatory omega-6 fatty acids—actually increases levels of inflammation in its consumers. And these inflammatory omega-6 fatty acids reduce the beneficial health impacts of a farmed salmon's omega-3s. In addition, farmed salmon are fed fish meal, the ubiquitous corn and soy, and are often artificially colored with added synthetic pigments to mask their naturally occurring, unappetizing pale gray color. By contrast, wild salmon eat an all-natural marine diet rich in krill and shrimp, which are rich in the carotenoid astaxanthin. It is astaxanthin that gives wild salmon their beautiful color, which ranges from pink to orange to red across the various species. Farmed salmon are fed a steady diet of antibiotics to grow, unlike wild salmon. Finally, the fish meal and fish oils fed to farmed salmon have a direct impact on levels of PCB (polychlorinated biphenyl, an industrial by-product that has been identified as a probable carcinogen in humans).

GREEN FOODS AND WEIGHT LOSS

When barley grass is made part of a proprietary formulation containing *Super CitriMax HCA*, CLA in the form of *Clarinol CLA*, and *green tea extract*, it helps promote specific physiological mechanisms involved in stimulating weight loss and lean body mass. When this formula is used in combination with a healthful diet and regular exercise program, it increases both energy levels and fat metabolism, reduces appetite, promotes lean body mass, and provides detoxification and antioxidant protection.

RECENT STUDY ON MAGMASLIM AND WEIGHT CONTROL

Certified nutritionist Deborah Arneson, director of nutrition consultants of Healing Quest Center, recently performed a study with two servings each of the proprietary formula MagmaSLIM in combination with Green Magma barley grass. The study showed the following results: an increase in energy levels, an overall reduction in body weight, and dramatic decreases in both body fat and total cholesterol. Liver function increased as well.

OTHER IMPORTANT LEAN-FOR-LIFE SUPPLEMENTS

- Carnitine and ALC enhance the sensitivity of insulin receptors, helping to decrease blood sugar and circulating levels of insulin. *Dosage information:* Carnitine—one or two 250-milligram capsules with a meal up to three times daily, or as recommended by your health care professional. ALC—one or two 500-milligram capsules daily in divided doses between meals.
- Maitake SX Fraction enhances insulin sensitivity for controlling blood sugar levels. *Dosage information:* Take one 100-milligram tablet three times a day between meals, as a dietary supplement or as recommended by your health care professional.

- Gamma linoleic acid (GLA) from borage oil improves cell sensitivity to insulin, reducing our chance of developing diabetes, heart disease, and excess body fat. *Dosage information:* Take one 1,000-milligram softgel with breakfast and one 1,000-milligram softgel with dinner as a dietary supplement or as recommended by your health care professional.

- ALA increases insulin sensitivity by increasing the body's ability to take glucose into the cells. *Dosage information:* Take one 50-milligram capsule with breakfast or with lunch and one 50-milligram capsule in the evening with dinner as a dietary supplement or as recommended by your health care professional.

- Co-Q_{10} enhances the metabolism, giving us greater energy and endurance and a greater ability to lose body fat, while preventing the energy decline seen in aging cells. Co-Q_{10} also works synergistically with other antioxidants to elevate cellular levels of vitamins C and E and glutathione and to help regulate blood sugar and enhance insulin sensitivity. Co-Q_{10} also maximizes the burning of foods for fuel, helping to normalize fats in our blood. *Dosage information:* Take one to three 10-milligram softgels daily with or after a meal as a dietary supplement or as recommended by your health care professional.

Each of these supplements offers many other benefits as well, and I highly recommend them for their anti-aging as well as their weight-control properties.

Although many neurochemical and hormonal signals control appetite, so do psychological, social, cultural, economic, and environmental factors. Understanding the biochemical mechanisms of why we gain fat and lose muscle is a major step toward eliminating these unwanted problems and their potentially life-threatening ramifications.

Supporting Our Support Structure

3

I f you're looking for a prime example of cellular rejuvenation, look no further than the bones of the body. New research shows that cellular rejuvenation of bone tissue and muscle mass is a very powerful new reality. Having and maintaining a strong, healthy body and beautiful skin throughout our lifetime depends on a multitude of factors, including the support structure under the skin itself, which consists of our bone structure and muscle tissue.

As this chapter will reveal, we are not limited to the genetic hand we are dealt any more than we are destined (or doomed, as the case may be) to lose 5 pounds of muscle and gain 10 pounds of fat with each passing decade, the norm in the developed world. And we don't have to lose precious bone mass, resulting in age-related falls, fractures, and progressive physical weakness and disability.

While it's true that some bone loss is inevitable as a natural result of aging, we don't have to just take it in stride. As you will see in this chapter, there are positive steps you can take to not only prevent bone loss and preserve the bone you have but to also build new bone—even after menopause.

That's because of *secret 3: Key nutrients taken in the right combinations not only prevent bone loss but also can actually stimulate new bone growth.*

Through a process known as remodeling, old bone is constantly replaced with new. Bone formation—the acquisition of bone mineral density (BMD)—peaks between the ages of 20 and 30. However, bone mass is maintained as we age through remodeling, the continuous breakdown and re-formation of bone. Old bone is *resorbed*, or broken down by cells called *osteoclasts*, and new bone is formed by cells called *osteoblasts*. Problems such as osteoporosis occur when there is more resorption than formation, resulting in a net loss of bone.

The Truth About Bone Loss

The age-related loss of bone mass known as osteoporosis, a disorder characterized by porous, fragile bones, is a serious public health problem for more than 10 million Americans, 80% of whom are women. Another 34 million Americans have osteopenia, or low bone mass, which precedes osteoporosis. When we have osteoporosis, the inside of the bones becomes porous from a lack of calcium. As the bones become weaker, they become fragile and susceptible to fracture, especially of the hip, spine, and wrist, although any bone can be affected.

When we think of osteoporosis, we envision a little old lady, stooped over from the advancing years. Unfortunately, this is a pretty accurate picture: By the age of 80, two thirds of all women will develop osteoporosis. Starting at about age 40, people typically lose about half an inch in height each decade. This rate increases after the age of 70, leading to a total loss of between 1 and 3 inches of height.

Height loss is natural and shouldn't be a cause of worry, unless it occurs rapidly. However, the loss of 2 or more inches in height during adulthood serves as a powerful predictor of osteoporosis in the hip, and thus the risk for hip fractures in elderly women, according to a new study conducted by the Ohio State University Medical Center. The finding has led researchers to recommend that primary care physicians routinely screen aging patients for height loss.

Women are much more likely to suffer from osteoporosis than men for the following reasons:

- Women have less bone mass than men from the start.
- Women tend to live longer than men.
- Women usually consume less calcium than men do.
- The rate of bone loss accelerates after menopause because the female hormone estrogen is needed to keep bones strong (and estrogen decreases after menopause—see box below).

SPECIAL NEWS FOR POSTMENOPAUSAL WOMEN

The most rapid rates of bone loss in women occur during the first 5 years after menopause, when the decrease in the production of estrogen results in increased bone resorption and decreased calcium absorption. In fact, women may lose as much as 3% to 5% of bone mass per year during the years immediately following menopause, with decreases of less than 1% per year after age 65. Two studies are in agreement that increased calcium intakes during menopause *will not* completely offset menopause bone loss. However, other studies show that nutritional supplements such as silicon in the form of choline-stabilized orthosilicic acid improves the bone health benefits of both calcium and vitamin D (more about this later in the chapter).

- If a woman's ovaries are surgically removed, more rapid bone loss may occur, because estrogen is made in the ovaries.

Contrary to popular assumption, however, men are not immune to bone loss either. Total bone mass peaks at age 35 for both men and women. Thereafter all adults begin to lose bone mass unless they take action to prevent it. According to information from the Osteoporosis and Related Bone Disorders—National Resource Center posted on a website of the National Institutes of Health (NIH; http://www.osteo.org), the following factors can put you at increased risk for osteoporosis:

- Personal history of fracture after age 50
- Current low bone mass
- History of fracture in a close relative
- Being female
- Being thin and/or having a small frame
- Advanced age (Osteoporosis is a major public health threat for 55 percent of people 50 years of age and older. The older you are, the greater the risk.)
- A family history of osteoporosis
- *For women only:* estrogen deficiency as a result of menopause, especially early or surgically induced; also women who stop menstruating before menopause because of conditions such as anorexia or bulimia, or because of excessive physical exercise
- *For men only:* low testosterone levels
- Low lifetime calcium intake
- Vitamin D deficiency
- An inactive lifestyle
- Use of certain medications to treat chronic medical conditions such as rheumatoid arthritis, endocrine disorders (i.e., an underactive thyroid), seizure disorders, and gastrointestinal diseases may have side effects that can damage bone and lead to osteoporosis. One class of drugs that has particularly damaging ef-

fects on the skeleton is glucocorticoids (a group of steroids that have metabolic and anti-inflammatory effects). The following drugs also can cause bone loss:

- Excessive thyroid hormones
- Anticonvulsants
- Antacids containing aluminum
- Gonadotropin-releasing hormones, used for treatment of endometriosis
- Methotrexate, used for cancer treatment
- Cyclosporine A, an immunosuppressive drug
- Heparin and cholestyramine, taken to control blood cholesterol levels

- *Cigarette smoking:* A study reported in the January–February 2001 issue of the *Journal of the American Academy of Orthopedics* shows that smoking impairs muscle, bone, and joint health. This places smokers at a much greater risk of developing osteoporosis. The best action a smoker can take to protect his or her bones is to quit smoking; if you quit, even later in life, you help limit smoking-related bone loss.
- Excessive use of alcohol
- Being Caucasian or Asian (although African Americans and Hispanic Americans are by no means free of risk)

Taking Action

Since we achieve 98% of our bone mass by the age of 20, good nutrition in childhood and adolescence is vital in helping to prevent osteoporosis in our later years. However, this advice is not much help if we are an over-40, thin, petite, Caucasian or Asian woman who has been dieting since she was 12. Fortunately there is hope, as more and more studies are showing the remarkable benefits of diet, exercise, and nutritional supplements.

The National Osteoporosis Foundation's advice for bone health includes

- A balanced diet rich in calcium and vitamin D
- Weight-bearing exercise (more about this in Chapter Seven, "Stress Reduction = Life Extension")
- A healthy lifestyle with no smoking or excessive alcohol intake
- Bone density testing and medication, when appropriate

How Our Food Choices Impact Bone Health

As we get older, remodeling and bone cell rejuvenation become even more important. But the discovery that they are possible is tremendously encouraging. A December 2005 study reported in the *Journal of the American College of Nutrition* found that "bone remodeling triples from age 50 to 65 in typical women" and that "high calcium intakes in postmenopausal and older women [return] remodeling to approximately pre-menopausal values and improve bone strength immediately."

Ideally, our diet will include foods rich in calcium, and the range of such foods is much broader than you might think. Calcium superstars include milk, cheese, yogurt, kefir, dark leafy greens, broccoli, canned sardines and salmon with bones, dried beans and peas, tofu, and sea vegetables (seaweed). While calcium supplements can be an adjunct therapy, the best strategy is to include calcium-rich foods at every meal. *Calcium supplements should not be considered replacements for a calcium-rich diet.* Supplements can be added, but the key benefits—from weight loss to bone building—have been shown to come from foods.

The Food and Nutrition Board of the Institute of Medicine of the U.S. National Academy of Sciences has recommended the following adequate intakes (AIs) for calcium:

AGE GROUP/ SPECIAL CONDITION		ADEQUATE INTAKE (MILLIGRAMS PER DAY)
Infants:	0–6 months	200
	7–12 months	270
Children:	1–3 years	500
	4–8 years	800
Boys:	9–13 years	1,300
	14–18 years	1,300
Girls:	9–13 years	1,300
	14–18 years	1,300
Men:	19–30 years	1,000
	31–50 years	1,000
	51–70 years	1,200
	> 70 years	1,200
Women:	19–30 years	1,000
	31–50 years	1,000
	51–70 years	1,200
	> 70 years	1,200
Pregnancy:	14–18 years	1,300
	19–30 years	1,000
	31–50 years	1,000
Lactation:	14–18 years	1,300
	19–30 years	1,000
	31–50 years	1,000

Note: On a food label, calcium is generally expressed as a percentage of the 1,000-milligrams-a-day U.S. recommended daily allowance. Therefore, 20% would provide 200 mg per serving.

Here are my top dietary recommendations for building and preserving bone:

YOGURT AND KEFIR

Yogurt and kefir are fermented milk products that offer many outstanding health benefits; I cannot urge you strongly enough to include several servings of yogurt and/or kefir in your daily diet. Since this chapter is about building and preserving bone, I will start with these benefits. Both yogurt and kefir are rich sources of calcium. However, yogurt, kefir, and other fermented milk products contain an iron-building glycoprotein known as *lactoferrin*, a substance that can rejuvenate bones on a cellular level. A number of important studies have concluded that lactoferrin may have a physiological role in bone growth and healing, and a potentially therapeutic role as an anabolic factor in osteoporosis.

In other words, the lactoferrin found in foods such as yogurt will stimulate new bone growth while preventing further breakdown of existing bone tissue. The lactoferrin enhances both the growth and the activity of osteoblasts (the cells that build bone). In fact, lactoferrin reduces the rate of bone cell death by 50% to 70% and decreases the development of osteoclasts, the cells responsible for breaking down bone. Thus, it is exciting to report that among the myriad of health benefits conferred by fermented milk products, preventing and reversing osteoporosis may be added to the list.

One other note related to bone health: The *Journal of Nutrition* published a study by Israeli researchers that found that lactobacillus, one of the probiotic (pro-life) bacteria found in yogurt, offers "remarkable preventive and curative" effects on arthritis. Because probiotic bacteria have beneficial effects in infectious and inflammatory diseases, principally in bowel disorders, they hypothesized that these bacteria would reduce inflammation found in arthritis. Hopefully research will continue and validate these early findings.

HEALTH FROM THE SEA

If you are looking for one of Mother Nature's most precious gifts, you will need to look to the oceans, rivers, and lakes of the world and not its gardens and farmland. Here you will find sea vegetables, wild ocean plants, and marine algae, which are enjoyed daily as staples and healing foods in many coastal parts of the world. Small amounts of sea veggies add a rich flavor and enhance the nutritional value of most dishes. Popular American sea vegetables are dulse, kelp, alaria, laver (from the East Coast), and sea palm (from the West Coast). Asian varieties include nori, hiziki, arame, kombu, and wakame. Maine Coast Sea Vegetables (www.seaveg.com) farms the pristine, clear, cold waters of the gulf of Maine for dulse, kelp, alaria, laver, nori, sea lettuce, and bladderwrack. According to the experts at Maine Coast, these tasty treats are fat free, low calorie, and one of the richest sources of minerals to be found in the entire vegetable kingdom because of their ready access to the abundance of minerals found in the ocean. The gentle wave action of the underwater currents ensures that the entire surface of the sea vegetable receives nourishment. It is also interesting to note that seawater and human blood contain many of the same minerals in very similar concentrations.

Sea vegetables are rich in minerals and trace elements, including calcium, magnesium, iron, potassium, iodine, manganese, and chromium, at levels much greater than those found in land vegetables. They contain the B vitamin folate, riboflavin, and pantothenic acid, and like flax and pumpkin seeds, they are rich in lignans, phytochemicals with cancer-protective properties. Sea veggies also provide vitamins, fiber, enzymes, and high-quality protein. Marine phytochemicals found only in sea vegetables have been shown to absorb and eliminate radioactive elements and heavy metal contaminants from our bodies. Other recent research demonstrates that sea vegetables inhibit tumor formation, reduce cholesterol levels, and possess antiviral properties.

Certain sea vegetables exert anti-inflammatory actions, while their rich magnesium and B vitamin content promote stress relief. Other health benefits include

- Protection from cardiovascular disease
- Relief from symptoms of menopause
- Lower levels of the heart-threatening chemical homocysteine
- Protection against migraine headaches
- Less severe asthma symptoms
- Lower blood pressure
- Better thyroid health
- Lower stress level

It's very easy to incorporate these superfoods into your diet. In Japanese restaurants, you will find that sheets of nori (dried black or dark purple seaweed, roasted over a flame until green) are wrapped around sushi or chopped and used as a topping. Other sea vegetables make tasty stocks for soups and sauces, refreshing salads, and add a delicate flavor to soups. But you can just as easily add small amounts of bite-sized pieces to your own favorite soups, salads, sandwiches, and stir-fries. Nori has a wonderful, almost salty flavor that can really put zing in a simple dish and can be added to recipes; for sources of sea veggies, see the "Resources" section.

Remember that dried sea vegetables are an extremely vital, wild food and provide highly concentrated nutrition. A little goes a long way; most recipes use less than ¼ ounce per serving. The legendary health and longevity of the rural Japanese people who follow the traditional Japanese diet, rich in sea vegetables, is testimony to the unparalleled health benefits of these gifts from the sea.

CANNED SALMON AND SARDINES

My readers know that I am perhaps the greatest living advocate on the health benefits of wild salmon and other cold-water fish, which are rich in omega-3. Here is another way to get their benefits, especially where bones are concerned: by eating wild salmon and sardines that come in cans. Canned salmon or sardines—provided they are canned with both skin and bones—not only are great sources of protein and omega-3 EFAs but also provide significant levels of dietary calcium.

If you think this is old news, it is. Back in 1995, the *Mayo Clinic Health Letter* reported that canned salmon was ranked number 7 of the 15 best calcium sources. However, this outstanding, easily absorbable form of calcium and other superior nutrients is often ignored—at our peril. Canning softens the bones and allows them to be easily combined with other ingredients. There is approximately *thirty times* more calcium in "traditional style" canned sockeye (with skin and bones) than in the salmon (and tuna) sold with these nutritional components removed.

According to nutritional analysis from Vital Choice Seafood, wild Alaskan sockeye salmon has 221 milligrams of calcium per 100 grams, which means that each 3.75-ounce can of *bone-in* sockeye (called traditional wild red) has 232 milligrams, or 23% of the RDA (1,000 milligrams) of calcium for adults between ages 30 and 51, and each 7.5-ounce can has 464 milligrams (46% of RDA). Canned sardines are also excellent calcium sources. Vital Choice's sardines have 234 milligrams of calcium (23% of RDA) per ¼-cup (62-gram) serving.

Many people are initially turned off by the *idea* of skin and bones in canned salmon, but after being enlightened about the superior flavor and nutritional advantages of traditional-style salmon almost everyone eventually comes to prefer it—including me. Among canned-salmon connoisseurs—especially in Europe and Japan—there is little or no demand for a skinless and boneless canned-salmon product.

In fact, when the Japanese initially learned that the bones were being removed from Vital Choice's canned salmon for other markets, they requested that their orders containing the skin and bones be canned separately, and ultimately purchased them all. True story!

Supplements for Rebuilding Bone

Although research has shown, as mentioned earlier, that the optimum method of obtaining cellular rejuvenating nutrients is through the foods we eat, diet doesn't always supply adequate amounts. Fortunately, there are several supplements we can take that reinforce bone remodeling to protect against bone loss, especially as we age.

THE NEW NEWS ABOUT VITAMIN D

Vitamin D attracted a great deal of attention in 2006. Scientists are finding that when we avoid sunlight all the time by slathering ourselves with sunscreen or avoiding the outdoors altogether, we lose our most effective source of vitamin D. When the body is exposed to the sun's UV light, it produces its own vitamin D. No one is saying that you should lie out on the beach and tan all day the way we used to before we knew about the dangers of skin cancer. All that's required is about 10 minutes a day in the summer, and about 15 in winter.

Unfortunately, between our sedentary lifestyle and our conscientious use of sunscreens, most Americans don't get enough vitamin D. Studies have shown that this vitamin's beneficial effects extend to reducing the risk of colon, breast, and prostate cancers. And it's long been known that vitamin D helps maintain strong bones. Older adults can also reduce their risk of falls by more than 20% by ensuring that they get enough vitamin D. A study recently reported in the *Journal of the American Medical Association* noted that "vitamin D may also improve muscle strength, thereby reducing fracture risk through falls."

Blood levels of vitamin D are low in at least one in five women who live in North America and northern Europe, and most postmenopausal women also get too little dietary calcium. But the former deficiency may be more important than the latter, according to new research results. In fact, recent research suggests that higher-than-

RDA intake of vitamin D is probably more important than RDA-level intake of calcium to bone health!

That's because there is actually a tightly intertwined connection between vitamin D, calcium, and a lesser-known (to the lay public) substance called parathyroid hormone (PTH). PTH regulates the amount of calcium in the bloodstream. When blood levels of calcium are low, the thyroid gland secretes more PTH, which raises the level of calcium by taking it from the bone. If this pattern continues, bones will eventually become brittle and prone to breakage.

Enter vitamin D. High blood levels of vitamin D inhibit secretion of PTH, thereby preventing the loss of calcium from bones. Conversely, low vitamin D levels prompt loss of calcium from bones and raise the risks of osteoporosis and fractures. This is one reason why most experts say the RDA for vitamin D (400 international units per day) is too low and should be increased to 600 to 800 international units per day or even higher.

The Food and Nutrition Board of the Institute of Medicine of the U.S. National Academy of Sciences has recommended the following AIs for vitamin D (the biological activity of 1 microgram of vitamin D_2 or vitamin D_3 is 40 international units):

AGE GROUP/ SPECIAL CONDITION		ADEQUATE INTAKE (MICROGRAMS PER DAY)
Infants:	0–12 months	5.0 (200 IU)
Children:	1–8 years	5.0 (200 IU)
Boys:	9–18 years	5.0 (200 IU)
Girls:	9–18 years	5.0 (200 IU)
Men:	19–50 years	5.0 (200 IU)
	51–70 years	10.0 micrograms (400 IU)
	> 70 years	15.0 micrograms (600 IU)

Women:	19–50 years	5.0 (200 IU)
	51–70 years	10.0 (400 IU)
	> 70 years	15.0 (600 IU)
Pregnancy:	14–50 years	5.0 (200 IU)
Lactation:	14–50 years	5.0 (200 IU)

IU = international units.

Scientists in Iceland have found that consuming more than 800 milligrams of calcium per day may be unnecessary for bone health if the body has enough vitamin D. Using food consumption records from more than 900 adults, the researchers determined that sufficient vitamin D levels can ensure an ideal level of PTH, even when calcium intake is less than 800 milligrams per day. However, taking as much as 1,200 milligrams of calcium per day will not be enough to maintain the ideal PTH if we are deficient in vitamin D.

The study is part of a growing body of work that points to the important role of vitamin D, and not just calcium alone, in bone health, a growing concern in North America and Europe as the population ages.

VITAMIN K — GOOD FOR THE BONES AND THE HEART

I recently met with Stephen Sinatra, M.D., a friend and colleague who, like me, enjoys staying abreast of the latest breakthroughs in health and science. Dr. Sinatra is board certified in both internal medicine and cardiology. He is also certified in anti-aging medicine and clinical nutrition, and again like me, frequently uses nutritional interventions in his cardiology practice, in conjunction with the more traditional therapies.

Because arterial plaque is the number-one enemy of a healthy heart, Dr. Sinatra devotes a lot of his research to finding ways to combat this threat, whether they are related to nutrition, nutritional supplements, or some other therapeutic strategy.

DIETARY SOURCES OF VITAMIN D

Fish are among the few good dietary sources of vitamin D. The chart below shows comparisons of several fish sources from Vital Choice. According to the company's research, sockeye salmon is the winner! Although albacore tuna also scores highly, use caution because of the possibility of mercury. Salmon, whether fresh, frozen, or canned, is a much safer choice.

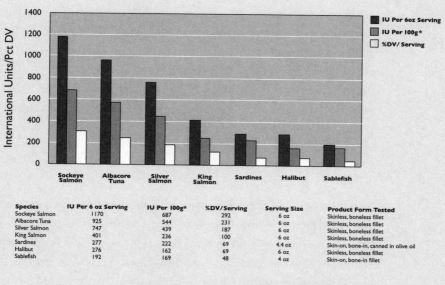

Vitamin **D** Content of Vital Choice Fish
Analysis conducted 6/05 by Covance Laboratories, Inc.

Species	IU Per 6 oz Serving	IU Per 100g*	%DV/Serving	Serving Size	Product Form Tested
Sockeye Salmon	1170	687	292	6 oz	Skinless, boneless fillet
Albacore Tuna	925	544	231	6 oz	Skinless, boneless fillet
Silver Salmon	747	439	187	6 oz	Skinless, boneless fillet
King Salmon	401	236	100	6 oz	Skinless, boneless fillet
Sardines	277	222	69	4.4 oz	Skin-on, bone-in, canned in olive oil
Halibut	276	162	69	6 oz	Skinless, boneless fillet
Sablefish	192	169	48	4 oz	Skin-on, bone-in fillet

*100 grams = 3.5 oz.

For more information go to www.vitalchoice.com

Most recently, he has been working with MK-7 (menaquinone-7), a form of vitamin K_2, which is made by the bacteria that line the gastrointestinal tract. As he reported in the July 2006 edition of his newsletter, *Heart, Health & Nutrition*, two animal studies showed that K_2 demonstrated plaque reversal in blood vessels. This is very promising; it appears that K_2 helps to decalcify hard plaque formations. Similarly, a 2004 Dutch study analyzed the K_2 intake of nearly 5,000 people and found a relationship between higher intakes of K_2 and reduced aortic calcification.

Most of us are familiar with vitamin K in the form of vitamin K_1, a fat-soluble vitamin that also plays an important role in blood clotting. Vitamin K_1 is found in cabbage, cauliflower, spinach, kale, turnip greens, and other dark leafy greens, cereals, soybeans, and other vegetables. However, the richest source of vitamin K_1 by far is nori, a popular sea vegetable. Roasted nori is most often used as a wrapper for making rolled sushi, while dried nori is a flavorful and nutrient-rich addition to soups, stews, sauces, and so on. Records show that nori and other seaweeds have been used for both food and medicine in China since 300 to 800 BCE. As mentioned elsewhere in this chapter, ounce for ounce, sea vegetables' nutrient value far exceeds that of their land-bound counterparts.

VITAMIN K FOR BONE HEALTH

In the 1990s, scientists discovered that vitamin K_1 can increase bone mineral density. Some studies have found a direct association between low dietary vitamin K intake and increased risk of hip fracture. For example, one study observed that women who consumed lettuce (such as romaine) one or more times daily had a significantly—45%—lower risk of hip fracture than did women who ate lettuce once a week or less. It now appears that foods rich in vitamin K_1 exert a protective effect. Other research demonstrates that vitamin K_1 may offer important protection from osteoporosis.

As excellent and important to both bone and arterial health as vitamin K_1 is, when it comes to bone health vitamin K_2 is the superior choice. In vivo (biological processes that take place within a living organism or cell) and in vitro (outside the body or in the laboratory studies) have shown that vitamin K_2 may directly act on bone metabolism. In vitro studies have demonstrated that vitamin K_2 inhibits bone resorption by, in part, inhibiting the production of bone-resorbing substances such as prostaglandin E_2 and interleukin-6.

In bone tissue, vitamin K_2 promotes calcium uptake. Low levels of vitamin K_2 have long been associated with an increased incidence of osteoporotic fractures and poor mineral density. Moreover, population-based analyses have consistently found widespread vitamin K deficiency.

The exciting synergy, as Dr. Sinatra points out, is that vitamin K_2 *adds* calcium to the bones, where it belongs, and *removes* it from the arteries, where is should not be. However it can be difficult to get adequate vitamin K_2 in our diets. Fortunately, there is an ancient dish that hails from feudal Japan and is still popular today. It is known as *natto* and is made from fermented soybeans. An interesting epidemiological study conducted in the cities of Tokyo and Hiroshima in Japan and in the British Isles measured natto intake and bone strength in women. The women in Tokyo ate the greatest amount of natto and had the strongest bones and lowest rate of fracture. The women in Hiroshima ate natto, but less than their Tokyo counterparts. They had weaker bones and a greater rate of fractures. The women in the British Isles ate no natto; their bones were by far the weakest and they had the greatest rate of fracture. Natto is unprecedented in its ability to support bone health. Because of its powerful smell and sticky consistency, natto is an acquired taste for many. For optimum value, do not heat or cook it, or you will destroy many nutrients. Experts recommend combining a little low-sodium tamari soy sauce and mustard with the natto—and this may be served atop a bowl of cooked oats or lentils. Others recommend mixing with a little yogurt, fresh fruit, and nuts. The good news is that eating natto two to three times a week is enough for it to confer its incomparable heart and bone benefits. As

Dr. Sinatra says, "The miracle of natto and/or efficacious formulations of vitamin K_2 are that a little goes a long way. Not only is K_2 much better absorbed than K_1 [but also] the half life is . . . much longer. K_2 stays in the blood for an extended period, and when . . . natto or . . . K_2 [is taken] as a supplement, it continues to build up in the body, accruing superior, long-term protection from thinning bones, fractures, and other bone-related problems." For the finest source of supplemental vitamin K_2, see the "Resources" section.

OMEGA-3S BUILD BETTER BONES

Salmon and sardines are also superior sources for the vitally important omega-3 EFAs, which play a starring role in this book because of their superior anti-aging properties. Luminous, radiant, wrinkle-free skin; improved mental faculties; weight loss; preservation of muscle mass; enhanced absorption of nutrients from foods; and a happy, positive mood are just a few of the benefits accrued by incorporating the omega-3s into our daily diets.

However, there is another reason to include these vital fats in our diet. We now know that we must also maintain the correct balance of dietary fats to prevent much of the bone loss associated with post-menopausal osteoporosis. Researchers at Purdue University and the Indiana University School of Medicine found that diets containing a low ratio of omega-6 fatty acids to omega-3 fatty acids had decreased bone loss. Unfortunately, most Westerners' diets are just the opposite—high in omega-6s (found in most vegetable oils, grains, and grain-fed beef) and low in omega-3s (found in such foods as salmon, sardines, nuts, and omega-3 eggs). That's just one more link in the chain connecting diet and degenerative disease in the developed world. The more our diets "progress" from the hunter-gatherer foods, eaten in their natural, unprocessed state, the more our mental and physical health declines.

Referring to a study published in the *Journal of Nutritional Biochemistry* in April 2006, researcher Bruce Watkins, professor and director of Purdue's Center for Enhancing Foods to Protect Health, stated, "Our lab and others have shown that omega-3 fatty acids help promote bone formation. We also have shown that higher intakes of omega-6 fatty acids lead to an increased production of compounds associated with bone loss."

Mark Seifert, a professor of anatomy and cell biology at the Indiana University School of Medicine and the study's coauthor, believes the bone-protective effects of omega-3 fatty acids may be linked to their previously established role in minimizing inflammation in the body. Seifert says, "We believe omega-3s may minimize bone loss with estrogen deficiency in association with their anti-inflammatory effects." I heartily concur with this concept.

And he goes on to say, "Many people don't realize it, but our bones are not static structures." This is very true—and important to remember if we are to successfully rejuvenate our bones on a cellular level. Inflammation is caused by a number of compounds, including a class of molecules called cytokines. These cytokines also stimulate the bone breakdown that is part of the bone-remodeling process. Watkins found that omega-3s change the behavior of cytokines in a way that is consistent with the role of omega-3s in mitigating cardiovascular disease.

As mentioned earlier, there are two types of cells that govern the bone-remodeling process—bone-resorption cells, which remove small portions of bone, and bone-building cells, which fill in the gaps. Estrogen blocks some of the inflammatory compounds associated with bone resorption, which may explain why osteoporosis typically progresses after estrogen levels fall with the onset of menopause. Watkins's earlier studies have shown that omega-3 fatty acids may reduce the production of these same inflammatory compounds, accounting for their bone-protective effect.

Dosage information: I suggest one 1,000-milligram softgel of wild sockeye salmon oil with or after a meal, up to three times daily, as a dietary supplement. To maximize benefits, higher doses may be taken and should be approved by your health care professional.

MAGNESIUM MAGIC

We don't always have to look for exotic substances in the field or in the test tube to discover proverbial magic bullets that can literally transform our lives. Such is the case with magnesium. Often overlooked, magnesium is a vital nutrient that has many critical functions. Numerous enzyme systems that are needed for the transfer of energy within our bodies require magnesium, which also plays a part in the normal functioning of muscles and nerves.

Magnesium is the fourth most abundant mineral in the body, and approximately 50% of total body magnesium is found in bone. Magnesium can be taken as a supplement; however, it is vitally important to include magnesium-rich foods in your diet. Good dietary sources include sea vegetables, peanuts, and green leafy vegetables such as spinach, collards, dandelion greens, peas, parsley, garlic, celery, cauliflower, and cabbage. Other good choices include Brussels sprouts, asparagus, avocados, blackberries, green olives, chives, kelp, soybeans, wild rice, oats, almonds, Brazil nuts, and sunflower seeds.

A recent U.S. study reported in the *Journal of the American Geriatric Society* found that increasing magnesium intake could increase bone density in the elderly and reduce the risk of osteoporosis. According to researcher Kathryn Ryder and colleagues, higher magnesium intake through diet and supplements was positively associated with total-body BMD in older white men and women. For every 100-milligram-per-day increase in magnesium, there was an approximate 2% percent increase in whole-body BMD.

Magnesium confers so many benefits that I recommend that you start making sure now that you have an adequate dietary intake. The National Institutes of Health's Office of Dietary Supplements (www.ods.od.nih.gov) contains excellent information on the importance of magnesium, including its impact on cellular rejuvenation. If we do not get enough magnesium, our bodily functions slow down at the cellular level, causing everything to become sluggish until we eventually experience whole-body fatigue.

Magnesium helps to

• Ease anxiety
• Stabilize mood
• Decrease the release of the stress hormone cortisol, known to disrupt sleep and promote the increase of abdominal fat (For more on cortisol, see Chapter Six, "Reversing Aging Through Exercise.")
• Prevent metabolic changes that may contribute to heart attacks and strokes
• Metabolize carbohydrates and influence the release and activity of insulin
• Regulate blood pressure, because of its natural muscle relaxant ability
• Ease muscle cramps

Dosage information: Typical doses of magnesium (expressed as elemental magnesium) range from 100 to 350 milligrams daily.

The Food and Nutrition Board of the Institute of Medicine of the U.S. National Academy of Sciences has recommended the following AI and RDA values for magnesium:

AGE GROUP/ SPECIAL CONDITION		AI OR RDA (MILLIGRAMS PER DAY)
		AI
Infants:	0–6 months	30
	7–12 months	75
		RDA
Children:	1–3 years	80
	4–8 years	130
Boys:	9–13 years	240
	14–18 years	410

Girls:	9–13 years	240
	14–18 years	360
Men:	19–30 years	400
	31–50 years	420
	51–70 years	420
	> 70 years	420
Women:	19–30 years	310
	31–50 years	320
	51–70 years	320
	> 70 years	320
Pregnancy:	14–18 years	400
	19–30 years	350
	31–50 years	380
Lactation:	14–18 years	360
	19–30 years	310
	31–50 years	320

SILICON — BONE BUILDER AND WRINKLE SMOOTHER

Silicon is a trace mineral found in connective tissue. A recent study presented at the American Society for Bone and Mineral Research conference suggests that silicon, in the form of choline-stabilized orthosilicic acid (ch-OSA), improves the bone health benefits of both calcium and vitamin D. Along with dietary sources and supplements of both calcium and vitamin D, I recommend taking Jarrow Formulas BioSil, a 2% silicon solution in the form of stabilized orthosilicic acid.

Dosage information: Take 6 to 20 drops of 6-milligram BioSil daily with or without food, dropped into at least ¼ cup water or beverage and drink immediately.

Results from a new clinical trial add to mounting evidence that ch-OSA supplementation supports physiological roles in bone health and type I collagen synthesis in human bone–building cells. (Collagen is a very important protein that our body uses to create skin, scar tissue, ligaments, tendons, and blood vessels.) The researchers concluded, "This study suggests that combined therapy of ch-OSA plus Calcium and Vitamin D is a safe, well-tolerated treatment that has a potentially beneficial effect on bone turnover, especially bone collagen, and possibly femoral BMD, compared to Calcium and Vitamin D alone." The femur (thigh bone) is the largest bone in the body. This study shows that this form of silicon can help improve femoral bone mass density, making it an important supplement to include for bone health.

Previously presented research suggests that ch-OSA helps build and maintain bone by regulating bone mineralization, helping to trigger the deposition of calcium and phosphate, reducing the number of osteoclasts (bone-destroying cells), and increasing the number of osteoblasts (bone-building cells). A recent epidemiological study also indicates that higher dietary silicon intake is associated with greater BMD in both men and premenopausal women.

This is very exciting news, for both bone health and skin health. As always, beauty, health, and strength from the inside out is both our goal and our reward.

4

The Skin We're In

Perhaps the most discouraging aspect of aging is aging skin, because the skin is our largest and most visible organ. But it isn't just aging skin that should concern us; it is also the aging of underlying tissue, such as the subcutaneous fat, musculature, and bone. This is the result of cellular degeneration, which produces abnormal structural changes and decreased function in our cells. It is this cellular degeneration that is responsible for the aging of all organ systems, not just the skin. As I've tried to emphasize throughout this book, what we see on the surface is a reflection of what is going on underneath it. And the signs of aging skin are a perfect example.

As we all know by now, there are many things we can do to make ourselves look better. There is a wide range of options available, from cosmetics to plastic surgery, that can temporarily disguise the damage caused by cellular degeneration. But my concern literally goes deeper than that; for lasting and dramatic changes, I am interested in reaching the very cells themselves, not only to stop the degeneration but also to repair and reverse much of the damage that has already occurred.

To achieve this, I emphasize three elements: (1) the anti-inflammatory diet with plenty of high-quality protein, (2) skin-supporting nutraceutical muscle protectors, and (3) targeted topical treatments augmented with electronic muscle stimulation (EMS).

The Shape of Things to Come

The first noticeable signs of aging in the face appear as fine lines and wrinkles, which may appear as early as our late twenties and early thirties. However, these harbingers of what is to come with the passing decades are not necessarily the true culprits in what make us look older. I have seen many young people in my practice aged 25 to 30 whose light complexion and overexposure to the sun have resulted in wrinkles—particularly in the eye area. But if I ask the average person to guess someone's age, they are usually fairly accurate—because it is not fine lines and wrinkles that give the face an aged appearance. We begin to look old when we lose convexities, which are defined as "shapes that curve or bulge outward." A young face is characterized by the bulging outward of our facial structures, such as the forehead, cheekbones, chin, and jawline. As we get older, we lose those outwardly bulging convexities. The result is a flat and drooping look to the face. The cause is the loss of underlying or subcutaneous tissue, especially fat and muscle. In general, our goal is to cut down on body fat, for both health and esthetic reasons. However, there is one important exception: the subcutaneous fat that is vital for keeping the face looking young.

As we age, the muscles in the face begin to elongate and subsequently sag. Sagging, drooping muscles are the true hallmark of an aging face—in fact, plastic surgeons remedy this by cutting the muscles to shorten them and "lift up" the face. However, this also flattens the muscle, so that even though the face will be pulled up, eliminating the drooping and sagging, the beautiful curves and convexities of a rounded, youthful muscle will not be present. The look of youth will be more illusory than genuine. Many surgeons are injecting the face with fat to remedy this problem. However, I believe a more natural, holistic approach is needed. To maintain a youthful face, we need to do more than just prevent wrinkles; we must maintain the contours and convexities of the face, which rely on both the underlying subcutaneous fat and muscle tissue.

That leads us to *secret 4: To make the face look younger, start by rejuvenating the underlying tissue.*

EAT YOUR WAY TO FIRMER SKIN

We all know that we are what we eat, and that includes how young we are. It may come as a surprise to learn that what we eat can help determine how young (or old) we look. However, we now know that certain categories of foods (enumerated in Chapter One, "Cellular Rejuvenation," and Appendix A, "The Anti-aging Kitchen") are vital to maintain and improve the processes of cellular rejuvenation. And, as we also learn in those chapters, protein is of major importance in stimulating cells to repair themselves. Since we cannot store protein in our body, we must take in high-quality protein every day. If our protein supply is inadequate or depleted, the body is forced to feed on itself. This results in the breakdown of both tissue and muscle. Without enough protein, the aging process is visibly accelerated.

The bad news is that this ongoing lack of protein is first noticeable in the face. And women, unlike men, are notorious for not eating enough protein. This is one of the reasons men often look younger than their female counterparts. Another reason has to do with testosterone, which helps regulate the thickness and oiliness of the skin. Most people are unaware of the fact that women's bodies also produce testosterone, which is essential to their health and well-being.

Although they produce far smaller quantities of this male hormone, below-normal levels in women have been associated with decreased or nonexistent libido. When women go through perimenopause and menopause, an imbalance in testosterone can cause noticeable changes in the skin—too much testosterone can lead to clogged pores and acne; too little can lead to dry skin. A third reason is that men have naturally thicker skin than women do, making it less vulnerable to the damaging effects of the sun and the environment (i.e., free radicals).

Therefore, it is even more important for women to choose the anti-inflammatory diet as their first line of defense against aging. Unfortunately, men have an advantage in this area as well. Women frequently crave sugary, starchy foods in an effort to increase levels of that feel-good hormone, serotonin. This strategy backfires, setting women up for a roller-coaster ride of food craving and overeating. As a rule, men tend to have higher levels of serotonin, making them less likely to binge on these types of foods. When we don't get enough protein, and we combine that with a diet of high-glycemic carbohydrates, our features take on a soft, doughy appearance. The sharp, contoured cheekbones and crisp jawline begin to lose definition.

As you can see, lack of protein, combined with the wrong carbohydrates, packs a one-two punch when it comes to destroying facial contours. In fact, once you know what to look for, you can spot a "high-carb, low-protein" diet person immediately—male or female. The inflammation caused by the high-glycemic carbs results in puffiness and swelling in the face and eye area. The glycation caused by the sugars and starches will eventually lead to deep wrinkles and sagging of the skin. This protein deficiency can be visible in both women and men as early as their twenties. The sharp definition, contoured cheekbones, and great jawline all become blurred.

Eating the wrong carbohydrates (the sugary, starchy foods) causes an inflammatory response that results in the glycation of collagen in the skin and all other organs, laying the foundation for the birth of wrinkles, sagging muscles, and loss of tone, elasticity, and resilience. To visualize this, think of the skin as a rubber band. When young, it will snap back into place if stretched. With cross-linking, the skin and its underlying structure lose the ability to snap back. This inflammatory response also contributes to overall puffiness, dullness, and loss of radiance.

The first critical step on the road to recovery is to ensure that you consume adequate protein throughout the day and limit your carbohydrate intake to colorful, nonstarchy fruits and vegetables, beans and legumes, and whole grains such as old-fashioned oatmeal. If you follow this simple formula, you will see the results almost immediately—and that even goes for women and men aged 40 and beyond. Whether you are 21 or 51, you can and will quickly see the difference.

A theme throughout this book and my entire body of work is the recognition of the deleterious effects of inflammation. Maintaining youthful facial contours and convexities, radiance, elasticity, and so on also relies on controlling inflammation—from the obvious, such as avoiding lying in the noonday sun, to the not-so-obvious: avoidance of anti-inflammatory foods, dehydration, and inadequate sleep.

FACING THE FACTS ABOUT INSULIN

Loss of muscle tone and muscle mass increases with weight gain and is also a normal, albeit unwelcome, occurrence of aging. However, we can counteract this. The end goal of following the anti-inflammatory lifestyle is to prevent an exaggerated insulin response, not only for the health reasons we have previously discussed, but for the sake of your appearance as well.

As you now know, cellular rejuvenation is the key to staying young, feeling young, and looking young. It affects our overall health and our ability to lose weight and maintain muscle mass, it keeps our infrastructure strong and secure, and it gives us a healthy, vibrant appearance. Cellular rejuvenation affects all the systems of the body, and they all affect each other. If you follow the suggestions in this chapter, for instance, because you're interested in improving your appearance, you'll automatically be influencing all aspects of your health. And vice versa—if you follow the recommendations throughout this book in order to improve your overall health, you'll find that your appearance has also improved dramatically.

One of the most important recommendations you can follow is found in secret 2, which, as we've learned, is about learning to control your blood sugar and insulin levels. The end goal of following the 7 Secrets lifestyle is to prevent a large insulin response, which in turn causes an inflammatory cascade and inhibits cellular rejuvenation. But insulin affects more than our ability to stay slim. It also affects our skin.

Insulin is a critical hormone. Too much of it circulating in the bloodstream will

- Accelerate aging both internally and externally
- Promote weight gain and obesity by putting a lock on body fat
- Shrink muscle mass in both face and body, resulting in a tired, droopy, sagging face, eye area, neck, and jawline and in the loss of that healthy toned look that comes from good muscle tone in the upper body, midriff, thighs, and so on

To prevent the aging effects of elevated insulin levels, take the following steps:

- Follow an anti-inflammatory diet.
- Avoid sugar and starchy foods.
- Eat the right fats to burn fat.
- Stabilize blood sugar and insulin levels.
- Eat your protein first at the start of every meal or snack.

Controlling blood sugar levels is the single most important anti-aging step we can take to make sure that we age beautifully, prevent wrinkling, preserve lean muscle mass, and, as we learned in Chapter Two ("Lean for Life"), eliminate unwanted body fat. In addition, we

THE ABCs OF STABILIZING BLOOD SUGAR

The following three foods are especially effective in stabilizing blood sugar, and eating them is a good way to keep insulin levels under control:

- *Apples:* Despite their relatively high sugar levels, apples actually exert a stabilizing effect on blood sugar, due in part to their high fiber content and to phloretin, a flavonoid-type, blood-sugar-stabilizing phytonutrient found exclusively in apples. A study in Finland found that eating apples can lower the risk of type 2 diabetes. The researchers attributed apples' antidiabetes effect to the antioxidant activity of quercetin, a major component of apple peels. This is another reason to buy organic, unsprayed fruit so that you can safely eat the skin.
- *Beans and lentils:* A meal with legumes raises blood sugar very slowly and moderately, and even moderates the blood sugar response to the next meal you eat, whether that next meal includes beans or not. When beans and legumes are eaten with relatively high glycemic foods (sugars, refined flour products) they still wield a potent stabilizing influence on blood sugar levels and subsequent insulin levels. Beans and legumes are excellent sources of fiber, which also helps to stabilize blood sugar. In addition, beans and lentils contain resistant starch (RS), fiberlike carbohydrates that increase the rate at which the body burns (oxidizes) body fat. They do not cause unhealthy spikes in blood sugar levels, and they prevent other, higher glycemic foods in a meal from doing so.
- *Cinnamon:* Scientists at the U.S. Department of Agriculture (USDA) have found that cinnamon keeps blood sugar levels on an even keel. The phytonutrient compounds responsible for cinnamon's beneficial effect on blood sugar control are the flavon-3-ol polyphenol class of antioxidants, which enhance the stabilizing effect of insulin on blood sugar and decrease insulin resistance in two ways: First, they activate enzymes that

stimulate insulin receptors. (Remember that when we are insulin resistant, our cells cannot sense the presence of insulin. By sensitizing these receptors, we are potentiating insulin's power to reduce blood sugar levels.) Second, they enhance the effects of insulin-signaling pathways within skeletal muscle tissue.

By increasing insulin sensitivity, the flavon-3-ol antioxidants in cinnamon decrease the harmful effects of high-glycemic carbohydrates, such as fluctuating blood sugar levels that cause carbohydrate cravings and the chronic inflammation that promotes obesity. Because flavon-3-ol antioxidants enhance insulin sensitivity, more of your blood glucose enters the cells where it belongs, and blood sugar levels stabilize, effectively stopping the inflammation and ending carbohydrate craving. Just ¼ teaspoon of cinnamon mixed in water or tea will do the trick. In fact, cinnamon will continue to help stabilize blood sugar for days—in one study, the group that took the cinnamon reported healthy blood sugar levels up to 3 weeks after consuming the cinnamon!

must have a moderate exercise program, get enough sleep (cellular repair takes place when we sleep), take nutritional supplements, and apply topical cellular rejuvenators with anti-inflammatory properties.

ANTIOXIDANTS + ANTI-INFLAMMATORIES = ANTI-AGING

Inflammation has been discussed many times throughout these chapters. However, it is extremely important to understand the mechanisms of chronic, pervasive, subclinical (invisible to the naked eye) inflammation and its role in aging skin. This inflammation can be triggered by sun exposure, harsh environmental exposure (such as extreme cold or heat), psychic/mental stress, environmental pollutants, chemicals, soaps and detergents, and even exposure to computer screens. Perhaps most disheartening is the fact that a recent article suggests that gravity itself exerts a pulling effect on the skin, creating inflammation.

Whether it is exposure to the noonday sun on a summer day or extreme mental stress, the end result is the same. Free radicals generate pro-inflammatory chemicals, leading to a cascade of events that result in low-grade inflammation. As we learned in Chapter One ("Cellular Rejuvenation"), the body has an endogenous (produced inside an organism or cell) antioxidant system consisting of enzymes and vitamins C and E that will scoop up these free radicals and help prevent further damage. However, in a few short minutes, the endogenous antioxidant system is quickly overwhelmed and the free radicals start their destruction. They begin by attacking the cell plasma membrane with the production of arachidonic acid, which then flows into the cell, creating inflammation, further free radicals, and eventual cellular breakdown. Like environmental stressors such as UV exposure, a pro-inflammatory diet will also result in free radical production because it creates a rise in blood sugar and insulin levels. The anti-

THE SPICE OF (LONG) LIFE

I highly recommend liberal use of the spice turmeric in your meals. This remarkable spice, an indispensable curry ingredient, is a powerful anti-inflammatory. And like alpha lipoic acid (see page 92), it inhibits the pro-inflammatory actions of nuclear factor kappa B, making it an outstanding wrinkle fighter. This alone is a great motivator to add a dash of turmeric to soups, omelets, and salads (not to mention the fact that turmeric also enhances the liver's ability to eliminate dangerous, carcinogenic toxins).

inflammatory diet will prevent the production and activation of inflammatory chemicals, preventing skin wrinkling, as well as the loss of muscle and convexities in both the face and body.

Neuropeptides: The Information Superhighway to Cellular Repair

The skin has abundant nerve endings whose role is to provide information to the brain. It is also composed of many different types of cells, such as fibroblasts and keratinocytes, as well as messengers such as hormones, neuropeptides, and neurotransmitters. When the skin is challenged by an environmental stressor such as the sun or by physical or mental stress, its responsibility is to provide information to all of the other organ systems in our bodies. In other words, the skin can function very much like the brain or the endocrine system in providing important data to the body.

When we are in an embryonic state, the layers of cells that eventually develop into skin are also responsible for making brain cells. This means that the skin and brain are very closely connected. I refer to this as *the brain–beauty connection*, and as you will learn, it clearly indicates that the skin is much more than just a protective barrier. The skin also has *receptor sites* for all the different types of messengers mentioned above. This means that the skin can not only *transmit* messages throughout the body but also *receive* messages by way of neurotransmitters, neuropeptides, hormones, and nerve impulses. This information was revelatory for scientists, who knew that the brain communicated with other organ systems but did not realize that the rest of the body was responding! This information superhighway communication system opened doors to a much greater understanding of the entire mind–body connection and its role in physical and mental health. This discovery is extremely relevant when we look not only at diseases of the skin but also at mental diseases and disorders.

By just stimulating the skin, you can actually *change* the chemistry in your brain. Conversely, your skin will show the result of anxiety attacks and depression.

This is of tremendous importance to dermatologists and their patients because historically many skin diseases have been categorized as having an unknown etiology (the cause or origin of disease). This has made many skin diseases notoriously difficult to treat. However, we know that these diseases have a significant inflammatory component and that diseases such as acne, psoriasis, and atopic dermatitis are all deeply affected and even precipitated by mental stress. Any acne sufferer will tell you that new lesions always appear right before an important event—and that is no coincidence. This adds a new level of truth to the aphorism "You are what you eat" and proves that you are also what you think and feel.

If we are to age successfully, looking and feeling good into advanced decades, we must remember these two simple yet incontrovertible facts: The foods we eat not only affect our physical health but also profoundly affect our mental attitudes and our sense of well-being, especially where stress is concerned.

When we experience stress, a neuropeptide known as substance P (SP) is released into both the skin and the brain. SP is a strong, pro-inflammatory molecule. When released into the skin, it starts a flow of pro-inflammatory chemicals, resulting in the activation or exacerbation of skin disease. SP can also slow hair growth and cause hair loss because of its ability to affect hair follicles. SP also affects the sebaceous glands (glands in the skin that produce sebum, an oily substance) by making them more active and by affecting their growth and creating the inflammation that can clog pores. It is interesting to note that the skin of acne patients has a much greater number of these SP-containing nerves than the average person. Thus we can see the brain–skin connection is a powerful one, mediated by neuropeptides, with the final common pathway, as always, being inflammation.

Topical Cellular Rejuvenators

In Chapter One ("Cellular Rejuvenation"), we discussed the superior mitochondrial rejuvenation properties of supplemental ALA. And so it is not surprising that topical ALA remains unsurpassed for its ability to rejuvenate the skin. In its natural form, ALA is fat soluble. However, it undergoes a fascinating transformation when it enters into the cell. Because it is fat soluble, it first enters the cell plasma membrane, composed of phospholipids (fats) and embedded proteins. The cell plasma membrane protects the cell and controls what moves in and out of it. ALA can enter this delicate portion of the cell and provide powerful antioxidant protection, making it an ideal substance for the treatment of skin. But the benefits of ALA go even further than the cell plasma membrane. Once inside the cell, ALA converts to DHLA, which is water soluble and can penetrate the water-soluble portion of the cell as well, which means that it can reach and protect all portions of the cell.

As we learned in Chapter One, ALA is found naturally in the mitochondria portion of our cells, as part of an enzyme system that helps energy production. Aging cells, whether in the skin or elsewhere in the body, need energy to maintain themselves. We know that a young cell is characterized by its energy. By taking supplemental ALA and by applying ALA topically to the skin, we deliver therapeutic amounts of this substance to help increase the energy for proper cellular metabolism, which is desperately needed by the skin cells for their cellular repair.

ALPHA LIPOIC ACID REPAIRS DAMAGED CELLS

ALA first concentrates in the cell plasma membrane, where it neutralizes free radicals. It then moves on to the watery interior of the cell, known as the cytosol, where it can also quell the activity of free radicals and prevent activation of other pro-inflammatory chemicals. The cytosol is filled with a gelatinous material, which houses the nucleus, the DNA, and substances known as *transcription factors*, regulatory proteins that control when genes are switched on or off.

These transcription factors act as tiny molecular messengers that can move to the nucleus of the cell to stimulate our DNA to replicate RNA (ribonucleic acid) and make important proteins for cell function. For our purposes, we want to concentrate on two important transcription factors, NFkB and activator protein 1 (AP-1). These transcription factors are not active in the cell unless free radicals are about to overwhelm the cell's defense mechanism. This is the state known as oxidative stress; when the cells are in a state of oxidative stress, these transcription factors are activated, where they wreak cellular havoc.

NFkB does its damage by migrating to the nucleus and attaching to the DNA, resulting in the production of pro-inflammatory cytokines—chemicals that are the so-called serial killers of the cellular world. ALA can prevent the activation of NFkB, thus preventing gene expression of other pro-inflammatory chemicals. Simply put, ALA effectively turns off a messenger system that can cause further damage to the cell.

The other transcription factor, AP-1, is even more mischievous, as it can either damage the cell or repair it. If AP-1 is activated by a pro-inflammatory event such as sunlight, it too migrates to the nucleus, where it causes the production of a variety of chemicals, including collagenase, which actually *digests* collagen. As the collagen is digested, it results in "microscars," which lead to wrinkles. However, when AP-1 is activated by the powerful anti-inflammatory ALA, the cell is instructed to *turn on* collagenases that only digest already damaged collagen, thus *repairing* wrinkles and scarring. ALA is truly a great gift for creating and maintaining youthful skin.

Alpha Lipoic Acid Counters the Effects of Menopause

A study published in the *Archives of Gerontology and Geriatrics* acknowledged that menopause is often accompanied by hot flashes and degenerative processes such as arteriosclerosis and atrophic changes of the skin (skin that is thin and wrinkled). These changes suggest an acceleration of aging triggered by estrogen depletion. Historically this lack of estrogen has been treated by hormone-replacement therapy (HRT). However, because of potentially deadly side effects of synthetic hormones, physicians are looking for safer alternatives that can counteract the unpleasant physical and aesthetic effects that often accompany menopause.

The reviewed data in the study support the concept that other antioxidants such as ALA and several others (including turmeric) may help to prevent antioxidant deficiency, thereby protecting the mitochondria from cellular degeneration. They also found that combinations of these antioxidants, both in the diet and applied topically for skin protection, may have favorable effects on the health and quality of life of women, especially those who cannot be treated with HRT, suffer high levels of oxidative stress, and do not consume a healthy diet that includes five daily rations of fresh fruit and vegetables.

I recommend supplementing with ALA every day, along with a liberal application of topical formulations of ALA for optimum cellular protection of the skin.

ALPHA LIPOIC ACID REVS UP CELLULAR ENERGY

We know that ALA is part of an enzyme complex in the mitochondria responsible for the conversion of food to energy. What we are now discovering is that ALA's ability to increase energy levels in the cell has a direct influence on the appearance of the skin.

Over the years, I have observed firsthand and also heard from people around the world that topical application of ALA has resulted in large pores' decreasing in size, giving the skin a smoother appearance. Just why this happens is not completely clear. Energy-deficient oil glands produce abnormal ratios of oils secreted on the surface of the skin. When the proportion of these oils is out of balance, the pores begin to clog. My theory is that ALA increases energy production in the oil gland, normalizing the oils secreted, resulting in a shrinkage of the pore size. It should also be noted that ALA, a powerful anti-inflammatory, will diminish inflammation within the pore and thus prevent pore clogging. As I have mentioned before, the primary event in a clogging pore for acne is invisible inflammation, still not recognized by many dermatologists. When abnormal oils are no longer clogging and stretching the pores, these tiny openings gradually normalize until they are invisible to the eye.

In addition to the decrease in wrinkles and pore size, puffiness in the eye area and the face (also known as edema) will respond rapidly to topical ALA applications because this edema is a result of inflammation. Other benefits will be a decrease in under-eye circles, a lessening of redness and uneven skin tone, and a return to a radiant, healthy glow. These benefits are all a result of ALA's capacity to regulate production of nitric oxide, which controls blood flow to the skin, rapidly transforming the complexion from dull, pasty, ashen, or pale to vibrant and glowing.

ALPHA LIPOIC ACID REVERSES GLYCATION

In the first two chapters, we discussed a condition known as *glycation*, which occurs when a sugar molecule attaches to a protein such as collagen. This is one of the very negative and cytotoxic (poisonous to the cell) effects of eating sugar, HFCS, other sweeteners, and starchy foods that rapidly convert to sugar. Glycation is very damaging to the skin because the skin is collagen-rich and the protein–sugar bonds cause the collagen to become stiff and inflexible. Glycation, also known as cross-linking, results in an aged appearance to the skin. We know that taking supplemental ALA can *prevent* the attachment of sugar to collagen. At the same time, ALA makes our cells more sensitive to insulin, thus allowing our body to metabolize sugar—to burn it up before it can attach to the body's proteins. This preventive action is key because once the sugar does attach to the collagen, the resulting protein–sugar bond becomes a veritable factory for producing free radicals and inflammatory chemicals. ALA not only prevents accelerated aging in the skin by protecting us from sugar's toxic effects but also quenches the pro-inflammatory events taking place. Contrary to what has been previously thought by scientists, there is now some evidence that under certain conditions, ALA *can reverse* the glycation that has already occurred.

Although I first wrote about ALA in the mid-1990s, new studies continue to reveal how important ALA is for women, both as a dietary supplement and when applied topically.

VITAMIN C ESTER: CONNECTIVE TISSUE REGENERATOR

Vitamin C ester is a nonirritating form of vitamin C, which is a well-known and highly regarded antioxidant with superior anti-inflammatory properties. As with ALA and dimethylaminoethanol (DMAE; see

SILICON AS WRINKLE SMOOTHER

As we learned in Chapter Three ("Supporting Our Support Structure"), silicon is a trace mineral found in connective tissue. A form of silicon known as choline-stabilized orthosilicic acid (ch-OSA) improves the bone health benefits of both calcium and vitamin D. In addition, improvements in type I skin collagen after supplementation with ch-OSA have been noted in an animal study. Similarly, a report on a clinical study presented at the sixty-third American Academy of Dermatology annual meeting (2005) confirms that ch-OSA also helps reduce the appearance of wrinkles and helps improve skin elasticity. The improvement in skin parameters is likely a result of the regeneration of damaged collagen fibers or the synthesis of new ones—all in all, very exciting and encouraging results.

pages 98–99), my findings in studies examining the effects of ascorbyl palmitate (vitamin C ester) on aging skin have been dramatic. When increased levels of this fat-soluble form of vitamin C are in the dermis, levels of both collagen and elastin increase. This facilitates a more youthful appearance by helping to reverse the thinning of skin seen both in the natural aging process and as a result of sun damage. Vitamin C ester is highly stable (unlike ascorbic acid, the unstable, irritating, and water-soluble form of vitamin C) and will maintain its efficacy over long periods of time. Its fat-solubility allows it to rapidly and easily penetrate the skin to deliver the therapeutic levels of vitamin C

WHERE SCIENCE MEETS ART: THE MAGIC OF FULLERENES

In addition to the powerful age-reversing benefits of antioxidants, light therapy, and EMS, we also have exciting, proprietary delivery systems available for the first time. One such delivery system is based on *fullerenes*, so named because the 60 atoms that make up their spherical molecule resemble Buckminster Fuller's geodesic domes, which are lighter than plastic yet stronger than steel. Also known as buckyballs, they were first identified in 1985 by three scientists who later received a Nobel Prize for the discovery. The fullerenes used in this delivery system are highly stable, microscopic, hollow carbon balls that function as a potent reservoir for the transport of the Perricone patented technology to the skin. Fullerenes deliver active ingredients to protect and nourish the skin around the clock. This revolutionary system brings the intriguing and transformative world of nanotechnology to the fine art and science of high-performance anti-aging skin care formulation.

needed to enable the fibroblasts, which are the cells that make connective tissue, to produce collagen and elastin. These collagen- and elastin-stimulating effects are magnified even more when vitamin C ester is added to formulations containing DMAE.

DMAE: ANTIOXIDANT CELL STABILIZER

DMAE is a precursor to the neurotransmitter acetylcholine (ACh) and is a nutritional substance with powerful anti-inflammatory properties. ACh is a stimulatory neurotransmitter that plays an important role in memory. Taking DMAE as a supplement has been shown to increase cognitive function by improving memory and problem-solving ability. ACh is also essential in the communication from one nerve to another and between nerves and muscles. For your muscles to contract, the message must be sent from your nerves to your muscles via ACh.

DMAE and ACh also appear to play an important role in maintaining muscle tone. As we age, our levels of ACh decline, resulting in reduced muscle tone. This process, as explained earlier, leads to muscles that become elongated and relaxed, instead of staying short and tight, so that we have a sagging face and body. We call this *loss of anatomic position*. DMAE, when applied topically, can provide optimum levels of nutrients required by the body to synthesize ACh. When this happens, it creates the powerful capability to increase skin tone within minutes of topical application.

The way to improve muscle tone is to increase ACh levels, and one of the best ways to do this is by introducing additional DMAE into your system. There are four ways to do this, and they work synergistically to provide optimum levels of DMAE in the body:

- Eat fish, the only significant dietary source of DMAE.
- Take DMAE in the form of a nutritional supplement.
- Apply a high-potency, rapidly penetrating DMAE topical lotion

to the skin on the face and body morning and evening after cleansing.

• Keep the muscles toned with exercise.

In conjunction with DMAE, we now have other new and exciting strategies to increase muscle tone in the face. Just as exercising the body makes us firm, well-muscled, and attractive below the neck, so it turns out that exercising the face can do the same above the neck. EMS to the face can help shorten elongated, drooping muscles to create a more youthful appearance, while helping to stimulate blood flow to the face, increasing circulation, and decreasing puffiness and pallor.

A SPICY SKIN REJUVENATOR

Although you'll read about this in detail in Chapter Six ("Reversing Aging Through Exercise"), you should know about an exciting new product—oil of oregano. According to Dr. Cass Ingram, a physician, researcher, and author of 20 books, including *Natural Cures for Killer Germs* and *The Cure Is in the Cupboard*, oil of oregano possesses vast microbe-destroying properties. It is, in other words, a natural antiseptic. It can be taken orally to kill a myriad of germs, fungi, bacteria, and parasites.

It also comes in a cream version called Oreganol P73 Cream, a powerful rejuvenating formula containing propolis (a resinous substance bees use to construct and maintain their hives), wild essential oils, and wild honey. Made with the highest-ranked antioxidants in the world, Oreganol P73 Cream's proven antiseptic powers cleanse the skin and are highly effective for skin disorders, bug bites, burns, cuts, abrasions, sunburn, warts, and skin lesions. For best results, use the cream daily on the affected area.

A New Concept in Facial Rejuvenation: Electric Muscle Stimulation

EMS is a procedure that contracts muscles by use of electric impulses. Physicians may use electrical muscle stimulators for patients who require treatment for conditions such as muscle atrophy (the progressive loss of muscle mass caused by reduction in the size or number of muscle cells), reeducation of muscles, increasing range of motion, joint replacement, and gait training, as well as for treating medical conditions that usually result from a stroke, a serious injury, or major surgery. The effect of using these devices is primarily to help a patient recover from impaired muscle function.

But can the positive effects of EMS be used for facial rejuvenation? For years patients in my practice and readers of my books have asked if these machines are effective, especially the devices designed for the face (many of which they had seen on television infomercials). Until relatively recently, I really could not answer their question. Because there had been no clinical studies published in the dermatology literature and I had no firsthand experience, I could not give an informed answer.

In theory the concept made sense. As mentioned earlier in this chapter, our aging muscles droop as the result of declining levels of ACh, the neurotransmitter that carries messages between the nerves and muscles. I reasoned that if we could make the muscles contract through electric stimulation, then with time and persistence, the muscle should begin to shorten and we would restore the rounded, convex musculature of the young face. I began to do some research.

ELECTRIC MUSCLE STIMULATION TO THE RESCUE

When it comes to increasing muscle size to where it can actually affect the appearance of the muscle (as in bulging biceps and washboard abs), the general consensus is that EMS is not effective.

However, these conclusions refer to the larger muscles of shoulders, arms, legs, and abdominals. Since the muscles on the face are much smaller in comparison, the concept seemed feasible, and I decided to put it to the test.

I purchased a number of these rather simple devices from a company whose representative appeared in a television infomercial. I then asked patients to begin using them, as instructed, over a period of 8 weeks so that I could determine whether these machines actually improved facial musculature. They eagerly complied, although they admitted that the process was somewhat tedious, as they had to work first one side of the face and then the other. It was slow going, but I did see some improvement. This inspired me to try two different topical formulations in conjunction with EMS to see if I could increase the benefits. The first lotion consisted of a combination of topical DMAE with ALA. I then formulated a second lotion combining DMAE and vitamin C ester.

ALL YOU NEED IS (A) GLOVE

I was determined to invent a superior device that would be easy to use and would also yield significant results in a timely manner. I developed an apparatus consisting of two gloves (one for each hand) attached to a central power unit. Electrodes were placed on the first two fingers of each glove, allowing the patients to treat both sides of the face simultaneously. This synchronicity offered significant benefits and improvement over the original handheld device, including the following:

- Cutting the session time in half
- Allowing the corresponding facial muscles on both sides of the face to synchronize and work together for optimum contraction and lift
- Enabling the user to pinpoint exact pressure points for effective muscle contraction

My next step was to produce a number of prototypes of the glove device and distribute them to patients. I also gave them topical lotion containing either DMAE and ALA or DMAE and vitamin C ester, with instructions to apply the lotion twice daily. They were to do the facial stimulation exercises approximately 5 or 6 days per week. My goal was significant clinical improvement, and I was not disappointed.

As the benefits of EMS and DMAE combinations continued to accrue with the passing weeks, I realized that a patient now had the tools, literally at her fingertips, to improve the symmetrical appearance of her face. By using EMS, it is possible to exercise both sides at once, or to exercise one side over the other. That flexibility provides the added advantage of helping to restore and even create something most people are not consciously aware of—facial symmetry.

Many supermodels, actors, and celebrities are renowned for their perfect faces. But what makes them perfect? In many cases, it is the appearance of symmetry. In recent years, as my practice has greatly expanded, I have begun to see many beautiful, famous faces on a regular basis. I expected to discover that the reason for their legendary beauty was a perfectly symmetrical bone structure. When I examined them, I found that it was not so much the bone symmetry that gave them that glamorous look but an increased amount of facial muscle mass and a healthy layer of subcutaneous fat. The combination of these two attributes gave their faces the greater convexities typically associated with the glamorous face.

Most of us are not so lucky. And as we age, we lose what convexity we may have once had. It was exciting to think that we might be able to level the genetic playing field through the combination of DMAE and ALA or vitamin C ester and EMS, allowing anyone to achieve that greater muscle mass that I have seen in the "beautiful people." Even if the average person is lacking in ideal bone structure and symmetry, all is not lost. We can compensate and increase the symmetry by building up the muscle on one side of the face.

MIA'S STORY

I first met Mia during a photo shoot in Los Angeles. A renowned, highly skilled photographer, Mia had a professionalism, warm personality, and sparkling sense of humor that turned a normally grueling and exhausting process into an enjoyable event. As we got to know each other, Mia revealed that she had been an extremely popular teenage model in the 1980s. However, because of the encroaching years and the media's relentless obsession with youth, she had begun to feel more comfortable behind the camera than in front of it.

A true artist, Mia understood the impact of lighting and angle in photographing the face. As a result, her photographs were evocative, glamorous, compelling, and also extremely flattering—much in the style of the great Hollywood photographers of the 1930s and 1940s. As we began to discuss the planes and convexities of the face, Mia turned pensive. "Dr. Perricone," she asked, "is there any way to tighten up a sagging face without invasive surgery?" I explained to her that I was currently researching that very question. "Let me know if you need any volunteers," she replied.

It was now Mia's turn to sit under the lights as I examined her face. Mia had been born with a strong bone structure, and even at age 42 she still had a very healthy and attractive layer of subcutaneous fat. However, her jawline and the lower cheek area, often referred to as jowls, had begun to sag. Mia appeared to be an excellent candidate for trying the electric stim glove. I was hopeful that with its regular use, she could lift the lower cheek area to eliminate the sagging and lift the brow area to give her eyes a more wide-open and less hooded look. I also wanted to see the area under the chin and along the jaw become firm, tightened, and toned.

Mia's Exercise Regimen

Mia's face was also on the thin side. For optimum results, we needed to accomplish two goals. First, lift the sagging muscles, and second, increase the amount of muscle mass in the face. Contrary to popular belief, it is not the bone structure that gives the striking look of glamour to a face—it is the muscle mass that creates the alluring contrasts of rounded muscles and deep hollows. I advised Mia to concentrate extra attention in the cheek area to recreate that youthful, apple-cheeked look. In addition, the left side of Mia's face had significantly less tone and more sag than the right side. I recommended that she start out exercising each muscle group for 60 seconds and then add an extra 30 seconds to the left side to help correct the asymmetrical look to her face. Eventually she would work up to 3 minutes on each exercise, always adding an extra minute to the left side.

Mia's Topical Regimen

Mia's skin was on the dry side, and like many of her generation, she had spent long, hot summers at the beach during her teens and early twenties. As a result, her skin showed signs of photo damage, including redness, uneven skin tone, and a thin, somewhat papery texture.

I gave Mia the DMAE–ALA lotion to be applied in the morning after her electric stim session. I also gave her a DMAE–ALA eye cream to be blended with the DMAE–vitamin C ester serum described below. This eye therapy combo was an important step in restoring tone, reducing the puffiness and dark circles, and thickening the very delicate and translucent skin around the eye while diminishing the appearance of fine lines, wrinkles, and crow's feet.

Mia was to apply the DMAE–vitamin C ester cream to her face, neck, and throat each evening. I advised Mia to faithfully adhere to the program, to follow the anti-inflammatory diet, get enough sleep, and stay well hydrated. I then arranged to evaluate the results in 4 weeks and again 4 weeks later.

In those first few weeks, I could immediately discern a greater radiance to her face due to ALA's ability to increase blood flow and circulation. I also observed a measurable decrease in the sagging of the upper and lower cheek area, jawline, and upper eyelid. I was convinced that the increased appearance of lift, firmness, and tone to the skin was of a greater degree than seen with DMAE alone. I was also very happy to observe that the upper eye area was regaining tone and contour—her eye appeared to widen as the brow was lifted, and the upper lid firmed up, eliminating that hooded look. In addition to the tightening, toning, and lifting, I noticed improvement in the surface of the skin, with an increased radiance and clarity and decrease in puffiness.

This improvement far exceeded the results of the electrical stimulation devices previously tested. I was also gratified to observe that the EMS appeared to enhance the anti-inflammatory effects of both of the topical formulations that were being used in conjunction with the EMS. The electric stimulation also appeared to be responsible for the skin appearing more plump and youthful. This was an exciting breakthrough because one of the hallmarks of vitamin C ester is its ability to thicken atrophic or thin skin, and this trait was obviously enhanced by the EMS. The vitamin C ester also gave the skin a porcelain-like appearance, while its ability to repair and rebuild natural collagen resulted in an overall improvement in skin tone, texture, and elasticity.

Mia's complexion was also transformed from somewhat dull, pale, and blotchy to radiant and vibrant, thanks to ALA's ability to regulate the production of nitric oxide, which controls blood flow to the skin. ALA also caused a significant decrease in pore size and normalized her skin, eliminating dryness and decreasing fine lines and wrinkles.

After 8 weeks I could see that the asymmetrical look to Mia's face was normalizing and her facial contours were becoming much more pronounced. Greatly encouraged by these early results, Mia vowed to stay with the EMS regimen, and as the months passed, the improvements continued to accrue—to our mutual delight.

THE MIGHTY REJUVENATION COMBINATION

DMAE's superior lifting and toning properties are partly attributable to its ability to increase the production of glycosaminoglycans, which form an important component of connective tissue including collagen and elastin. However, I suspected that the electrical stimulation was greatly enhancing these effects. Over a period of months, I began to observe an overall improvement in facial structure, which could be a result of an actual increase in bone density caused by the electric stimulation. Clinical studies are needed to confirm this observation.

Although therapeutic intervention with EMS and anti-inflammatory antioxidants DMAE–ALA and DMAE–vitamin C ester is only in its infancy, all of the indications point to a marked decrease in wrinkles; virtually no detectable sagging; a lifting and tightening of the eye area, brow, and jawline; a thickening of the dermis; and an increase in muscle mass, resulting in the restoration of the convexities associated with the younger face.

It was gratifying to know that the DMAE–EMS combinations were winning ones and able to achieve far greater results than either when used alone. However, it is important to remember that as with any exercise program, we need to be consistent. It can take decades for our faces and muscles to lose their tone and elasticity, and a natural approach will take longer to achieve the desired results. But the exciting news is that we now have the means to naturally increase tone, decrease sagging, and, at the same time, achieve greater muscle mass, thereby rejuvenating and enhancing the youthful and attractive convexities and contours of the face.

Light Therapy—Tomorrow's Technology Today

For many years dermatologists have used light to treat a wide variety of skin diseases. Psoriasis and various forms of eczema retreat when exposed to sunlight. Certain forms of cancer are also treated with a combination of UV light and psoralens, photosensitizing chemicals administered orally or topically to increase the skin's reaction to light for a therapeutic effect. Now, light therapy, also known as phototherapy, is emerging as an important treatment for aging skin and inflammatory skin diseases such as acne.

A study reported in the *British Journal of Dermatology* evaluated the use of blue light and a mixed blue and red light in the treatment of acne vulgaris (the most common form of acne). One hundred and seven patients with mild to moderate acne vulgaris were randomized into four treatment groups: blue light, mixed blue and red light, cool white light, and 5% benzoyl peroxide cream. After 12 weeks of active treatment, a mean improvement of 76% in inflammatory lesions was achieved by the combined blue–red light phototherapy; this was significantly superior to that achieved by blue light alone, by the benzoyl peroxide, or by the white light. The researchers concluded that phototherapy with mixed blue–red light, probably by combining antibacterial and anti-inflammatory action, is an effective means of treating acne vulgaris of mild to moderate severity, with no significant short-term adverse effects. This is very exciting news because inflammation is at the root cause of both acne and the signs of aging.

SEEING THE LIGHT: NONLASER LIGHT THERAPY

Although laser therapy is perhaps the best known form of light therapy, lasers cause a certain amount of tissue destruction. Lasers may leave the patient with an inflammatory response that lasts for weeks or months, thereby accelerating the aging process. An important focus of my research has been the use of nonlaser light therapy for the improvement and prevention of aging skin.

To this end I have devised a light apparatus with anti-inflammatory properties that treats and repairs damaged and aging skin, both for use in a clinical setting and for cosmetic purposes.

I have long taught that skin inflammation and aging are closely related phenomena. In fact, they are so intrinsically linked by the processes involved with both that aging is sometimes described dermatologically as a *chronic low-grade inflammatory condition*. As we know, both inflammation and aging are initiated in part by free-radical damage, which takes place mostly within the cell membrane. Most of Chapter One ("Cellular Rejuvenation") is devoted to methodologies to stop the free-radical damage occurring in the cell and reverse damage that has already occurred. The problem is that many different types of free radicals are generated simply by normal metabolism, as well as through UV sun exposure, exposure to other forms of ionizing and nonionizing radiation, environmental factors such as pollution or exposure to chemicals in the home or workplace, and stresses such as infection or extreme exercise. In fact, it is almost impossible to avoid free radicals. To make matters worse, the body's endogenous antioxidant defense systems are quickly overwhelmed by the unending onslaught.

This means that scientists have to be on a continuous quest for new and better antioxidant anti-inflammatories. Fortunately, therapeutic results accruing from the use of light therapy for these purposes are opening up a whole new category of age-reversing options.

THE RAINBOW CONNECTION

While the visible light we receive from the sun is a mixture of all the different colors of the spectrum, it appears almost white in color. When the air bends the light, a rainbow is created, causing the various wavelengths of light to become visible. Researchers are now discovering that different wavelengths of light have therapeutic effects on the skin. For example, when blue light, which is characterized by a wavelength of 400 to 500 nanometers, is applied to the skin at certain frequencies, lengths of time, and intensity, clinical improvement is noted and the skin develops a much smoother appearance. This blue light also possesses anti-inflammatory capability.

During my research, I made a startling discovery: Visible short-wavelength blue-violet light, which is of a wavelength that typically doesn't penetrate skin well, can impart smoothness and radiance to exposed skin surfaces, resulting in a vibrant, healthy skin appearance. It can also resolve erythema (redness or inflammation of the skin due to capillary dilation), such as that produced by the UV effects of sunlight.

Scientific studies have shown that light irradiation on skin and other tissues may increase the growth and proliferation of cells, including the acceleration of wound healing and healing of skin grafts. This is important because the ultimate result of skin aging is that while individual cells enlarge, the total number of cells decreases by at least approximately 30%. This results in the loss of the regularity of tissue structure. Other benefits of this light treatment are the control of bacterial infection and the treatment of neoplastic (the conversion of normal cells into tumor cells) tissue, pigmentations (including tattoos), psoriasis, and, as mentioned, acne.

To capitalize on these positive effects, I created a thin, pliable mask comprised of LEDs (light-emitting diodes) for application directly to aging, damaged, or blemished skin on the face and neck. I have been very encouraged with the results and can see that visible light therapy for the treatment of aging skin (as well as acne) offers a technologically advanced, safe, and highly effective solution to a variety of skin problems. Prior to this technological advance, these conditions could be resolved only by costly, invasive therapies or powerful pharmaceuticals, both of which have potentially dangerous side effects. The outstanding anti-inflammatory effects offer short- and long-term anti-aging benefits, helping to reverse many signs of aging as well as the rapid healing of unsightly acne lesions. The many benefits of this new light therapy will help ensure a significantly more youthful, radiant, clear, unblemished, and healthy skin on both face and body.

SKIN-BRIGHTENING AGENTS

One of the most common complaints from my patients, particularly women, is the darkening of the skin, especially on the forehead, cheeks, and chin, that occurs with the passing years. This condition is known as melasma. Although it can affect anyone, melasma is particularly common in women, especially pregnant women and those who are taking oral contraceptives or HRT medications. When melasma occurs in pregnant women, it is known as chloasma, or the mask of pregnancy. This condition occurs in half of all women during pregnancy. The brown color often fades in winter and gets worse in the summer. In fact, sunlight is a major factor in the development of melasma.

The current available treatments for melasma consist of applying topical bleaching agents such as hydroquinone, Retin-A, and kojic acid. These therapies are less than satisfactory because they require a fairly lengthy period of treatment and are not totally effective.

However, it is not just people suffering from melasma who are in need of a skin brightener. Asian skin may be characterized by a lack of radiance. Many of my Asian patients are constantly searching for skin-brightening agents. Many of my darker-skinned patients also suffer from dark patches if there is the slightest bit of inflammation present in their skin. Topical ALA has been of some help for these patients, because of its powerful anti-inflammatory activities—but something stronger is called for if we are to successfully resolve this problem.

TETRONIC ACID

Since I first wrote about tetronic acid in *The Perricone Prescription*, new research has come to light that has exceeded even my own lofty expectations. I believed then as I do now that tetronic acid could be an effective lightening agent for the skin. Tetronic acid is nontoxic and is much less irritating than other agents.

I have found that molecules that are derivatives of tetronic acid are significantly more powerful in their ability to protect the cell. Working with these derivative molecules, I was able to develop an entirely new type of skin brightener—one that acted as a powerful antioxidant and anti-inflammatory. This is an important step forward, as our goal is to stabilize the cell plasma membrane and prevent the production of inflammatory chemicals, which trigger the production of free radicals.

When tested, this form of tetronic acid demonstrated a remarkable ability to decrease pigmentation of the skin, including sun spots, age spots, uneven color, and melasma. These positive results could be seen within 30 minutes of application. Current treatments, such as hydroquinone and kojic acid, as well as those available via prescription through your physician's office, can take months before they produce any results—and the results are marginal at best.

This new anti-aging, anti-inflammatory molecule can deliver substantially better results in under an hour—making it the fastest acting of any skin brightener discovered to date.

5

Sex for Life

Restoring and maintaining sexuality into midlife and beyond has always been a concern, but it had never gotten
the kind of attention it has since the appearance of Viagra in the mid-1990s. For obvious reasons, we all want to
restore or maintain a good sex life. But it turns out that good sex is a
two-way street. If we are in good health, we are likely to enjoy better
sex. More remarkably, it turns out that enjoying a healthy and robust
sexuality likewise confers many health and potential longevity benefits. A white paper (a short treatise whose purpose is to educate industry customers) published by the Katharine Dexter McCormick
Library, Planned Parenthood Federation of America (and available at
www.plannedparenthood.org), states what many of us have known
intuitively, that sexual activity may enrich our well-being in many
ways, including fostering happiness, enhancing immunity, promoting
longevity, managing and alleviating pain, and improving reproductive

health. Some studies even suggest that sexual activity may be associated with reducing the risk of the two leading causes of death in the United States: heart disease and cancer.

That leads us to *secret 5: A robust sex life enhances cellular health.*

More Sex, More Life

An interesting study with a 10-year follow-up from the aforementioned white paper conducted in Caerphilly, South Wales, examined the relationship between frequency of orgasm and mortality. From 1979 to 1983, 918 men aged 45 to 59 were recruited for the study. The men were given a physical examination, including a medical history and blood pressure, electrocardiographic, and cholesterol screenings.

At the 10-year follow-up examination, it was found that the mortality risk was 50% lower among men who had frequent orgasms (defined in this study as two or more per week) than among men who had orgasms less than once a month. Even when controlling for other factors such as age, social class, and smoking status, a strong and statistically significant inverse relationship was found between orgasm frequency and risk of death. The authors of the study concluded that sexual activity seems to have a protective effect on men's health.

To that end, another study reported in the white paper monitored 252 racially diverse men and women in North Carolina over the course of 25 years to determine what factors were important in determining life span. Three of the factors studied were frequency of intercourse, past enjoyment of intercourse, and present enjoyment of intercourse. For men, frequency of intercourse was a significant predictor of longevity. While frequency of intercourse was not predictive of longevity for women, women who reported past enjoyment of intercourse did have greater longevity. Current enjoyment of intercourse had no correlation with longevity for either women or men. These results are noteworthy. Even though we cannot know their exact cause from this study, they strongly suggest a positive association between sexual intercourse and pleasure and how long we live.

Heart Disease and Stroke

Further analysis of the Caerphilly study (which included only men) examined the relationship between engaging in sexual intercourse and experiencing heart disease and stroke. Researchers found that even when adjusting for age and other risk factors, frequent sexual intercourse—two or more times a week—was correlated with lower incidence of fatal coronary events. At a 10-year follow-up examination, the men who reported an intermediate or low frequency of sexual intercourse—less than once a month—had rates of fatal coronary incidents twice that of those who had reported a high frequency of sexual intercourse. However, a Swedish study of both men and women found that mortality was higher among men who had ceased having sexual intercourse at earlier ages. No association was found between sexual intercourse and mortality for women.

Using similar methods, researchers found that frequent sexual intercourse did not result in an increased risk of stroke. This finding is particularly important, because there is a prevailing belief that frequent sexual intercourse may cause strokes—even though this is untrue.

More fascinating facts from the white paper on the benefits of sex include the fact that sexual expression may lead to a decreased risk of breast cancer; research has also shown that sexual activity and orgasm may bolster the immune system in women and men.

The sexual and reproductive health of women and men is directly influenced by their sexual experiences. It has been found that sexual activity can have positive effects on

General Physical Well-Being, Because Sex . . .

- *Improves sleep* because orgasm causes a surge in oxytocin (a hormone best known for inducing labor, but also associated with human attachment and bonding) and endorphins that may act as sedatives.
- *Increases fitness* by burning calories and fat. It has also been suggested that people with active sex lives tend to exercise more frequently and have better dietary habits than those who are less sexually active.
- *Cures wrinkles!* A study conducted during a 10-year period and involving more than 3,500 European and American women and men examined various factors associated with youthful appearance. A panel of judges viewed the participants through a one-way mirror and then guessed the age of each study subject. Those women and men whose age was regularly underestimated by 7 to 12 years were labeled "superyoung." Among these superyoung people, one of the strongest correlates of youthful appearance was an active sex life. On average, superyoung participants reported engaging in sexual intercourse three times a week in comparison with the control group's average of twice a week. The superyoung were also found to be comfortable and confident regarding their sexual identity.

Sexual and Reproductive Health, Because Sex . . .

- Protects against endometriosis
- Enhances fertility
- Regulates the menstrual cycle
- Relieves menstrual cramps
- Protects against early delivery in pregnancy
- Supports prostate health
- Relieves chronic pain
- Helps to relieve migraines

Psychological, Emotional, Social, and Spiritual Health, Because Sex . . .

- Improves overall quality of life
- Decreases risk of depression and suicide
- Reduces stress
- Increases self-esteem
- Enhances intimacy
- Improves social health
- Increases stability of relationships
- Heightens spirituality

More Sex, More DHEA

In past books, I have written about the hormone DHEA (dehy-droepiandrosterone) and its anti-aging benefits. DHEA is manufactured in the adrenal glands. The hormone breaks down in the body into testosterone and estrogen in both men and women.

However (as you will learn in Chapter Seven, "Stress Reduction = Life Extension"), I never recommend taking this over-the-counter supplement without specific instructions and monitoring by your primary health care provider because of possible negative side effects. According to Ray Sahelian, M.D., author of *DHEA: A Practical Guide*, the supplement can trigger heart palpitations and irregular heartbeats—possibly even a heart attack.

Fortunately, there is a more natural way to elevate levels of DHEA, which decline with age, and that is an active sex life. Research with middle-aged men suggests a relationship between the levels of the DHEA, which is released with orgasm, and a reduction in the risk of heart disease. Testosterone, which is the hormone important to the sex drive in both women and men, has also been shown to help reduce the risk of heart attack and to reduce harm to the coronary muscles when heart attack does occur.

With such a plethora of benefits, it is good to know that there are natural ways to help maintain a healthy sexual response as we age. These include many therapeutic strategies that act as mitochondrial rejuvenators to elevate mood, increase intellectual capacity, enhance the immune system, and improve sexual performance. (These are not mitochondrial toxins, which can accelerate aging, such as Viagra. According to the *New York Times*, in 2005 the FDA approved new labeling for Viagra, Cialis, and Levitra—the three most popular drugs for erectile dysfunction—to warn men about a possible link of these drugs to a rare form of blindness.)

Pheromones—the Sweet Smell of Romantic Success?

Our sense of smell is a highly important function of both the body and the emotions. In fact, relating the association of different smells with an emotional reaction is not fiction—it is an actuality. This is because our olfactory receptors are directly connected to the limbic system, the most ancient and primitive part of the brain, considered to be the seat of emotion. The limbic system is a kind of mini brain that largely controls emotions and behavior and influences our feelings, from happiness to misery and love to hate. It is also crucial for learning and memory. The human limbic system shows little difference from that of primitive mammals; it is also where inherent responses required for survival as a species are thought to originate.

Scientists have discovered that there are two sets of receptor cells in the nose; the main set detects general odors. The other set is seen almost as a separate structure and is known as the vomeronasal organ, or the VNO. Although it was first discovered nearly three centuries ago, its function was not known until much more recently. In fact, it was considered a vestigial organ in humans; that is, it might have been important at one point in humankind's evolution but is no longer functional. However, in the mid-1970s it was learned that this theory was incorrect and the VNO was recognized as a sensory organ that produced pheromones in mammals, including humans.

THE NEUROPEPTIDE CONNECTION

Some pheromones are hormone-like substances that ca[...] neuropeptides, which are peptides (short chains of amino [...] leased by neurons (brain cells) that act as inter-cellular messe[...] of these messengers are extremely important. We now know [...] not just the major neurotransmitters such as serotonin, dopamine, and norepinephrine that control our moods and our brain. There is a fine-tuning performed by neurotransmitters and an even *finer tuning* performed by neuropeptides, including the pheromones. This vast intracellular network, made up of the endocrine and nervous systems, controls the rate at which our brain, skin, and organ systems age.

Unlike hormones, which act on the same individual, the pheromones' chemical messages are relayed between members of the same animal and insect species. First discovered in insects in 1959, pheromones are used to attract members of the opposite sex, to mark trails and territory, and as warnings. Each insect (or animal) has its own complex chemical pheromones, which act as a stimulus to other individuals of the same species for one or more behavioral responses.

In humans, pheromones are found on the skin. In a series of experiments, scientists collected skin cells and placed them in vials in the laboratory. When the vials were uncorked, it was discovered that the lab workers became more social and cooperative. The scientists believed that these pheromones were affecting behavior. This led to a lot of research into pheromones, and it was found that the pheromones directly activated the VNO, affecting a whole host of human emotions.

LIKE ATTRACTS LIKE—AND OPPOSITES ATTRACT

So what is happening here? The major histocompatibility complex (MHC) is a very important group of genes that control aspects of the immune response. The products of these genes, the histocompatibility antigens (antigens are foreign substances that cause the immune system to make a specific immune response), are present on every cell of the body and serve as markers to distinguish "self" from "non-self" cells. If, for example, we receive an organ transplant, our MHC recognizes that it is foreign and will reject it. One of the keys to successful organ transplants is suppression of the MHC.

Studies with mice found that mice nest with other mice that have genes that are compatible with their own MHC because they feel safe with these mice. However, once the mice reach puberty, they feel a desire to mate with mice that have MHC genes very different from their own. The logic of this becomes immediately apparent; by mating with partners whose MHC genes are unlike our own, we create a more diverse gene pool.

A study involving human subjects, conducted in Switzerland by Claus Wedekind, consisted of 44 men and 49 women. The men were given T-shirts and instructed to wear the T-shirts to bed for two consecutive nights to ensure that the T-shirts were totally saturated with pheromones. They were also given scentless soap and other toiletries and told to use them exclusively.

At the end of the experiment, the T-shirts were put into a box and rated, on the basis of smell scent—pleasant or unpleasant—by women. A number of boxes were filled with clean T-shirts to act as a control. The women preferred the scents of the T-shirts worn by men with a dissimilar MHC gene. Many of the women commented that the scents reminded them of boyfriends or husbands.

Another interesting observation was made when pheromones were placed on the upper lip of women as they reached midlife and were experiencing diminished sexual desire. Not only did their libido revive but they also reported an increase in well-being and self-esteem. Women who were prone to panic attacks reported a significant decrease in the attacks. Another double-blind study was conducted with 20 women, each receiving the pheromone treatment three times per week. All participants reported a higher rate of sexual contact with their mates. Similar studies with men also showed a higher rate of sexual relations when they were exposed to the pheromones.

As interest in pheromones began to accelerate, *ABC News* conducted an informal test on human synthetic pheromones. They chose two sets of identical twins; one set of twins was male and the other set was female. One female twin and one male twin were given an unscented pheromone spray. The other twins were given a witch hazel spray containing no pheromones.

Fast-forward to a Manhattan singles bar. Upon arrival, the twins were instructed to separate and gravitate to different areas of the bar. They were also instructed not to make the first move toward any members of the opposite sex. Interestingly, the men received about equal attention from the women in the bar, the pheromone-wearing twin notwithstanding.

But it was a different story with the female twins. The non-pheromone-wearing twin proved to be quite popular; she was approached by 11 men. However, the twin wearing the pheromones was approached by a whopping 30 men—just about triple the number of men who approached her identical twin. And while the pheromones appear to increase a person's sexual attraction, they also increase self-confidence, thus making people feel more attractive and adding to their overall allure and attractiveness. Morgan's story clearly illustrates the many benefits of pheromones when added to a fragrance rich in therapeutic botanical essences.

Planting the Seeds for Sexual Health

For thousands of years indigenous peoples have relied on native plants for food, shelter, medicine—just about all of their basic needs. And so it should come as no surprise that there is also a long history of plants being used for sexual health as well.

Unfortunately, the world of botanicals and their unique healing and restorative properties has not received significant study in the United States. It may be due to the fact that many Americans have lost touch with the ancient, time-honored cultures whose connection to

MORGAN'S STORY

Morgan was a high-powered New York–based investment banker, following in the footsteps of her father and grandfather. At 42 she was pretty much at the top of her game and consistently outperformed the majority of her coworkers.

However, as is often the case, the monetary and career success came at a price. Morgan was exhausted—and even worse, she found herself losing interest in both her professional and private life.

Morgan was very active on the charity and fund-raising circuit, and it was at one of these dinner events that I found myself seated next to her. "I have long been an admirer of your books and PBS specials," Morgan said to me after we were introduced by a mutual friend and colleague. "In fact," she added, "I have been rereading all of your books in an attempt to recharge my batteries." She confided that she had regular annual physicals and knew that she was not suffering from any health problem. I gave Morgan my phone numbers and told her to call my office and arrange an appointment. At the very least I could get her on a solid program of good nutrition and supplements that would increase her energy very quickly.

As I recorded her case history several weeks later, she explained her dilemma in greater detail. "I'm not sure if my problem is mental, emotional, or physical," Morgan said. "I just can't seem to get up any enthusiasm—for work or play. I'm afraid I'm driving away my husband as well. We used to enjoy each other's company. We both have such busy schedules, getting together was always like a special date, even after ten years of marriage. But lately I find myself withdrawing emotionally and avoiding all forms of intimacy."

Morgan was not the first patient I have had suffering from a general malaise and loss of libido. In fact, she appeared to be an ideal candidate for a special neuropeptide fragrance I had formulated. The formula consisted of a combination of pheromones and aromatic oils of special spices and botanicals. I instructed Morgan to apply the fragrance to her pulse points, as she would a normal fragrance. I then told her to apply a drop or two on her upper lip. It is here that all relationship to a "normal" fragrance ends. The upper-lip application would ensure that the fragrance reached her olfactory receptors, a direct pathway to the limbic portion of the brain.

Morgan left with a vial of the neuropeptide fragrance and instructions to call me in 2 weeks. I was eager to learn of her progress, as prior results had been very positive. However, I was quite surprised when I saw Morgan's name in my appointment book a scant 5 days later.

"Dr. Perricone, I couldn't wait to thank you," Morgan said excitedly as she entered my office. "I have to admit I tried this fragrance with a strong dose of healthy skepticism but have since become convinced that it is nothing short of miraculous."

After our initial appointment Morgan had gone home to get ready for a dinner date that evening with her husband. She dutifully applied the neuropeptide fragrance as instructed. About 20 minutes later, just as Morgan was sitting down at her table, she felt a sudden sense of well-being sweep over her. "It was the best evening I've had in years," she told me. "And it wasn't just the lovely bottle of champagne. I felt like I was on a first date. Our conversation sparked and we were laughing all evening. I never felt so self-confident or attractive. I have to admit that I was even flirting with my husband—after a decade of marriage!"

Best of all was the renewed love and shared intimacy that they enjoyed later. "It has been a whirlwind week," she added. "I applied the neuropeptide fragrance again the next morning before leaving for the office, and by the time I arrived I felt the euphoria I experienced last night returning. I knew that I had a very hectic and stressful day ahead of me but found myself looking forward to each challenge; my mind was crystal clear and I was able to handle difficulties that had previously seemed unsolvable." She laughed and added, "I also noticed that my male colleagues were particularly attentive, much more so than usual!"

Many of my patients have shared similar stories of their experiences with the neuropeptide pheromone fragrance. The good news is that it is not just a mood enhancer and libido booster, as important as those assets are. The right combination of pheromones and botanicals can greatly enhance memory and mental clarity, lift depression, increase self-confidence, and increase one's attractiveness to the opposite sex. Additionally, because the limbic portion of the brain controls autonomous body functions, these fragrances can also lower blood pressure, increase blood flow to the brain and thus eliminate the confusion that sometimes plagues older people, increase problem-solving skills, reduce levels of the stress hormones cortisol and adrenalin and actually slow the aging process. Women in particular report that men become much more attentive and responsive. This should come as no surprise, as it is well known in scientific circles that many different odors play an important role in mammalian reproductive biology.

Unfortunately we cannot stop aging and the loss of many of the drives and motivations we had in our younger days. Fortunately with the help of neuropeptides and pheromones and the right blend of rejuvenating fragrances, we can restore a lost libido and that wonderful sense of joie de vivre that often accompanies youth.

the plant world ensured their survival—our own native Americans notwithstanding. And it may also be the financial factor: Pharmaceuticals are hugely profitable, while herbs and botanicals are not. Fortunately, there are many internationally renowned botanical experts hailing from other countries and continents whose ongoing research complements thousands of years of history and lore. Chris Kilham, explorer in residence at the University of Massachusetts Amherst, has traveled the world in search of these experts and the safest and most efficacious of these plants. He chronicles them in his book *Hot Plants*.

Three of the most widely researched botanical remedies are described below. All of them provide benefits ranging far beyond improved sexuality.

Tongkat Ali to Increase Testosterone Levels

Tongkat ali (*Eurycoma longifolia*), which translates to "Ali's walking stick," is the popular folk name for a slender, medium-size tree reaching 10 meters in height. Documented use of tongkat ali, a native of Malaysia, lower Burma, Indonesia, and Thailand, dates to the 1700s.

Tongkat ali root contains a treasure trove of phytonutrients, including powerful antioxidants. It also has antiviral and antimalarial properties and helps fight high blood pressure. A scientific collaboration between Malaysian researchers and pharmaceutical researchers in the United States has identified considerable anticancer activity in tongkat ali.

Tongkat ali boosts testosterone production, the primarily male hormone produced by the testicles, which is responsible for the development and the release of sperm, male physical characteristics, and sex drive. Small amounts of testosterone are also produced in women by the ovaries and the adrenal glands. Testosterone levels begin to decline in men by approximately 2% per year, starting around the age of 30. By age 45 a man may have a scant 60% of the testosterone he had at age 25, and by the age of 50 this will have further declined to 55%. Varying factors will influence this decline. For example, exercise—particularly weight lifting—will increase testosterone levels. On the other hand, poor lifestyle choices, such as smoking and excess use of alcohol, will accelerate the decline.

The decline in testosterone levels is also linked to decreased muscle mass, energy, and feelings of well-being. Although women have much lower levels of testosterone to begin with, their levels also decline with each passing year, resulting in decreased libido and increased body fat.

Tongkat ali appears to increase testosterone production in both men and women, which may help to halt many of the signs of aging. Benefits include improved energy and sexual function, reduction in body fat with increase in lean muscle, and reduced risk factors associated with cardiovascular disease.

WHAT THE STUDIES SHOW

One of the world's leading experts on tongkat ali is Dr. Johari Saad, a prominent scientist in the Malaysian scientific community whose field of expertise is nutritional biochemistry, protein and enzymology, and natural product biochemistry (use of natural products in traditional medicine). His body of research has had a tremendous impact on the Malaysian herbal industry, and his many awards bear testimony to his legacy in the field of herbal medicine. He is much sought after for national and international seminars on herbal medicine and has published more than thirty articles in local and international biochemical journals.

Dr. Saad found in his animal studies that a water-soluble extract of tongkat ali not only increased testosterone levels, energy, and muscle mass but also inhibited sex hormone–binding globulin, allowing more free testosterone (the active, available testosterone in the body) to remain in the blood.

Another highly regarded researcher studying tongkat ali is Dr. Ismail Tambi, head of the Specialist Reproductive Human Research Center at the National Population and Family Development Board in Malaysia and chief editor of *Manual of Sexual and Reproductive Health*. As one of the foremost experts on reproductive health in Southeast Asia, Dr. Tambi works with both men and women on sexual health, reproductive disorders, and fertility problems. He is also the leading medical expert on the effects of tongkat ali root extract on humans.

In his work with men, Dr. Tambi has found that use of tongkat ali extract significantly increased testosterone production. Dr. Tambi states, "I was very skeptical at first about this type of thing, using some plant to change hormone levels. But I did some work with it, and tongkat ali turned out to be highly potent. In our studies, we found that tongkat ali extract increased the serum level of testosterone considerably. . . . Men found that tongkat ali boosted their sex drive quite a lot. I think that for low libido, tongkat ali extract is very valuable. I have seen this result for myself and can say that this plant really works. It certainly should boost libido in women as well, as testosterone is essential to a woman's sexual desire. Women have used tongkat ali for a very long time in this culture."

Dr. Tambi conducted the PADAM study, in which he investigated partial androgen deficiency in males. The testosterone levels of all participants increased when given 100 milligrams of standardized tongkat ali extract daily. Ninety-one percent reported an improvement in libido, 73% reported improvement in sexual function, and 82% reported psychological improvement relative to overall sexuality. Dr. Tambi further reported that while testosterone does decline with age, tongkat ali can reelevate the level of this important sex hormone.

Dr. Saad, Dr. Tambi, and other experts recommend that you read the label of the tongkat ali products and make sure that they contain 100 milligrams of concentrated, standardized water-extracted tongkat ali daily for men, and 50 milligrams for women, standardized to approximately 22% glycoproteins. (See the "Resources" section for more information about where to get this and other botanicals mentioned in this chapter.)

MACA TO ENHANCE FERTILITY

Maca is the edible root of the Peruvian plant *Lepidium meyenii*, traditionally employed for its purported aphrodisiac and fertility-enhancing properties. Maca grows exclusively in the central highlands of the Peruvian Andes, at altitudes between 10,000 and 15,000 feet. Interestingly, it is the only cruciferous plant native to Peru (the plant family that includes cabbage, bok choy, collards, broccoli, Brussels sprouts, kohlrabi, kale, mustard greens, turnip greens, and cauliflower). Cruciferous plants contain potent anticancer phytonutrients called indoles and glucosinolates. In fact, population studies indicate that ounce for ounce, the anticancer properties of cruciferous vegetables are greater than those of other fruits or vegetables, including foods with higher antioxidant levels.

Collectively, indoles and glucosinolates stimulate the immune system's cells and messenger chemicals (cytokines), boost liver enzymes that whisk carcinogens out of the body, and block enzymes that promote tumor growth—particularly in the breasts, liver, colon, lungs, stomach, and esophagus.

Maca has been used for its nutritional and tonic properties by native Peruvians for more than 2,000 years—predating the arrival of the Inca civilization. It was believed that maca increased both energy and fertility in both humans and animals.

REVEALING RESEARCH

In twenty-first–century Peru, maca is considered a highly nutritious food and as such is made into blender drinks, cakes, cookies, porridge, and other dishes. Nutritional benefits notwithstanding, maca is most popular for promoting a healthy libido and enhanced sexual function. One of the world's leading researchers into the use of maca for enhancing healthy sexual function is Dr. Qun-Yi Zheng, who received his B.S. in chemical engineering from China's Hunan University and his Ph.D. in synthetic organic chemistry from the University of Colorado at Boulder. He has also been a postdoctoral research associate at Cornell University.

Dr. Zheng is a leading expert in the standardization of botanical extracts. His extensive résumé includes many scientific papers and publications and thirteen pending or current patents, many of which are related to his work in enumerating, isolating, and characterizing various anticancer constituents from natural products such as taxol and artemisinin.

At PureWorld Botanicals (now Naturex), Dr. Zheng and his team of analytical chemists analyzed maca to discover what compounds might be attributable to its reputed ability to boost libido, enhance sexual function, and increase overall energy. They discovered two previously unknown groups of novel compounds in maca, the macamides and macaenes. And though these compounds occur in very small quantities, their effects are significant.

The researchers conducted a series of controlled animal experiments, the results of which were published in the medical journal *Urology*. Rodents fed a proprietary extract of maca known as Maca-Pure, which contains a concentration of macamides and macaenes, demonstrated greatly increased energy. The animals also exhibited a striking increase in sexual activity as compared with non-maca-fed animals, or those fed lesser amounts of macamides and macaenes. Another study by Dr. Zheng, published in the 2002 American Chemical Society proceedings, found that MacaPure significantly improved stamina in the animals studied.

As interest in maca continued to grow, it caught the attention of one of the world's preeminent ethnobotanists, Dr. Michael Balick, vice president and chair, botanical science research and training, and director and philecology curator, Institute of Economic Botany at the New York Botanical Garden. Dr. Balick teamed with Roberta A. Lee, M.D., medical director of Continuum Center for Health and Healing at Beth Israel Medical Center in New York, whose clinical and research interests include ethnomedicine, to publish an important article entitled "Maca: From Traditional Crop to Energy and Libido Stimulant" (see "Resources" section). The doctors interviewed Dr. Zheng and the manufacturer of MacaPure, Natalie Koether, who stated that they were not positioning maca as an herbal Viagra because Viagra acts more on mechanical function. Maca acts more on the libido, a more natural and less potentially harmful methodology.

Today the use of maca is on the increase for boosting libido, enhancing energy, and improving sexual function. Many physicians, both here and in Peru, are incorporating maca in their practices. Hugo Malaspina, M.D., a cardiologist practicing complementary medicine in

Lima, often recommends maca for women experiencing premenstrual or menopausal symptoms. Dr. Malaspina believes that there are different medicinal plants that work on the ovaries by stimulating them; he believes that maca can *regulate*—as opposed to *stimulate*—ovarian function. Aguila Calderon, M.D., the former dean of the faculty of human medicine at the National University Federico Villarreal in Lima, also prescribes maca in his medical practice. He has found it useful for erectile dysfunction, menopausal symptoms, and general fatigue and has found that maca's high levels of easily absorbable calcium, magnesium, and silica make it very useful in treating the decalcification of bones in both children and adults. For optimum results, make sure that the MacaPure you purchase is labeled as 400 milligrams standardized to contain 0.6% macaenes and macamides. Follow the label directions for correct dosages.

RHODIOLA TO DESTRESS

Rhodiola rosea is classified as an *adaptogen*, a term that applies to herbs that maintain health by increasing the body's ability to adapt to environmental and internal stress, a topic we will discuss at greater length in Chapter Seven ("Stress Reduction = Life Extension"). Our society suffers from astronomically high levels of stress—both mental and physical—making the need for effective adaptogens unprecedented. Adaptogens generally work by strengthening the immune system, nervous system, and/or glandular systems. One of the finest adaptogens is *Rhodiola rosea*, a very exciting plant that appears to have been used as early as 77 BCE by Greek physician Dioscorides. The plant continues to be recognized for its outstanding healing properties. It is interesting to note that *Rhodiola* hails from Siberia, just like a potent form of another adaptogen, Siberian ginseng. It may be the tremendously harsh environment in Siberia that gives its native plants such exceptional properties in adapting to strenuous circumstances!

Rhodiola's Myriad Benefits

Rhodiola has been found to increase physical endurance, enhance physical productivity, prevent altitude sickness, and treat fatigue, depression, anemia, nervous system disorders, and various infections. Studies done in humans, animals, and cells in test tubes have verified that the plant has antifatigue, antistress, anticancer, antioxidant, and immunity-enhancing effects. *Rhodiola* also appears to accelerate weight loss and protect against heart disease. It has also been found that *Rhodiola* has sexually stimulating effects; it has been used to increase libido and to treat impotence.

Rhodiola rosea contains a group of novel compounds that have not been found in other plants, including rosin, rosavin, and rosarin, known collectively as rosavins. Each of these has been studied, and each appears to make a significant contribution to the plant's unrivaled antistress properties. *Rhodiola* also contains the agent salidroside and other protective antioxidants that inhibit the cellular deterioration process of oxidation.

Healthy sexual function may be attributable to equal parts mental and physical health. Chronic stress and exhaustion will take its toll on all biological functions, including sexuality and reproduction. When we experience stress, the levels of a variety of substances are increased in our bodies, including adrenaline, opioids, and catecholamine, a chemical in the brain that affects mood and appetite. If high levels of these substances stay in circulation in the body, they can damage both nervous system and glandular function, including the sex glands. One substance in particular, known as corticotropin-releasing hormone, originally named corticotropin-releasing factor (CRF) and also called corticoliberin, is a polypeptide hormone and neurotransmitter. It is involved in the stress response and can impair sexual function. *Rhodiola rosea* lowers levels of stress hormones, including CRH, thereby helping to restore normal function to the body.

In human clinical studies, a standardized powdered extract was used in many cases. That extract was standardized to 3% rosavins and 0.8% salidroside. Participants in studies took between 150 and 200 milligrams of the extract daily. Follow the directions on the label for the correct dosage.

As we can see, there are many different strategies available to help maintain a healthy sexuality, regardless of chronological age. Even more important is understanding that a healthy and active sex life impacts our physical and mental health.

6

Reversing Aging
Through Exercise

Scientists long ago established that exercise greatly reduces both the incidence and severity of age-related degenerative diseases. But we don't just want to live longer; we want to extend the number of our *healthy* years. We want to stay fit and active with the capacity to enjoy life to its fullest. Gerontologists refer to this as our health span—as opposed to our simple life span—and universally agree that exercise is a crucial component to extend and improve them both.

Throughout this book I have presented strategies that will help to regenerate the body on a cellular level. Now we are ready to use the power of exercise to do so much more than make us look good. The right exercise will strengthen our bones and muscles, improve and restore physical and emotional balance, relieve stress, and improve physical, mental, and emotional health. But to achieve these goals we need to incorporate specific types of exercise. Disciplines such as yoga, tai chi, and chi kung (also known as qigong), for example, may not seem strenuous enough, yet they yield unparalleled physical, mental, emotional, and spiritual benefits.

And thus we come to *secret 6: The right form of exercise will restore balance, unity, and harmony between mind and body.*

This secret is in many ways contrary to most forms of Western-style sports or exercise, which are, for the most part, based on muscular exertion and increased oxygen consumption. The speed of the cardiac pump is accelerated during this kind of exercise. The muscles need more oxygen, which is supplied by a sharp rise in respiratory rates. This in turn leads the heart to intensify its efforts even more, increasing perspiration and the elimination of toxins. In other words, typically Western forms of exercise make our heart and lungs work hard. The principal aims of this kind of exercise are building good muscle tone and increasing endurance.

While these goals are worthy and important, we need to be careful when performing vigorous physical exercise. Too much exertion increases oxygen demand beyond the optimum level, resulting in the production of inflammatory free radicals that accelerate cellular degeneration (and thus the aging process). Ironically, the wrong type of exercise will backfire by accelerating the aging process. Because our desire is cellular rejuvenation on all levels, it is encouraging to discover that there are forms of exercise that will help us achieve that goal. And there is a vital role for aerobic types of exercise, as long as they are not overdone.

Strong Body, Strong Mind

I have long been impressed with the physical and mental health benefits of Asian martial arts. From the aggressive forms such as aikido, karate, and judo to the more gentle, meditative movements of tai chi and chi kung, practitioners gain much more that physical fitness. For example, practitioners of tai chi (a form of movement that has a med-

EXERCISE, HEART HEALTH, AND COGNITIVE DECLINE

The NIH Cognitive and Emotional Health Project has determined that exercising the body, controlling blood pressure, and keeping the heart healthy can also keep the brain in good cognitive and emotional shape. Investigators at the NIH reviewed a significant number of factors that could have an effect on brain health. They concluded that the same factors that affect cardiovascular health have an important impact on the cognitive and emotional health of people 65 and older. We define *cognitive* as the mental process by which knowledge is acquired; this includes thinking, reasoning, remembering, imagining, and learning. These functions go far beyond knowing where we left the car keys. They are critical to our overall mental and physical well-being—in fact, our very existence depends upon these faculties.

The following factors were most often associated with cognitive decline:

- Hypertension
- Age
- Diabetes
- Stroke or transient ischemic attacks
- Infarcts or white-matter lesions on brain imaging
- Low mood scores
- Higher body mass index

The chairperson of the study, Hugh Hendrie, M.B., Ch.B., D.Sc., a professor of psychiatry at Indiana University School of Medicine, stated: "Based on our review of cardiovascular risk factors, the link between hypertension and cognitive decline was the most robust across studies."

"This article points to the possibility that healthier living can significantly contribute to reducing the numbers of sick and mentally declining older people, and reduce health care costs," said William Thies, Ph.D., vice president for medical and scientific affairs of the Alzheimer's Association.

Cognitive decline is debilitating to the person and the community. If physical exercise can protect us from it, and it appears that it can and does do so, we need to incorporate it into our daily lives both individually and on a large scale, to prevent a dependent, deteriorating society.

No health care system in the world could handle an en masse onslaught of millions of sick and aging people—but we could face such a scenario if we don't take action now. In 2006, the first crop of baby boomers turned 60—approximately 2.8 million men and women. As the approximately 76 million baby boomers age over the next two decades, it becomes everyone's personal and collective responsibility to adopt a lifestyle that will keep us healthy and active, both mentally and physically.

itative quality similar to yoga) have found that it restores both physical and emotional balance. It appears that tai chi can increase strength while instilling a calm and harmonious sense of well-being. It is presumed to work by improving the flow of internal energy (or *qi*) throughout the body.

As a physical exercise, tai chi benefits the entire body, increasing muscle strength and enhancing balance and flexibility. People who practice tai chi are also said to exploit the strength of yin (the Earth) and the energy of yang (the heavens) through exercises designed to express these forces in balanced and harmonious form. Dr. Chenchen Wang, a physician at Tufts–New England Medical Center, examined 47 studies on tai chi in English and Chinese medical journals and analyzed the effect of the practice on healthy people as well as those with assorted health conditions. According to Dr. Wang, "Overall, these studies reported that long-term tai chi had favorable effects on the promotion of balance control, flexibility and cardiovascular fitness and reduced the risk of falls in the elderly. Benefit was also found for balance, strength and flexibility in older subjects, and pain, stress and anxiety in healthy subjects."

The flowing movements of tai chi serve as a moving meditation that reduces stress and provides a way to cultivate body and mind. Many thousands of individuals have found tai chi's massage-like movements to be an effective therapy for a wide range of health problems, including poor circulation, headaches, high blood pressure, arthritis, back pain, breathing difficulties, and digestive and nervous disorders, to name but a few.

The Power of Chi Kung

HEALING THE BODY, STRENGTHENING THE MIND

I find the Chinese form of exercise known as chi kung particularly intriguing for the astounding benefits it brings to the practitioner on all levels. Like tai chi, chi kung combines movement with a meditative focus and has been proven to restore both physical and emotional balance. Chi kung is an ancient physical discipline that means "energy mastery." It is more than 5,000 years old—its origins lost in antiquity— and yet it survives today. Chi kung uses deliberate movement, slow breathing, mental concentration, and visualizations. According to an exceptional book titled *Chi Kung* by Dr. Yves Réquéna, chi kung is based on movements made without muscular exertion or an increase in heart and breath rate. In fact, unlike Western forms of exercise, in the practice of chi kung, breathing slows down.

According to Dr. Réquéna, who is also an acupuncturist, phytotherapist, and director of the European Institute of Chi Kung, when sedentary people begin practicing chi kung (no matter what their age), even their stiffened joints become gently relaxed. In addition, the circulation of energy throughout the entire body is increased, without causing undue sweating or fatigue. Consequently, overall health improves without the stress-producing effects of strenuous exercise.

Chi kung reinforces stamina, strengthening the joints and providing energy and strength for brief and intense muscular exertion. Moreover, it strengthens the practitioner's capacity for concentrating and encourages the development of visualizing the most perfect or efficient action for any given situation. The ability to visualize ideal situations, circumstances, and outcomes is a very powerful tool and can give us much greater control of our lives than we would have otherwise. As with all disciplines, the more you practice it, the more proficient you will become and the greater success you will achieve.

I encourage you to learn chi kung regardless of age or physical condition because it will prevent much of what has been considered the normal signs of aging. In fact, the age-related physical and mental deterioration that occurs with passing decades is far from normal—it is actually preventable and reversible. Regular practice of chi kung will enable you to remain vital into your seventies, eighties, and nineties. Master practitioners of Eastern martial arts are known to attain very advanced ages while maintaining their suppleness of movement and a state of perfect mental and physical health, outperforming students many decades their junior.

Chi kung can act as a lifeline when stiffening joints and tightening muscles diminish an individual's physical capabilities and flexibility. When the cardiovascular system is failing, respiration is weakened, or physical disabilities confine an individual to an armchair or walking with a cane, chi kung is our most powerful and effective path to physical rehabilitation. The energy that is created through chi kung practice provides immediate sensations of well-being. Practitioners experience significant physical improvement, which will immediately slow, stop, and even reverse the aging process.

SOOTHING THE SPIRIT AND LENGTHENING LIFE

But the benefits of chi kung reach even further to make it an invaluable and holistic means for achieving perfect mental and physical health. It turns out that chi kung has a calming effect on the nervous system and is therefore beneficial in the treatment of anxiety, insomnia, and depression. It has been scientifically established that chi kung stimulates the immune system, helping to alleviate dangerous inflammatory conditions. By increasing vital energy, chi kung helps the body's struggle against disease by virtue of strengthening the body's defenses. When vital energy is increased, so is longevity, because cellular regeneration is accelerated and the normal wear and tear on the body is slowed down.

Chi kung also encourages the revelation and realization of personal potential. No matter what you do professionally and creatively, the practice of chi kung will greatly enhance your abilities by increasing the powers of concentration. And no matter how stressed we may be, chi kung helps us to relax, regardless of the situation. The practice of chi kung will not only contribute to an expanded life span but will also ensure that we live in peak mental, emotional, and spiritual form.

Slowing down the aging process allows us to conserve and also recover important physical and intellectual capabilities. People new to chi kung often ask how all of these benefits are accomplished. Simply put, it is the combination of *movement, breathing, visualization, and focus* that results in physical and spiritual renewal. An added bonus is the stress relief that comes from meditation and quiet contemplation. I believe that the finest health insurance you can have is the practice of chi kung.

Chi kung is not designed to build up muscle but rather to increase flexibility, balance, and strength. Strength and muscle size do not necessarily go hand in hand. Bodybuilders may have huge muscles, but they build them for bulk. Serious weight lifters will not have muscles that look as large, but they will be stronger.

To build muscles by lifting weights or practicing T-Tapp—which I recommend because chi kung does not build muscle mass—wait at least 2 hours after practicing chi kung. In Dr. Réquéna's highly recommended book, you will find clear illustrations demonstrating how to perform the simple, easy-to-follow chi kung movements. For more information, see the "Resources" section at the back of this book.

From East to West: the Benefits of Weight Training

One of the seemingly unavoidable pitfalls of aging is unwanted weight gain. In fact, it is such a widespread problem that I made it the focus of my previous book, *The Perricone Weight-Loss Diet*, and also devoted an entire chapter to it in this book. This is not because of the aesthetics of being overweight—it is because excess fat is highly toxic to the body and therefore highly aging as well.

Traditionally women tend to gain weight in their hips and men gain weight in their abdomen. However, as they get older, women are particularly subject to weight gain in the abdomen. And it often seems that no matter how carefully they control their diet, it becomes more and more difficult to lose this weight with each passing year. But there is good news on the horizon. According to a recent University of Pennsylvania study, weight training is especially effective in helping to eliminate central obesity, or excess fat in the abdomen.

Funded by the NIH, the study found that just two 1-hour sessions of weight lifting per week can bring down the chances of age-related fat buildup in the abdomen. As we know, there are two types of fat: subcutaneous (under the skin) and visceral (found in the abdomen and surrounding our vital organs). Central obesity is visceral fat and is considered the most dangerous because it surrounds vital organs and is metabolized by the liver, which turns it into blood cholesterol. Visceral fat also puts pressure on the heart and the arteries, increasing the chances of heart trouble. In fact, physicians refer to this type of fat as "toxic fat" because it produces a veritable factory of inflammatory chemicals, increasing the risk for heart disease, strokes, and diabetes.

COURTING DISASTER FROM TOO MUCH CORTISOL

A lot of the blame for this visceral fat can be attributed to chronic stress and the effects of stress-induced cortisol production. Cortisol stimulates fat and carbohydrate metabolism for fast energy (the fight-or-flight response), thereby stimulating insulin release to keep pace with the rising blood sugar levels. The result is an increase in appetite. If we experience chronic stress, with chronically high levels of cortisol, we may end up hungry all the time, resulting in overeating and unwanted weight gain.

Even more to the point, cortisol also influences where that weight will be deposited. A fascinating study on the effects of the release of cortisol during acute and chronic stress in nonoverweight women was published in the journal *Psychosomatic Medicine* in 2001. The study demonstrated that this excess cortisol contributes to the deposition of visceral fat, particularly in the abdomen. Women used to worry about the size of their hips; however, when it comes to the health dangers of extra weight, it is preferable to have it on the hips as opposed to the stomach. Interestingly, the cause-and-effect process flows both ways: It has been proven that women (and men) who store their weight in the abdomen also have higher cortisol levels and higher stress levels than those whose weight is stored on the hips.

I have long been a fan of weight lifting and resistance training in conjunction with some form of aerobic exercise, such as running, walking, and biking. Unfortunately many women shy away from working with weights, fearing that they will bulk up like their male counterparts. This is not the case. To begin with, women do not have the same physical capacity as men do for increasing the size of their muscles. This is because the average woman has approximately 10 times less of the muscle-building hormone testosterone than the average man. In addition, female muscle produces less tension per unit volume, and each muscle fiber has a smaller cross-sectional area. What women need to know is that these factors make it harder for female muscle to grow as large as male muscle, so instead of bulking up, women doing weight lifting will have an elegant, attractive, and sculpted body.

While the average woman will not be developing the large bulging muscles of her male counterpart, she will, however, significantly increase her strength and muscle tone. The actual shape of the body may also be significantly enhanced by weight training in women because of the changes that occur in the all-important ratio of fat to muscle. We know that muscle burns more calories than fat does and that increased muscle enables us to burn excess calories even while resting. (For more tips on how to successfully build and maintain muscle while eliminating body fat, refer to *The Perricone Weight-Loss Diet*.) But building muscle can also tighten and tone our bodies in ways that simple weight loss cannot.

Weight-training exercises will also slow age-related functional degeneration—again highlighting the outstanding anti-aging benefits of exercise. Traditionally, three 45-minute weight-training workouts per week (Monday, Wednesday, and Friday) is considered ideal. For optimum benefit, rotate weight training with other forms of exercise. It may take as long as 6 weeks to begin to see noticeable physical changes, but don't despair. Stay with it because the beneficial and highly visible changes are well worth the effort. Some of the incomparable benefits include

- Development of muscular strength, speed, and power
- Visible and significant changes in body composition (the more toned muscles we have, the more energy and calories we burn)
- Improvement in posture
- Increase in lean body tissue
- Enhanced athletic performance
- Repair and strengthening of muscles after injury
- Increased metabolic rate, resulting in decreased body fat
- Protection and maintenance of bone density to prevent osteoporosis
- Decrease in pro-inflammatory, toxic abdominal fat
- Improvement in self-esteem and sense of accomplishment

Another benefit of weight training and increased muscle mass is the decreased risk of type 2 diabetes. Muscle is metabolically active, enabling it to use blood sugar, which decreases the need for insulin, removing the burden on the pancreas.

But remember the other side of the coin: Overexercising is pro-inflammatory. Overexercising can trigger the release of cortisol, promoting unwanted weight gain (especially in the abdomen), break down muscle tissue, and accelerate the rate at which we age. Before starting a weight-training program (if you are completely new to this form of exercise), consult your physician and/or professional trainer to make sure you are training at the right level, to avoid injury and to ensure that you are performing the exercises correctly.

The National Institute on Aging website (www.niapublications.org) is an outstanding resource on all forms of exercise and even includes drawings and animations of actual exercises in the following categories:

- Resistance
- Endurance
- Balance
- Stretching

T-Tapp—10 Minutes to Turn Back Time

A Rehabilitative Approach

I recently had the good fortune to learn about a program called T-Tapp, an innovative wellness workout that incorporates many different elements to build balanced muscle tissue along with strength and flexibility. Created by fitness expert Teresa Tapp, T-Tapp takes a preventive, rehabilitative approach to fitness—one that will stabilize your spine and strengthen your joints while helping to build stronger bones and a healthy cardiovascular system.

Teresa's mantra of "Less is more" is in direct contrast to the old adage of "No pain, no gain." I heartily embrace her approach, because as we discussed earlier, overexercising is counterproductive to our goal of a lean, lithe, well-toned body. Teresa encourages people to start with what she refers to as a boot camp of 4 to 14 consecutive days (depending on how quickly a person needs to see results). She then recommends performing the workout every other day. Her program also coordinates nicely with running, walking, yoga, Pilates, chi kung, and tai chi.

Although the movements used in T-Tapp appear simple, they are actually quite complex. Each exercise involves five to seven muscles, with each muscle fully activated at both ends (origin and insertion), as opposed to traditional exercises that work only one attachment and the belly of the muscle. This strategy means that your body will build the long, lean, beautifully sculpted muscles that act like spandex to cinch in, uplift, tighten, tone, and resculpt your body. The primary focus is to "move your machine" so your body can rebuild neuro-kinetic connections (neuro refers to the brain or nerves or the nervous system; kinetic pertains to motion), maximize muscle mechanics, and improve metabolic function, all of which results in the loss of inches and fat without excessive exercise or dieting.

T-Tapp focuses on the spine not only for core muscle development but also for better alignment and bone density. These exercises are designed to provide sustained stimulus (pull or tug) where the muscle attaches to the bone, to help promote new bone growth as well as help prevent bone loss. These are all factors that lessen the chance of the types of injury that often increase with age. In addition, the T-Tapp program is very beneficial for anyone with lower back, hip, knee, upper spine, neck, or shoulder problems.

The T-Tapp workout is unique in that it teaches you how to actually use your own body as a machine. This means that it requires no additional equipment, just 4 square feet of space (allowing us to get in a full workout even when traveling), and is extremely low impact, making it protective of joints. When T-Tapp's series of movements are performed in the correct sequence, they are designed to fatigue your muscles layer by layer, thereby developing muscle density from the inside, resulting in the rapid loss of inches.

As long as you achieve your personal maximum in performing the exercises, you will never need to increase the level or duration of your workout to achieve the highest level of fitness. The program works regardless of your age or fitness level. To learn more about T-Tapp, consult the book *Fit and Fabulous in 15 Minutes* by workout creator Teresa Tapp or visit the T-Tapp website at www.t-tapp.com.

IMPORTANT CELLULAR BENEFITS

Throughout this book, I have emphasized the importance of controlling blood sugar and insulin levels as one of the premier cellular rejuvenation strategies available to us. Yet another benefit of the T-Tapp program is that it helps your body to maintain better blood sugar balance. The use of comprehensive, compound muscle movement combined with isometric contraction and lymphatic pumping burns glucose quickly and continues to do so even after you stop exercising. The program is also designed to work your brain's cognitive abilities as you process both left and right movements simultaneously. Not only is this feature important for maintaining healthy brain function as we age but it also provides significant cognitive benefits to young people.

T-Tapp has also been designed with an emphasis on lymphatic function. Our lymphatic vessels carry lymph, a colorless, watery fluid originating from the tissues. The lymphatic system transports infection-fighting cells called lymphocytes and is involved in the removal of foreign matter and cell debris, making it a key part of the body's immune system. T-Tapp offers the dual benefit of helping your body maximize metabolic processing, while simultaneously reducing inflammation. Those suffering from an autoimmune disease such as chronic fatigue, lupus, or fibromyalgia report great benefits from doing the T-Tapp workout. Cancer patients undergoing chemotherapy or radiation report fewer side effects such as edema and nausea. Hormonal changes, such as puffiness, cramps, hot flashes, weight gain, and mood swings (whether due to a monthly cycle or menopause), are significantly de-creased in program practitioners.

The following very special "Ten Minutes to Turn Back Time" anti-aging T-Tapp workout was created by Teresa Tapp exclusively for this book. The exercises have been adapted from her book *Fit and Fabulous in 15 Minutes* and custom-tailored to increase their cell-rejuvenating benefits.

TEN MINUTES TO TURN BACK TIME

Step 1: *Warm-Up Shoulder Rolls*

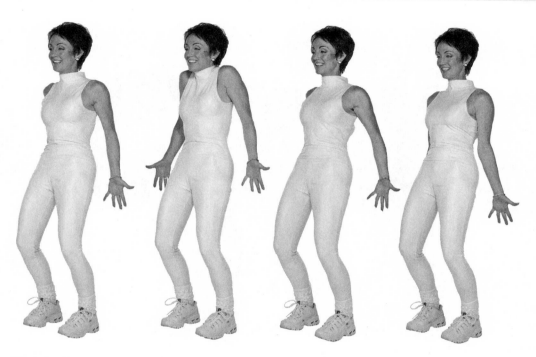

Assume the T-Tapp stance: Stand with your feet hip width apart and toes forward. Then bend your knees, tuck your butt under, and bring your shoulders back in alignment with your hips. Last of all, push your knees out toward your little toes (KLT position). Then flip your palms forward, stretch your fingers wide, and twist your palms away so your thumbs point back as far as you can. You should feel your shoulders rotate back and upper back muscles tighten. Then inhale big and reach down during exhale.

Now roll your shoulders up, back, and down 4 times, keeping your hands below your waist and your thumbs back. Reverse and roll your shoulders up, forward, and down 4 times. Then finish with one more set of 4 shoulder rolls back.

Step 2: *Tuck, Curl, and Scoop*

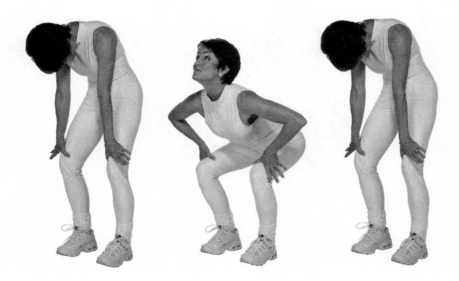

Push your hands into your knees with your thumb on the inside and fingers on the outside of each knee. While pushing, tuck your butt under and curl your back until your arms are straight. Inhale deeply during curl (counts 1 through 4) and exhale as you reverse, scooping out your spine and arching your butt up (counts 5 through 8).

FORM CHECK: Tuck your chin in and pull your shoulders back at top of curl and stretch your chin up during the scoop. Keep your knees bent in KLT position at all times. Repeat 4 times, but on the fourth curl, stop when your arms are straight (count 4) and proceed to step 3.

Step 3: *Spine Roll-Up*

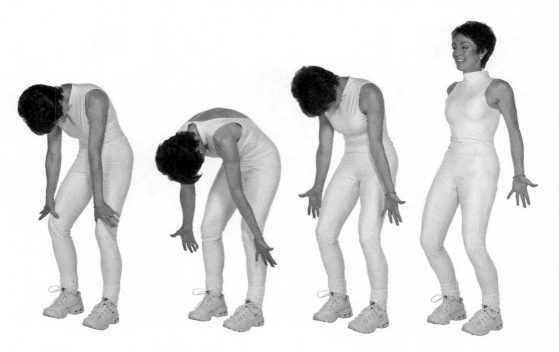

Flip your palms forward and tuck your butt under at the same time you reach down (count 5). Then use your laterals to pull your shoulders back and roll your spine up, one vertebra at a time (counts 6 through 8). Finish with 2 shoulder rolls back (counts 1 through 4).

FORM CHECK: Keep your knees bent and pushing out at all times (KLT).

Step 4: *Chest Press Plié Squats*

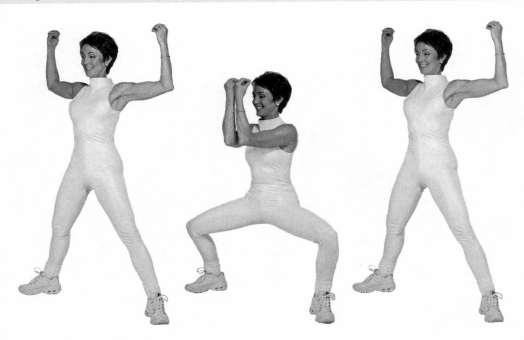

Place your feet shoulder width apart, with your toes turned out at a 30-degree angle or less. Press your fingertips and thumb together and lift your elbows up until they are level with your shoulders. Then bring your wrists into alignment with your elbows, and then open all the way back behind your ears. Hold this position for 2 counts while you inhale and exhale.

FORM CHECK: Keep your ribs up and your shoulders back in alignment with your hips and tuck your butt under to press your lower back flat.

Continue to push your knees out while you lower your body and bring your elbows forward without releasing your shoulders (counts 1 and 2). Your elbows should feel as if they are pressing against weight. Continue to push your knees out while you straighten your legs and bring your elbows back behind your ears (counts 3 and 4).

FORM CHECK: Keep your knees turned out when your legs straighten and tuck your butt harder as you come up against gravity. Keep your shoulders back and your lower back flat (no arch) at all times. Do not drop your elbows below shoulder level. *Tip:* To achieve optimal body alignment, practice against a wall. Repeat for a total of 8 plié squats. Take a water break and proceed to step 5.

Step 5: *T-Tapp Twist Stretch*

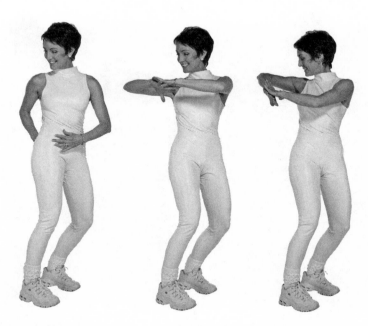

Resume the T-Tapp stance (toes forward, knees bent, butt tucked under, shoulders back, and knees in KLT). Now press your lower back against your hand at the same time you push into your stomach with your other hand. You should feel your abdominal core muscles tighten even more, as well as your hip and gluteal muscles. Focus to maintain this muscle activation to help isolate your lower body from your upper body during the twist. Now place your arms just below your collarbone, with your elbows level with your shoulders. It is important to establish isometric activation of your upper back and shoulder muscles too, especially the latissimus dorsi and trapezius.

Inhale big and push your left knee out even more to help stabilize your hips while you exhale and reach back with your right elbow as far as you can and hold (counts 1 through 4). Then relax and release your twist but do not lower your right elbow or release your T-Tapp stance (counts 5 through 8). Repeat—but this time during exhalation, increase the intensity of your tuck; push and reach while you look back at your right elbow to your best ability (counts 1 through 4). Then inhale bigger (counts 5 and 6) and exhale bigger (counts 7 and 8) while reaching to maximize your spinal stretch and lymphatic flow. Relax and return your upper body forward and do 2 shoulder rolls back with your palms forward.

FORM CHECK: Never allow your reaching elbow to drop lower than your shoulder! Repeat to the left side and proceed to step 6.

Step 6: T-Tapp Twist, Reach, and Roll

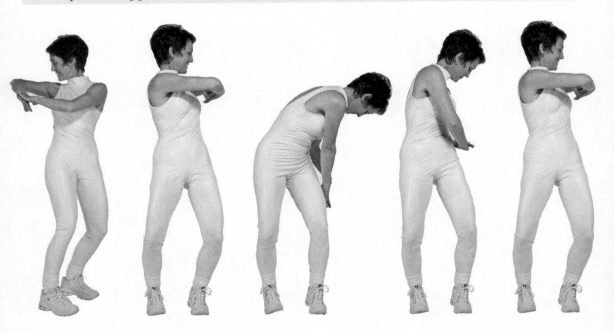

Twist your upper body to the right and pulse for 2 counts without moving your lower body. Now twist all the way over to your left side in 1 count until your shoulders are square to the side (count 3). Continue to tighten your tuck and push your right knee out as you reach down, aiming toward the back of your heel (count 4). Then keep tucking and pushing your knees out while you slowly roll up, keeping your upper body in a spinal twist position (counts 5 through 8).

FORM CHECK: Relax your head on count 4 and keep reaching down during the roll-up. Look at the side-view image for details. *Side view of step 6—reach and roll:* Your shoulders should be level and your head relaxed. Weight distribution should be equal—do not shift weight when reaching down!

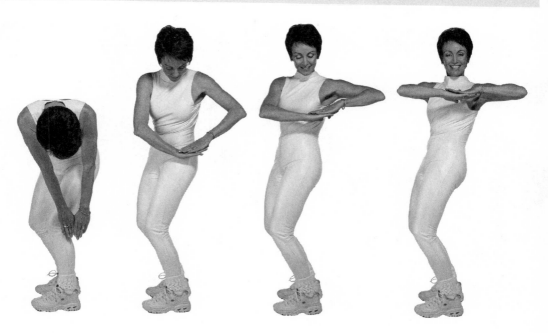

Repeat the sequence for a total of 8 repetitions, 8 counts each, but on the eighth repetition, do not roll back up. Instead, during counts 5 through 8, move your upper body from side to front, touch your fingertips on the floor, and relax your head. (Keep your knees out!) Inhale and exhale and proceed to step 7.

Step 7: *Release, Relax, and Roll*

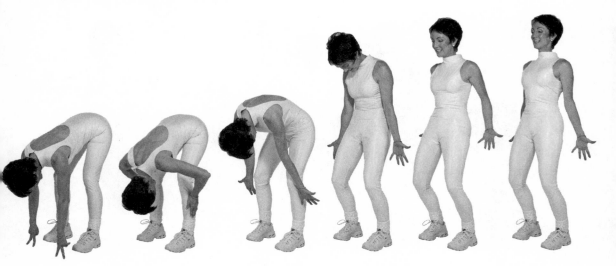

Place your hands on the outsides of your calves. Push your hands in while you push your knees out to tighten your muscles. Maintain this isometric tension while you gently rock your head 4 times. Keep pushing while you tuck and curl your spine until your arms are straight. Then flip your palms forward and reach down while you tuck your butt under (count 5). Then use your latissimus dorsi to pull your shoulders back and roll all the way up, one vertebra at a time (counts 6–8). Finish with 2 shoulder rolls back.

Repeat steps 6 and 7, twisting to your left for a total of 8 repetitions, 8 counts each. Then take a water break and proceed to step 8.

Step 8: *Hoedowns Front Lift/Touch*

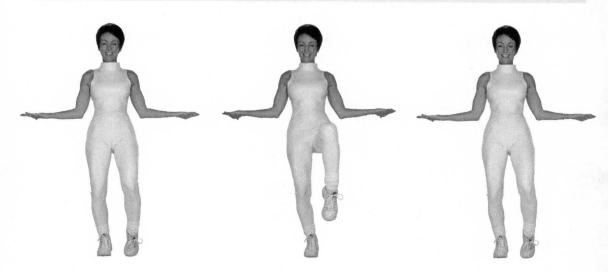

Assume the T-Tapp stance but shift your weight to your right leg. Keep your right knee bent in KLT position, your butt tucked under, and your ribs up while you extend your hands out to the sides of your body with your palms up and thumbs back. Now push your elbows forward and pull your hands back to your best ability. You should feel your shoulders pull back and every muscle tighten in your upper back. Inhale and exhale—ready, begin: Lift your left knee up in alignment with your left shoulder (count 1) and then tap your toes to the floor (count 2). Repeat for a total of 4 lifts and taps (8 counts).

FORM CHECK: Try not to move your upper body when lifting your knee. Keep your butt tucked and your right knee bent in KLT at all times. Proceed to step 9 without stopping.

Step 9: *Hoedowns Side Lift/Touch*

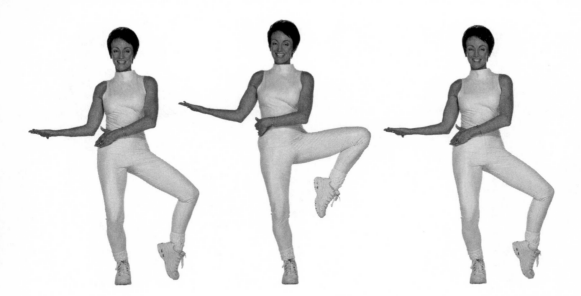

Without stopping, lift your left knee up and out to the left side as you bring your left hand across your body to the right (count 1) and tap your toes to the floor (count 2). Repeat for a total of 4 lifts and taps (8 counts).

FORM CHECK—SIDE VIEW OF HOEDOWNS SIDE LIFT/TOUCH: Linear alignment is important during lifts and taps. In addition to aiming your knee toward the shoulder while lifting, also keep your foot pointed and in alignment with your knee. *Tip:* Pointing toe intensifies activation of abdominal muscles.

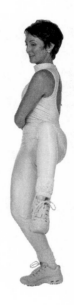

REPEAT STEPS 8 AND 9 AS FOLLOWS:

Two sets of 4 lifts and taps (8 counts front, 8 counts on left side, twice), 2 sets of 2 lifts and taps (counts 1 through 4 front, counts 5 through 8 left side, twice), and 1 set of 4 single lifts and taps (counts 1 and 2 front, counts 3 and 4 left side, 4 times)—all without stopping.

Then while inhaling and exhaling, do 1 shoulder roll back and reset starting position to repeat the same sequence on other side (2 sets of 4, 2 sets of 2, and 1 set of 4 single lifts and taps with right knee).

Then inhale big, exhale bigger, and repeat the entire sequence (left side, then right side) for a total of 2 sets of Hoedowns.

You Did It!

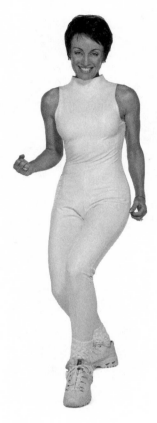

Now take a water break and
have a great day.

The various disciplines discussed in this chapter will greatly improve both physical and mental health. They will also help us to control public enemy number 1 in the causes of accelerated or premature aging: stress. In the next chapter, we will explore additional proven methods to fight the negative effects of stress.

Stress Reduction = Life Extension

It seems that the news about the negative effects of stress becomes grimmer with each passing day. Stress impacts our physical health in ways we never dreamed possible. Mental or emotional stress can no longer be considered in the mind—that is, as existing separately from the body. Stress manifests in myriad ways that make clear the direct connection between mind and body.

As the mind–body connection has become accepted in mainstream medicine, an entirely new branch of medicine has emerged, known as *psychoneuroimmunology*. In true holistic fashion, this exciting new area of research brings together knowledge from multiple fields of study in endocrinology, immunology, psychology, neurology, and other fields.

Psychoneuroimmunology holds great promise in many ways. It has the potential to integrate the systems of the body into a unified view of how the body works and interacts with itself and its environment. This integrated vision also allows us to recognize that cellular rejuvenation can take part on all levels of the mind and body. Perhaps most important, we can learn to control negative emotions and thought processes that upset the delicate balance of health and well-being and play no small part in the development of disease. This leads us to *secret 7: Controlling mental and physical stress is the key to a long, healthy, and happy life.*

Setting Stress in Motion

To understand how the mind directly impacts the body, we need to have a little background. Organs that produce hormones are called endocrine glands. (While the brain and kidneys also produce hormones, they are not considered endocrine organs, since this is a minor part of their function.) In Greek, *hormone* means "to set in motion"; hormones are made by endocrine glands to control or set in motion another part of the body.

The endocrine system works hand in hand with the nervous system. In fact, the *endocrine* and *nervous systems* are so closely linked that they are more accurately viewed as a single *neuroendocrine system*, which performs several critical tasks:

- Maintains the body's internal steady state or homeostasis (nutrition, metabolism, excretion, water and salt balances)
- Reacts to stimuli from outside the body
- Regulates growth, development, and reproduction
- Produces, uses, and stores energy

The neuroendocrine system is designed to help ensure each individual's safety from external or internal threats, and the hormones most responsible for this task are called stress hormones.

THE STRESS HORMONES

In my previous books I have written extensively about the hormones insulin and cortisol, also known as the death hormones. Both of these hormones are necessary for good health, but when their levels are elevated, they cause serious damage, including diseases such as diabetes and obesity. Stress hormones are important—they can give us the extra burst of energy needed to get out of the way of an oncoming automobile or other impending deadly threat. However, in today's world they are called into play too often, placing the neuroendocrine system under particular strain. The physical ramifications of negative emotions are alarming and far reaching. And while caregivers appear to be at particular risk, as detailed later in this chapter, none of us is immune to stress and its effects. Cell phones, e-mail, and other technological gadgets ensure that we almost never have a minute's peace to unwind and lower our stress levels.

At elevated levels, insulin and cortisol are inflammatory agents. Many of us suffer an excess of both of these hormones, the first from too many sugars and other carbohydrates in our diets, the second from too much stress and caffeine. Fortunately we can modify our behavior to eliminate their negative effects. Giving up sugars and starchy foods will help keep our insulin levels normal. Eliminating coffee will help control our cortisol levels. A study conducted at Duke University found that the effects of morning coffee consumption can exaggerate the body's stress responses and increase stress hormone levels all day long and into the evening. This is a high price to pay for that morning jolt to our systems.

Stress can affect us even at the very beginning of our lives. According to the *Wall Street Journal*, recent studies show that women who experience high levels of stress or anxiety during pregnancy increase their risk for delivering prematurely or delivering infants with low birth weights or other health problems, including respiratory and developmental complications. In addition, maternal stress during pregnancy is believed to affect the formation of the important hypothalamic-pituitary-adrenal (HPA) axis. A major part of the neuroendocrine system, the HPA axis controls reactions to stress and plays an important role in the regulation of body processes, including digestion, immunity, and energy use.

There is also increasing evidence that suggests that the detrimental effects of glucocorticoid (GC) hypersecretion (overproduction of steroids), which occurs when the HPA axis is activated, results in a number of diseases, including obesity, Alzheimer's, AIDS, dementia, and depression. Fortunately there are some targeted nutritional supplements, described later in this chapter, that can help keep the all-important HPA axis in balance.

How Cells Get Old Before Their Time

We all know that dealing with heavy stress can make us feel older than we really are. But a recent study at the University of California at San Francisco suggests that it isn't just a feeling—stress actually *accelerates* the rate at which cells age. It's an established fact that stress precipitates premature aging, but until recently the exact mechanism behind this has been unclear.

According to this study, stress affects telomeres, strips of DNA at the end of chromosomes that appear to protect and stabilize the chromosome ends. (A chromosome is a threadlike structure of DNA and associated proteins that is found in the nucleus of a cell.) Chromosomes carry genetic information in the form of genes. These key pieces of DNA are also involved in regulating cell division. Each time the cell divides, the telomere shortens, until eventually there is nothing left, making cell division less reliable and increasing the risk of age-related disorders.

Scientists took blood samples from 58 premenopausal women to carry out DNA analysis of telomeres. They also measured levels of an enzyme called telomerase, which helps build and maintain telomeres in immune cells.

Nineteen of the women in the study had healthy children and the rest had children with chronic illnesses. Being a caregiver is a highly stressful situation, and it was not surprising when the researchers discovered that women who had reported higher levels of psychological stress—those who were caring for sick children—had shorter telomeres. In fact, the difference was equivalent to more than a decade of additional aging when compared with the women who had lower stress levels.

The high-stress group also had lower levels of telomerase in their immune cells. According to Elissa Epel, Ph.D., leader of the research team, this finding implied that the immune cells would not function as well and could die sooner. It was also found that the high-stress women had greater levels of oxidative stress—cumulative damage caused by free radicals. Laboratory studies have confirmed that oxidative stress speeds up the shortening of the telomeres.

The researchers further stated that it was not clear exactly *how* stress affected telomeres, but they suggest that changes in stress hormone levels could have an effect.

STRESS HAS TEETH

It isn't just mothers of children with chronic illness who experience high levels of stress-related health problems. A fascinating study published in the journal *Psychosomatic Medicine* found that caregiver spouses of patients with Alzheimer's disease develop gingivitis, an inflammatory gum disease, at *twice* the rate of their noncaregiver counterparts. Since there was little difference in oral hygiene between the two groups in the study, the researchers believe the difference might have been related to stress. (The authors of the study also note that the relationship between chronic stress and severe gum disease was first noticed in the soldiers in the trenches during World War I, hence the rather graphic term *trench mouth*.) Gum disease is serious enough in and of itself. It can lead to serious bone destruction and tooth loss. But as we will find out, it may also precipitate serious life-threatening diseases.

Lead investigator Peter Vitaliano, Ph.D., of the University of Washington School of Medicine in Seattle, stated: "On a practical level, [the study's results] speak to relationships between chronic stress and oral health in the general population and suggest that these are independent of oral care. They show that caregivers are at risk for oral health problems and not just physical health problems."

The investigators not only evaluated the study subjects' gum disease but also measured the key components of metabolic syndrome:

- Blood insulin levels
- Obesity
- Intra-abdominal fat

The caregiver spouses scored higher on *all three* of these measures, placing them at great risk for type 2 diabetes.

Our Immune System: The Key to Cellular Rejuvenation of the Brain

New research shows that immune cells contribute to maintaining the brain's ability to preserve cognitive ability and cell renewal throughout life. It has been generally accepted, until recently, that each individual is born with a fixed number of nerve cells in the brain. As these cells gradually degenerate and die during the person's lifetime, they cannot be replaced. This is especially alarming when we realize that chronically high levels of stress-induced cortisol, so common in the world of today, cause the brain to shrink.

However, this theory was disproved when researchers discovered that certain areas of the adult brain *do* retain their ability to support and promote cell renewal (neurogenesis) throughout life, especially under conditions of mental stimuli and physical activity. The hippocampus, which supports certain memory functions, is one such area.

MORE REASONS TO FLOSS YOUR TEETH

In addition to the deleterious effects of stress on health, including oral health, the American Academy of Periodontology has also linked periodontal (gum) disease to heart disease. One theory they put forth is that oral bacteria produced by the gum disease can affect the heart when the bacteria enter the bloodstream, attaching to fatty plaques in the coronary arteries (heart blood vessels) and contributing to clot formation.

Coronary artery disease is characterized by a thickening of the walls of the coronary arteries because of the buildup of fatty proteins. Blood clots can obstruct normal blood flow, restricting the amount of nutrients and oxygen required for the heart to function properly. This may lead to heart attacks.

Another possible reason they put forth is that the inflammation caused by periodontal disease increases plaque buildup, which may contribute to swelling of the arteries. Researchers have found that people with periodontal disease are almost *twice* as likely to suffer from coronary artery disease as those without periodontal disease. Periodontal disease can also worsen existing heart conditions. This may well be another important link between stress and heart disease—a cause and effect: stress exacerbates gum disease, which can then lead to heart disease.

Additional studies have also linked gum disease and stroke. Researchers have found that the risk for stroke is 2.8 times greater for individuals with periodontal disease than those without periodontal disease. It is clear that there is a significant inflammatory component linking all of these syndromes and diseases, which is immensely important when we realize that inflammation directly impacts the progression of gum disease, heart disease, and atherosclerosis.

A team of scientists, led by Professor Michal Schwartz of the Neurobiology Department of the Weizmann Institute of Science in Rehovot, Israel, one of the world's top-ranking multidisciplinary research institutions, has come up with new findings that may have implications in delaying and slowing down cognitive deterioration in old age. These findings showed that the primary role of the immune system's T-cells (white blood cells responsible for the body's immunity) is to enable areas of the brain such as the hippocampus to form new nerve cells and maintain cognitive function. We still don't know how the body delivers the message instructing the brain to step up its formation of new cells. However, animal studies have shown that exposure to an environment rich with mental stimulations and opportunities for physical activity leads to increased formation of new nerve cells in the hippocampus. (As with muscle, it appears that the phrase "Use it or lose it" also applies to brain power.) When the scientists experimented with mice that lacked T-cells and other important immune cells, significantly fewer new cells were formed.

According to Professor Schwartz, "These findings give a new meaning to 'a healthy mind in a healthy body.' They show that we rely on our immune system to maintain brain functionality, and so they open up exciting new prospects for the treatment of cognitive loss."

Knowing that the immune system contributes to the renewal of nerve cells has potentially great significance for aging populations because aging itself is associated with a decrease in immune system function. Aging is also associated with a decrease in memory skills and the formation of new brain cells. Therefore, by manipulating and boosting the immune system, it might be possible to prevent or at least slow down age-related loss of memory and learning abilities.

Stress and Cholesterol

Previous studies have established that stress is linked to increased heart rate and weakened immune systems. Now researchers have

WARNING: DEADLY MICROBES ON THE RISE

Eating healthful food, living a cellular-rejuvenating lifestyle, exercising, and reducing stress is of no use if we are unlucky enough to fall prey to an antibiotic-resistant, potentially deadly organism. And the chances of this happening are increasing exponentially.

Serious epidemics are occurring globally. Unfortunately for all involved, modern medicine is often incapable of stopping them. Fifty-one million people die worldwide every year; 31 million of these deaths are due to communicable diseases alone. And it isn't just happening in less-industrialized countries. A recent article published in the *Journal of the American Medical Association* reported that 80,000 people die each year from infections contracted while in American hospitals. Although billions of dollars are spent annually on research for drugs and procedures to combat these problems, pharmaceutical firms have been unable to create drugs quickly enough to keep pace with the growing threat of microbial resistance.

Fortunately, the scientific community is beginning to recognize that powerful, broad-spectrum eradicators of these deadly microbes already exist in nature. In fact, they have been with us since antiquity. Before the development of modern antibiotics, doctors and folk healers prescribed a wide range of natural antiseptics. However, although a number of botanicals do possess antimicrobial action, many are potentially toxic. Only those that have been extensively tested for both safety and efficacy should be used.

Thanks to the pioneering work of Dr. Cass Ingram, a physician, researcher, and author of 20 books, including *Natural Cures for Killer Germs* and *The Cure Is in the Cupboard*, help is now at hand through the powers of *oil of wild oregano*, the premier natural antiseptic validated by modern research.

According to Dr. Ingram, oil of oregano possesses vast microbial-destroying properties. As Ingram asserts, "Oil of oregano's antiseptic powers are immense. . . . It inhibits the growth of the majority of bacteria, something that prescription antibiotics fail to accomplish." In the case of parasites, oil of oregano has had success neutralizing worms, amoebas, and protozoans.

Dr. Ingram's claims have been supported by peer-reviewed research conducted at major medical universities, including Georgetown University and Cornell University, as well as the Tennessee Food Safety Initiative funded by the FDA. Additionally, Dr. Roby Mitchell of Amarillo, Texas, has shown that Oreganol P73, the tested and recommended form of wild oil of oregano, is effective against virulent, methicillin-resistant *Staphylococcus aureus* (MRSA), which causes a variety of problems, from superficial skin lesions to deep-seated infections. MRSA is a major cause of hospital-acquired infections of surgical wounds and infections associated with in-dwelling medical devices. This deadly pathogen is fully resistant to antibiotics, and there is no known medical cure—yet it is completely destroyed by the Oreganol P73 form of oil of oregano.

In a series of preclinical studies, Dr. M. Khalid Ijaz showed that Oreganol P73 alone and in combination with the oils of cumin, sage, and cinnamon (OregaRESP) markedly reduces the virulence of human influenza virus A2 and the avian flu. This study follows earlier experiments showing that these two products can completely block replication of human coronavirus, the pathogen associated with severe acute respiratory syndrome (SARS) and a cause of the common cold. According to Dr. Ingram, "Oregano oil is both oxidative, which means it kills germs, and antioxidative, which means it protects cells simultaneously. This makes it the most magnificent natural medicine in the world."

As Michael A. Schmidt, Lendon H. Smith, and Keith W. Sehnert write in *Beyond Antibiotics*, "One of the advantages essential oils have over antibiotics is that bacteria *do not develop resistance* to essential oils. It seems almost too good to be true, but it appears that many of the antibacterial plant oils work by interfering with the bacteria's ability to breathe. The bacteria literally suffocate to death."

Oreganol P73 is both a potent natural antibiotic and a powerful free-radical fighter. As a concentrate it ranked at more than 3,000 units on the ORAC scale (the U.S. Department of Agriculture measurement of the antioxidant potency of foods, which, as noted in Chapter One ["Cellular Rejuvenation"], rates blueberries at 2,400 ORAC units and strawberries at 1,540), making Oreganol P73 indispensable for any anti-aging regimen. And just as with salmon, the wild variety proved to be more powerful than the farm-raised variety.

Oreganol P73 is also recommended for people suffering from almost any kind of recurring infection, as well as a whole range of ailments, from those that affect the sinuses to those that affect the digestive system, including bronchial allergies, asthma, bronchitis, colds, congestion, flu, sore throats, sinusitis, gum disease, diarrhea, intestinal gas, colitis, heartburn, and other digestive problems. As we saw in Chapter Four ("The Skin We're In"), Oreganol P73 Cream is also amazingly helpful in treating skin conditions such as eczema and psoriasis. Oil of oregano can also provide immediate help against bee stings and many venomous bites until medical attention can be reached. It can be taken sublingually (drops of the oil under the tongue), in capsule form, and applied topically. For more information on this remarkable, one-of-a-kind therapeutic substance, see the "Resources" section.

discovered that elevated stress levels appear to raise cholesterol levels over the long term. This is alarming because an elevated cholesterol level is a major risk factor for heart and circulatory disease, the number-one killer of both men and women in the United States.

A team of researchers, led by Professor Andrew Steptoe from University College London, put forth three hypotheses on how stress increases cholesterol levels:

- Stress may encourage the body to produce more energy in the form of fatty acids and glucose, requiring the liver to produce and secrete more LDL-C so that they can be transported to the other tissues of the body.
- Stress interferes with the body's ability to rid itself of excess cholesterol.
- Stress triggers a number of inflammatory processes that also increase cholesterol production.

Stress-Fighting Supplements

The Life Extension Foundation (www.lef.org) has compiled the latest news and research on targeted nutritional supplements and herbal adaptogens that can, along with exercise and meditation, help many individuals manage stress-filled lives. According to information found there, the following supplements may help keep the HPA axis in equilibrium, reduce elevated cortisol levels, and help optimize health. (For more information on the Life Extension Foundation, see the "Resources" section at the back of this book.)

VITAMIN C

Along with its beneficial effects as a connective tissue regenerator (as we saw in Chapter Four, "The Skin We're In") and in maintaining proper immune system function, vitamin C has been shown to help modulate high levels of cortisol brought about by stress. A study in 2001 examined the effects of supplemental vitamin C on high cortisol levels brought about by physical stress in marathon runners. In a randomized, placebo-controlled study, ultramarathon runners were given either 500 milligrams a day of vitamin C, 1,500 milligrams a day of vitamin C, or a placebo 7 days before a marathon, the day of the race, and 2 days after the race. Researchers found that athletes who took 1,500 milligrams per day of vitamin C had significantly lower post-race cortisol levels than those taking either 500 milligrams a day or placebo.

Another study reported in the journal *Psychopharmacology* reviewed evidence showing that vitamin C can reduce high cortisol levels brought about by psychologically induced stress. In a randomized, double-blind, placebo-controlled trial, researchers gave 3,000 milligrams per day of vitamin C or a placebo to 120 volunteers who were subjected to psychological stress through the Trier Social Stress Test, which consists of 15 minutes of psychological stress induced via a mock job interview, followed by a mental arithmetic challenge. Subjects who took vitamin C had lower blood pressure, subjective stress levels, and cortisol levels compared with those who were given placebo. *Dosage information:* Take 1,000 to 3,000 milligrams of vitamin C per day.

Omega-3 Fish Oil

In several earlier chapters, we learned how important it is to get enough omega-3 fatty acid in our diet for overall health, weight loss, and bone strength maintenance. In a number of clinical tests, fish oil has also been shown to reduce cardiovascular risk in women and men. Now, preliminary research has shown that fish oil may also help individuals cope with psychological stress and lower their cortisol levels. In a study published in 2003, researchers gave seven study volunteers 7.2 grams per day of fish oil for 3 weeks and then subjected them to a battery of mental stress tests. Blood tests showed that these psychological stressors elicited changes in the study subjects' heart rate, blood pressure, and cortisol levels. After 3 weeks of fish oil supplementation, however, the rise in cortisol levels secondary to stress testing was significantly blunted, leading the authors to conclude that supplementation with omega-3 fatty acids from fish oil "inhibits the adrenal activation elicited by a mental stress, presumably through effects exerted at the level of the central nervous system."

Thanks to a flood of research reported in recent years, we now know that the omega-3 EFAs in fish help prevent or ameliorate a wide range of mental disorders and disturbances, ranging from depression, bipolar disorder, and Alzheimer's disease to aggression, memory loss, and learning difficulties. In fact, it appears clear that these and many other conditions result from or are exacerbated by America's dietary deficiencies of omega-3s and not solely from environmental or genetic risk factors.

Now, the results of a new clinical study add to existing evidence indicating a close connection between low intake of omega-3s and angry, aggressive behavior. Emerging clinical evidence—including landmark studies funded by the NIH—suggests that low dietary levels of omega-3s—specifically, the omega-3 fats called EPA (eicosapentaenoic acid) and DHA (docosahexaenoic acid), which are found only in fish and marine organisms—promote anger, depression, and aggression.

The good news is that the preponderance of available clinical evidence shows that taking supplemental marine omega-3s may help alleviate all of these psychological disorders. The study in question took place at a Veterans Affairs facility in Brooklyn, New York, and involved 24 male outpatients with a history of substance abuse and aggressive behaviors. The study subjects were randomly assigned to two groups: one received 3 grams (five capsules) per day of purified fish oil containing 2,250 milligrams of EPA, 500 milligrams of DHA, and 250 milligrams of other omega-3 essential fatty acids. The second group received a placebo. The 13 patients who received the fish oil enjoyed a significant and ongoing decrease in their anger scores on psychological tests.

Unfortunately the average American is woefully deficient in these miracle fats. We have long known that people with the "type A" personality run a significantly greater risk of stroke and heart attack, and the possibility that low levels of the omega-3s may be an important contributing factor offers new hope for the proverbial hothead. Just the simple addition of high-quality fish to the diet and of fish oil capsules taken daily may help alleviate many of these unwanted feelings and behaviors.

It might seem hard to believe that something as simple as a fe meals of fish or capsules of fish oil could confer such huge health ar cosmetic benefits. But the available evidence indicates that humai evolved and thrived on diets high in omega-3–rich seafood, which why marine omega-3 fatty acids make up much of the fat in our brain cell membranes and are such critically important anti-aging nutrients and agents of good mental health.

It well may be that our depressed, overweight society—plagued by inflammatory "lifestyle diseases" such as arteriosclerosis, diabetes, Alzheimer's, obesity, and cancer—is suffering unnecessarily. Never before in human history have diets been so low in omega-3 fatty acids and so high in inflammatory omega-6 fatty acids. In fact, it is estimated that omega-3 intake has dropped by about half since the 1950s, while intake of inflammatory, cancer-promoting omega-6 fats has risen even more sharply. This is a preventive-health disaster of epic proportions. This crucial imbalance needs to be rectified if we are to regain and maintain optimal mental, physical, and emotional health.

To address this fatty acid imbalance, you need to take two simple steps: First, cut way back on omega-6-rich vegetable oils (corn, soy, canola, safflower, etc.)—which are abundant in most processed, frozen, and fast foods—and switch to heart-healthy EVOO, which is high in non-inflammatory monounsaturated fats and potent anti-inflammatory antioxidants. Second, add fatty cold-water fish such as wild salmon, sardines, anchovies, trout, sablefish, and herring to your diet at least three times per week and take fish oil capsules daily. *Dosage information:* Take 1 to 4 grams per day.

PHOSPHATIDYLSERINE

Another supplement that has been shown to be useful in combating the deleterious effects of stress is phosphatidylserine. This phospholipid (any of a variety of phosphorous-containing fats) constitutes an essential part of the cellular membrane. Beginning in the 1990s, studies showed that phosphatidylserine can cut elevated cortisol levels induced by mental and physical stress. In one early study, 800 milligrams per day given to healthy men significantly blunted the rise in cortisol caused by physical stress. Another article reported that even small amounts of supplemental phosphatidylserine (50 to 75 milligrams administered intravenously) could reduce the amount of cortisol responding to the physical stressors. In that study, eight healthy men had their blood drawn before and after physical stress induced by riding a bicycle ergometer (a stationary bike). While all study subjects showed increased cortisol levels, pretreatment with the 50- or 75-milligram dose of phosphatidylserine significantly diminished the cortisol response to the physical stressor.

Finally, a study reported in 2004 examined phosphatidylserine's effects on endocrine and psychological responses to mental stress, using the Trier Social Stress Test described earlier. This double-blind study followed 40 men and 40 women, aged 20–45, for three weeks. The subjects were given either phosphatidylserine (either 400 or 600 milligrams daily) or a placebo before taking the Trier Social Stress Test. Phosphatidylserine was effective in blunting the cortisol response to stressors, with those taking 400 milligrams daily (but not, surprisingly, 600 milligrams) of phosphatidylserine showing a significantly decreased cortisol response. The authors concluded that phosphatidylserine helps dampen the effects of stress on the pituitary-adrenal axis and may have a role in managing stress-related disorders. *Dosage information:* Take 300 to 800 milligrams per day.

DHEA

While cortisol levels stay the same or even increase as we age, levels of another vitally important hormone, DHEA, decrease with each passing year (as we learned in Chapter Five, "Sex for Life"). This relationship between cortisol and DHEA has led some to suggest that these adrenal hormones may play a significant role in the aging process and its associated negative health effects. A recent article in the *European Journal of Endocrinology* examined age-related changes in the HPA axis. The authors showed that the cortisol-to-DHEA ratio increases significantly as people age and is even higher in elderly patients who suffer from dementia. Supplemental DHEA, however, enhances the brain's resistance to stress-mediated changes, maintains functional abilities, and protects against age-related diseases. The authors concluded, "The changes of the hormonal balance [between cortisol and DHEA] occurring in aging may contribute to the onset and progression of the aging-associated neurogenerative diseases." *Dosage information:* Take 25 to 50 milligrams per day. Any hormone supplementation should be monitored by your physician; it is best to consult your physician before adding supplemental DHEA to your regimen to make sure that it is right for you.

Adapting with Herbal Adaptogens

Plant-derived adaptogens can be very useful in combating the mental and physical rigors of our modern lifestyle. Adaptogens work by modulating the levels and activity of hormones and brain neurochemicals that affect everything from cardiac activity to pain perception. The following three adaptogens have proven to be particularly effective stress relievers:

- *Rhodiola rosea:* Introduced here in Chapter Five ("Sex for Life"), this herb, also known as golden root and Arctic root, has been used for centuries in traditional Asian and European medicine and is revered for its ability to increase resistance to a variety of chemical, biological, and physical stressors. It remains a popular plant today in traditional medical systems in eastern Europe and Asia but is lesser known in the United States.

  Studies in cell cultures, animals, and humans have revealed *Rhodiola*'s many remarkable benefits: It fights fatigue and stress, it enhances immunity and protects against cancer, and, as we've discussed, it is also sexually stimulating. It even protects against the damaging effects of oxygen deprivation. *Rhodiola rosea: A Phytomedicinal Overview,* published by the American Botanical Council (http://www.herbalgram.org), is an excellent and comprehensive review of this remarkable plant. It was compiled by three highly regarded experts, Richard P. Brown, M.D., Patricia L. Gerbarg, M.D., and Zakir Ramazanov, Ph.D., D.S., and is recommended for further reading.

Multiple studies from the former Soviet Union have demonstrated *Rhodiola*'s effectiveness in combating both physically and psychologically stressful conditions. One study in particular demonstrated *Rhodiola*'s amazing ability to significantly reduce stress in a single dose. This study was unique in that it examined the effects of a single-dose application of adaptogens for use in situations that require a rapid response to tension or to a stressful situation. They found that *Rhodiola* was extremely effective in controlling stress generated by the part of the stress system known as the sympathoadrenal system. This is significant because, as the study points out, the traditional stimulant drugs used for controlling stress have the potential to become addictive. Users often develop a tolerance, making it necessary for them to take larger and larger doses of the drug. This behavior can easily lead to unintentional drug abuse, have a negative effect on sleep, and cause rebound hypersomnolence or come-down effects. Not only does *Rhodiola* produce no negative side effects but it also effectively increases both mental and physical performance, the researchers found.

Put simply, *Rhodiola* prevents adrenal burnout and all of the negative ramifications that arise from adrenal depletion, which can occur from excessive long-term stress, insufficient sleep, insufficient consumption of protein, insufficient consumption of vitamin C, overuse of caffeine and other stimulants, high intake of sugary or starchy foods, chronic illness, and so on. Chronic stress is the worst culprit in adrenal depletion.

Many studies indicate that *Rhodiola* is useful as a therapy in conditions such as decline in work performance, sleep disturbances, poor appetite, irritability, hypertension, headaches, and fatigue resulting from intense physical or intellectual strain, influenza and other viruses, and other illness. *Dosage information:* Take one 250-milligram capsule of *Rhodiola rosea* root extract, standardized to 3% rosavins (7.5 milligrams) and 1% salidrosides (2.5 milligrams).

- *Ginseng:* This herb has also been used throughout Asia since antiquity. It is important to note that ginseng is the name given to three different plants used as adaptogens. The most widely used is *Panax ginseng*, also known as Korean, Chinese, or Asian ginseng. *Panax quinquefolium*—or American ginseng—is also considered a "true" ginseng. However, Siberian ginseng (*Eleutherococcus senticosus*), while commonly referred to as ginseng, is not a true ginseng but a closely related plant. Yet no matter what the genus or species, all three of these plants have experimental evidence backing their adaptogenic claims. Animal studies have shown that ginsenosides, bioactive compounds in ginsengs, improve the sensitivity of the HPA axis to cortisol. In addition, studies suggest that all three plants provide protection against both physical and psychological stresses.

- *Ginkgo biloba:* For the last 5,000 years, leaves of the ginkgo tree have been used to treat various medical conditions. While ginkgo is currently used to help combat the debilitating effects of memory decline and dementia, emerging evidence suggests that it may be useful in treating the impact of stress and elevated cortisol levels. A recent double-blind, placebo-controlled study published in the *Journal of Physiology and Pharmacology* examined ginkgo's effects in modulating cortisol and blood pressure levels in 70 healthy male and female study subjects. When exposed to physical and mental stressors, study subjects who were given 120 milligrams per day of a standardized ginkgo extract saw smaller increases in their cortisol levels and blood pressure than did their counterparts who were given a placebo.

Exercising Stress Away

In the previous chapter, we learned about the power of exercise to influence cellular rejuvenation and the mind–body balance. We now also know about the powerful protective effect that exercise exerts over the stress hormones that threaten us with cellular degeneration.

Two forces are at work against us when we don't get enough exercise. First is the fact that human beings were built to be in motion. We evolved as hunter-gatherers, not as couch-sitting television watchers. Our systems were meant to be used by a physically active body. When that body is constantly sedentary, our systems do not perform at peak capacity and waste products are not eliminated as efficiently as they should be.

The second force that is at work against us is our body's natural fight-or-flight response. Our stress hormones were designed to help us defeat stressors in the form of physical threats to our safety or else run away from them. Today, our stressors are more often psychological than physical—but the production of stress hormones remains the same. They are not dissipated through fighting or fleeing; instead, they continue to circulate through the body, wreaking havoc on our cells.

Regular exercise is the best way to remove these toxic byproducts of the stress response. As long as it is not overdone, exercise relieves everyday stress, enhances immune system function, boosts circulation, and improves our ability to get a good night's rest (of primary importance, since we know that most cellular repair takes place while we sleep). One other note on sleep: a fascinating study has recently been completed showing the importance of sleeping in total darkness for many health reasons, including breast cancer reduction. It was found that women who worked night shifts, such as nurses and flight attendants, had a 60% higher rate of breast cancer. The research, conducted at the National Cancer Institute and National Institute of Environmental Health Sciences, revealed a disquieting finding: Exposure to light during the hours of sleep appears to aggressively promote breast cancer by shutting off the production of melatonin, a hormone produced by the pineal gland. This hormone, which is naturally produced by the body during the hours of darkness, is known to be a strong immune system booster. Its presence also impedes the growth of cancer tumors by as much as 80%, according to research findings.

We Have the Power

One of the truly positive aspects of growing older is the wisdom and serenity it can bring to our lives. And with that wisdom and serenity comes the power and knowledge to ensure that the choices we make have our best interests at heart. When we are young we are reckless, taking our health for granted, burning the candle at both ends, and making decisions that we later come to regret. We also feel that we have all the time in the world. When we reach our thirties, forties, and beyond, we realize that time is both precious and finite. We are now ready to take better control of our lives and focus on meaningful goals that are beneficial and for the long term.

As you have read in this chapter, stress is very physical in its many manifestations, and what is described here is no doubt just the tip of the proverbial iceberg. We have learned just how "wholistic" stress and negative emotion are—leaving no part of the body untouched. But we are not helpless, defenseless beings, subject to the whims and caprices of the world, slaves to mental and emotional stress. We have many teachers willing to provide the tools we need to maximize our physical and mental potential. Most of all, we need to realize and accept that we are powerful entities with great abilities to both create and destroy ourselves, our realities, and our universe. If the negative states of mind can do this much harm, might not learning how to de-stress and concentrate on positive thoughts and emotions be capable of producing even greater benefits? If this is true, and it is, then it stands to reason that reducing stress and learning to focus on positive emotions must hold the key to a brighter, happier, and healthier future for us all. It is up to us to light the way for the generations following in our footsteps.

The Anti-aging Kitchen

When it comes to food and anti-aging, convenience is a concept that cuts both ways. Yes, it makes our lives easier in many ways. It saves us time. It gets us out of the kitchen when we might prefer to be doing other things. And often, it tastes really good—even though we know it's really bad for us.

However, when we take a closer look at convenience foods—those that are packaged or frozen or come from fast-food outlets and even many restaurants—we begin to realize that convenience may be doing us more harm than good. This is because it is both cheaper and easier for food processors and makers of restaurant and fast-food meals to use many ingredients that are detrimental to our health. In fact, one may question whether they even deserve to be classified as food in the first place, since they were created in the laboratory and do not exist in nature (e.g., high-fructose corn syrup, hydrogenated fats, artificial sweeteners, colors, flavor enhancers, whipped food top-pings).

In addition, not only are the prevailing cooking methods in fast-food outlets (such as deep frying) dangerous because of the high levels of unhealthy fats that they produce but also the excessively high heats used to fry carbohydrates produce toxic by-products such as acryl-amide (a chemical with a variety of industrial uses). Foods such as French fries and potato chips contain large quantities of acrylamide.

Choose the Right Cooking and Salad Oils

It might not seem like a big deal whether you choose corn oil or olive oil in which to sauté your greens or dress your salad, but in fact, it is a very big deal.

Fat is one of the nutrients that we require in our body along with proteins, carbohydrates, and vitamins. The building blocks of fats and oils are called fatty acids, to which we have been previously intro-duced. The fatty acids known as EFAs are the fats that we can't make in our body; we have to obtain them from our food. These EFAs can be in omega-6 form, and that is called linoleic acid, which, as we have learned, is ubiquitous in the American diet. Then there is the omega-3 form of EFA, ALA. This is found naturally in fish such as wild salmon, in fish oil, and in grass-fed beef. Although olive oil has only a small amount of the essential fatty acids, it has a tremendously beneficial effect on our bodies and is an important food to include in our daily diets. Olive oil does contain some linoleic acid (omega-6) and some ALA (omega-3); however, it also contains about 75% of a nonessential monounsaturated fatty acid called oleic acid.

Oleic acid is a member of the omega-9 family. Unlike the omega-3 and omega-6 fatty acids, omega-9 fatty acids are not classed as EFAs. This is because they can be created by the human body from unsatu-rated fat and are therefore not essential in the diet. However, this statement is somewhat misleading. Oleic acid helps ensure that the vitally important omega-3 EFAs penetrate the lipid bilayer of the cell membrane. As we have learned, it is the role of the cell membranes to make sure that nutrients and oxygen get into the cell, that destructive free radicals are kept out, and that waste and carbon dioxide are eliminated. Therefore it makes sense to include superior sources of oleic acid (such as EVOO) in our diet to ensure that these vital functions are occurring. Oleic acid's ability to enhance absorption of EFAs will maintain the fluidity of the cell plasma membrane, thus keeping the cell supple and flexible. This is absolutely necessary for beautiful, youthful skin and a healthy body. In fact, there is also some very good evidence that olive oil can lower triglyceride levels, lower blood pressure, decrease the stickiness of platelets, and decrease heart attacks and their attending complications.

The next time you reach for the "fat-free" salad dressing, remember these facts. Olive oil enhances the absorption of all fatty acids, deficiencies of which will result in a wide variety of health problems, including

- Eczema (an inflammatory condition of the skin characterized by redness, itching, and oozing vesicular lesions, which become scaly, crusted, or hardened)
- Hair loss
- Liver problems
- Kidney problems
- Erratic, confused thinking
- Susceptibility to infection
- Delayed wound healing
- Sterility in men
- Miscarriages
- Arthritis-like conditions
- Heart and circulatory problems
- Depression

The Omega-6–Omega-3 Dilemma

WHICH OILS?

The cheap, heavily refined vegetable oils used most frequently by consumers—and by the makers of packaged, prepared, and restaurant foods—are high in inflammatory omega-6 EFAs and very low in anti-inflammatory omega-3 EFAs. These include corn, soy, canola, sunflower, safflower, peanut, and cottonseed oils.

While canola and soybean oils are often promoted as sources of omega-3s, they contain far greater proportions of omega-6s. Accordingly, they only add to the gross overload of omega-6s in the standard American diet, which delivers 25 to 40 parts omega-6 to 1 part omega-3. In contrast, EFA researchers recommend, with virtual unanimity, that people consume about 3 parts omega-6 to 1 part omega-3. In fact, our current consumption of omega-6 is twice what it was in 1940. Conversely, our consumption of omega-3s has shrunk by more than 50% since the mid-1800s.

Excessive amounts of omega-6 are unhealthy because they promote inflammation and can cause increased water retention and elevated blood pressure, as well as contribute to long-term diseases such as heart disease, cancer, asthma, arthritis, diabetes, and depression.

GETTING THE RATIO RIGHT

It is simply impossible to achieve the preferred 3:1 omega-6–to–omega-3 dietary EFA ratio by consuming omega-3 fish oil in absurdly enormous amounts. Practically speaking, the proper EFA ratio can be attained only by cutting back drastically on your intake of standard vegetable oils. I recommend eliminating them altogether because omega-6 EFAs are prevalent in the Western diet in other forms, such as grain-fed meat. As mentioned elsewhere in this book, if animals are in the pasture feeding on grass (their natural diet), the meat will be high in anti-inflammatory omega-3s. Unfortunately, most people are eating grain-fed meat, a much less healthy choice and one that contributes to the omega-3 deficiency.

I prefer oils low in inflammatory omega-6 EFAs and high in monounsaturated fatty acids, which help lower LDL (bad) cholesterol and raise HDL (good) cholesterol, while helping normalize triglyceride (blood fat) levels. Monounsaturated fatty acids also help cell membranes incorporate beneficial omega-3s and may reduce the risk of insulin resistance and aid blood sugar control in diabetes.

I recommend five alternatives, in descending order of preference:

- *EVOO* averages 75% monounsaturated omega-9 fatty acids and, unlike any commercially available oil, it is rich in potent antioxidants with proven benefits to vascular health.
- *Macadamia nut oil*, like olive oil, is dominated by monounsaturated fatty acids, including omega-9 oleic acid and omega-7 palmitoleic acid, and boasts a higher "smoke point" than EVOO (410° Fahrenheit versus 310° Fahrenheit), which means that it resists breaking down under higher temperatures. It is also more versatile than olive oil, since it has a near-neutral flavor.
- *High-oleic safflower and sunflower oils* come from plants bred to be high in oleic acid, the same monounsaturated fat that predominates in olive oil. Regular safflower and sunflower oils are undesirable, as they are high in inflammatory omega-6 EFAs and low in monounsaturated fats. Like macadamia nut oil, safflower and sunflower oils are more versatile than olive oil, since they have a near-neutral flavor.
- *Avocado oil* is high in monounsaturated fatty acids but is costly and hard to find.
- *Unrefined canola (rapeseed) oil* is fairly low in omega-6s, contains a substantial amount of omega-3 fats, and is high in monounsaturated fatty acids. While regular rapeseed oil contains toxic levels of erucic acid, canola oil comes from a rapeseed hybrid that contains less than 2% erucic acid. There is little credible evidence that canola oil poses more dangers than its supermarket shelf mates. However, it

has been around for only a few decades and tends to produce an unpleasant flavor when heated, so I see it as an oil of last resort.

The fatty acids in the most commonly used cooking oils—soy, canola, sunflower, safflower, and cottonseed oils—consist primarily of the pro-inflammatory omega-6 EFA called alpha-linoleic acid (75% to 90%), with most of the remainder consisting of monounsaturated omega-9 fatty acids (10% to 15%). And these oils contain only small proportions of omega-3 EFAs (alpha-linolenic acid) relative to omega-6 EFAs (alpha-linoleic acid). The only ones relatively low in omega-6 EFAs are olive, high-oleic safflower, and canola oils.

You should also know that standard refined vegetable oils typically contain substantial amounts of dangerous trans-fatty acids, created when manufacturers seek to extend their products' shelf lives by subjecting them to a process called deodorization, which will turn about 5% of a vegetable oil's fragile omega-3 and omega-6 EFAs into trans fats. New research shows that trans fats may lead to inflammation inside arteries, creating complications for people with heart disease, diabetes, and other diseases.

VEGETABLE OIL	OMEGA-6 EFAs (%)	OMEGA-3 EFAs (%)	MONOUNSATURATED FATTY ACIDS (%)	SATURATED FATTY ACIDS (%)
Safflower (HO)	14	1	77	8
Safflower	78	0	13	9
Sunflower	8	1	82	9
Corn	71	1	16	12
Soybean	57	1	29	13
Cottonseed	54	8	23	15
Canola	54	0	19	27
Olive	21	11	61	7
Peanut	9	1	75	15

EFA, essential fatty acid; HO, high-oleic.

A Special Note on Coconut Oil

Coconut oil has long been regarded as an unhealthy fat in the United States, although it is enjoyed liberally in many other countries, especially where the coconut palm naturally flourishes. In those countries it is a key daily dietary component.

However, here in the West we are beginning to rethink this narrow-minded stance, as there are solid scientific arguments that contradict prior opinion. Coconut oil is a saturated fat, and a healthy diet should consist of no more than 6% saturated fat out of total fat intake. However, most of what we consume in the United States consists of artery-clogging long-chain saturated fats derived from animals. The plant-based medium-chain fatty acids or medium-chain triglycerides (MCTs) tend to digest quickly, producing energy and stimulating the metabolism. A number of studies have found that the MCTs in coconut oil neither are as readily converted into stored fats as long-chain fats are nor can be readily used by the body to make larger fat molecules. It now appears that if we replace unhealthy fats such as margarine, shortening, and conventional vegetable oils with coconut oil, we will not only store less body fat but also increase our metabolism. The fatty acid profile of coconut consists primarily of caprylic and lauric acids, which support immune function. Researchers have also discovered that the lauric acid fraction in coconut oil has antiviral and antimicrobial properties.

Coconut oil is practically tasteless, which means that it will not adversely affect food flavors.

Pro-aging Foods to Avoid

Conventional convenience foods usually pack a trio of undesirable elements that combine to undermine health:

HYDROGENATED AND PARTIALLY HYDROGENATED OILS

To make hydrogenated oils (so-called vegetable lard), the EFAs in vegetable oils such as cottonseed or soy are transformed, by catalytic conversion, into saturated fatty acids. The purpose is to make the oils in processed foods much more resistant to oxidation (rancidity) during months spent on the shelf or in a freezer. When vegetable oils are hydrogenated, the remaining unsaturated fatty acids get changed from their normal *cis* form to the *trans* form. Unfortunately, these human-made saturated and trans unsaturated fatty acids promote inflammation, arteriosclerosis, and cardiovascular disease.

SUGARS AND STARCHES

Human beings are programmed by millennia of evolutionary pressures to seek out sugars, which are the most readily usable form of fuel for the cells in our brains and muscles. Fortunately, other than occasionally stumbling on a honeycomb our hunter-gatherer forbearers didn't find sugars to be readily available, much to their benefit. Unfortunately, the opposite is true for people today; food manufacturers and restaurateurs add sugars and other toxic, pro-aging forms of sweeteners to foods in various guises. Sadly, this common practice has ruined Americans' palates, beginning in infancy, and habituated us to expect sweetness not just from pastries and candies but also from foods and beverages of all kinds. Perhaps the quickest way to accelerate the aging process is to eat foods or drink beverages that convert rapidly to sugar upon ingestion.

SYNTHETIC ADDITIVES

I cannot see the logic in ingesting synthetic additives in any form. *Synthetic* means "artificially produced and not of natural origin." What are the potential short- and long-term risks of these chemicals? In general, synthetic additives are used entirely for the convenience of food manufacturers and retailers, to extend shelf life or replace costlier natural preservatives (potent antioxidants from rosemary, etc.), flavors, and colors (pigments that exert strong antioxidant effects).

Drink to Me Only

People ask me all the time whether it is okay for them to have a drink. They also want to know if there is one type of alcohol that is less damaging than others.

I do not have any problem recommending a glass of red wine with a meal, because (unlike white wine) it provides the very powerful anti-aging antioxidants called flavonols we learned about in Chapter One ("Cellular Rejuvenation"): blue-red-purple pigments that help protect the body in many ways.

As Plato said, exaggerating a bit perhaps, "Nothing more excellent or valuable than wine was ever granted by the gods to man." Recent studies show that drinking one glass of red wine every day may have certain health benefits, in part because of its high antioxidant content:

- Protection against certain cancers
- Protection against heart disease
- A positive effect on cholesterol levels and blood pressure

If you like wine, I suggest that you drink just one glass, and always with a meal, rather than before, to blunt the inflammatory and liver-stressing effects of alcohol.

Hard Liquor: A Pro-inflammatory Aging Accelerator

Drinking hard liquor, as opposed to a glass of wine with dinner, causes many problems in the body in terms of inflammation. Alcohol is detoxified by the liver. In hard liquor, the alcohol content is very high.

The metabolic products of alcohol are undesirable molecules known as aldehydes. In addition to causing an inflammatory response, aldehydes also cause damage to various portions of the interior cell. If you are going to drink hard liquor, remember that the sugars in mixing juices or sodas also exert pro-inflammatory, skin-aging effects, so avoid them and use pure water or seltzer instead. In summary, enjoying red wine in moderation is acceptable—probably even healthful—but forgo the martinis and cosmopolitans.

CAN THAT NIGHTCAP: HOW ALCOHOL DISTURBS SLEEP

Since sleep is so important to rejuvenation of the skin and the entire body, it is essential that we do whatever we can to enhance the sleep experience. To that end, it's best to make sure that you *never* drink alcohol on an empty stomach and that you stay well hydrated by drinking plenty of water.

A few alcoholic beverages in the evening may initially make us drowsy, but very soon the alcohol precipitates a burst of norepinephrine, a hormonelike neurotransmitter secreted in response to excitement or stress. Hours after taking a drink, a burst of norepinephrine can disrupt your sleep cycle or even cause you to awaken. This will not only result in a very poor night's sleep but also leave your skin looking mottled and dull the next day.

DRYING OUT: WHY ALCOHOL IS NO BEAUTY AID

While the results of many scientific studies indicate that a small amount of alcohol can confer cardiovascular health benefits, there are a great many dangers associated with excessive alcohol consumption, including skin damage.

People generally think that alcohol is bad for the skin because it makes us dehydrated. They believe that they can counteract this by drinking large quantities of water. However, while it is important to rehydrate, alcohol creates inflammation throughout the body, including the skin, resulting in effects that far outlast dehydration. Alcohol alters the blood flow to the skin and produces an unhealthy appearance for days following overindulgence. This effect can manifest as dullness, enlarged pores, discoloration, a red and blotchy complexion, puffiness around the eyes, loss of contours, sagging, and lack of resilience. These negative effects occur because alcohol causes small blood vessels in the skin to widen, allowing more blood to flow close to the skin's surface. In addition to a flushed skin color and feeling of warmth, this dilation of blood vessels can break facial capillaries. Alcohol also dehydrates the skin, and dry skin is more prone to fine lines than skin that is well hydrated.

When we are young, we can escape some of the physical, visible manifestations of excess alcohol—that is, they won't appear as severe as in older people because the young enjoy greater physical resiliency. But the effects are cumulative and will catch up with us. When we combine alcohol- and sun-induced damage, we are setting the stage for accelerated aging and destruction of the skin, including breakdown of the collagen needed to maintain firmness and elasticity.

Anti-aging Arsenal: Foods to Keep on Hand

The number-one priority in planning the anti-aging kitchen is making the right food choices. "As natural as possible" is a good rule to follow. One way to shop for healthy foods is to avoid most of the middle supermarket aisles. Instead, focus on the perimeter of the store, where you can find the fresh vegetables and fruit, the seafood, poultry, and dairy, as well as bulk herbs and spices, beans and legumes, nuts and seeds, and imported cheeses. By stocking your pantry, fridge, and freezer with the right foods, you'll increase your odds of eating right. These are some of my favorite anti-aging foods:

ALLIUM FAMILY

- *Best bets:* Onions, garlic
- *Good choices:* Chives, leeks, shallots, scallions

HANGOVER REMEDIES FOR INSIDE AND OUT

Should you overindulge in alcohol, drinking fresh, pure water and taking the right blend of nutritional supplements can help repair the internal and external damage that greets you the following morning. I recommend drinking a 10- to 12-ounce glass of water and taking 1,000 milligrams of vitamin C, 1,200 milligrams of *N*-acetyl cysteine, 100 milligrams of ALA, 1,000 milligrams of glutamine, 500 milligrams of pantothenic acid, and a B-complex supplement. Coffee is not an antidote to alcohol; in fact, it will leave you feeling even worse! The green foods introduced in Chapter One ("Cellular Rejuvenation") help neutralize the effects of the aldehydes that may be responsible for the damaging effects of alcohol on the liver—as well as that unpleasant feeling called a hangover that we get in the morning after drinking the night before. Curcumin, the substance that gives the spice turmeric its distinctive yellow color, stops the changes caused by excessive alcohol consumption that lead to liver damage. I recommend mixing ¼ teaspoon with a little water. This amazing spice will also lower blood sugar and provide superior antioxidant protection.

And following a bout of excess alcohol, targeted topical treatments— such as formulas featuring vitamin C ester, DMAE, and ALA—will enhance your appearance in several ways:

- Maintain that fresh, rosy look of youth and health
- Revive dull, lifeless skin
- Minimize skin discoloration and redness
- Reduce puffiness around the eyes
- Reduce dark circles under the eyes
- Decrease the appearance of fine lines and wrinkles
- Protect the skin from free-radical damage

- *Anti-aging benefits:* Rich in sulfur compounds and anti-inflammatory antioxidants that enhance cardiovascular health, destroy infectious microbes, and reduce the risk of stomach cancers

RICH COLD-WATER FISH

There's no easier or healthier meal than one provided by opening a can of tuna, sardines, or wild salmon. And if you're thinking, *But how can I keep fresh fish on hand?* be aware that frozen fish is usually much better than "fresh" fish, which is often anything but fresh! Most "fresh" fish spend several days or weeks on ice in a fishing boat's hold and untold hours or days more before hitting the supermarket display case, where they may linger for days before being sold. In contrast, fish destined for freezing are cleaned and flash-frozen within a few hours of harvest, a practice that preserves them in a truly fresh state. By choosing frozen fish, you can keep a good variety in the freezer. Once thawed, it will taste like you caught and cooked it within a few hours of reeling it in. To speed the process, just immerse frozen fish, in the watertight bag it came in, in cool water for 1 to 2 hours, until it is flexible.

- *Best bets:* Wild salmon (sockeye, king/Chinook, Coho/silver, pink, chum). Sockeye offers the highest omega-3 levels of any fish

  Note: Wild salmon offer a far healthier nutritional profile, compared with their farm-raised cousins. Both kinds are high in the anti-inflammatory omega-3 fatty acids sorely lacking in Western diets, which enhance mood, mental function, weight control, and heart health. But unlike wild salmon, farmed salmon are also high in the inflammatory omega-6 fatty acids found in extreme excess in the standard American diet. A clinical study from Norway indicates that eating farmed salmon raises blood levels of inflammatory chemicals associated with increased risk of cardiovascular disease, a sadly ironic situation, given the heart-healthy reputation of fish in general.
- *Good choices:* Sablefish ("black cod"), sardines, anchovies, herring, tuna, North Atlantic mackerel, trout, bass, shrimp, mussels, oysters, halibut

Pregnant and nursing women and young children should observe the consumption guidelines from the FDA and Environmental Protection Agency, and take fish oil capsules from a trusted and reputable supplier, to ensure adequate intake of long-chain marine omega-3 EFAs, which appear to enhance brain and eye development in fetuses and infants.

North Atlantic mackerel is relatively low in mercury, but avoid mackerel from the Gulf of Mexico or the south Atlantic, which are sometimes called Spanish or king mackerel.

Canned light tuna is relatively low in mercury, while young, low-weight, troll-caught Pacific albacore tuna are very low in mercury (see the "Resources" section). Pregnant and nursing women and young children should minimize their intake of (or avoid altogether) standard canned albacore tuna.

- *Anti-aging benefits:* Rich in omega-3 fatty acids, which enhance mood, mental function, and cardiovascular health and may help control weight, reduce the risk or severity of Alzheimer's disease, and inhibit the growth of common cancers

FAVORITE FRUITS

- *Best bets:* Apples, berries, grapefruit
- *Good choices:* Pears, peaches, plums, prunes, cherries, oranges
- *Anti-aging benefits:* Rich in fibers and anti-inflammatory antioxidants that enhance cardiovascular health; may reduce the risk of certain cancers

"BACK TO MONO" FRUITS: AVOCADO, OLIVES, COCONUT, ACAI

Mono fruits contain healthy monounsaturated fats.

- *Anti-aging benefits:* High in fiber, anti-inflammatory antioxidants (olives and acai), and anti-inflammatory/antiadiposity fatty acids, which inhibit inflammation and may help control weight

HOT CALORIE BURNERS: CHILI PEPPERS, CAYENNE, CHILI POWDER

- *Anti-aging benefits:* High in fiber and anti-inflammatory antioxidants that may inhibit appetite and help control weight

NUTS AND SEEDS

- *Best bets:* Almonds, pistachios, walnuts, filberts, pumpkin seeds, sesame seeds and sesame butter (tahini), flaxseed, sunflower seeds
- *Anti-aging benefits:* Rich in fiber, healthy anti-inflammatory fats, and anti-inflammatory antioxidants that may help control weight

LOW-FAT PROBIOTIC DAIRY: YOGURT, KEFIR, PROBIOTIC MILK

- *Anti-aging benefits:* Rich in calcium, whey protein, and beneficial bacteria, a combination that boosts bone health and immunity and enhances weight control. Greek yogurt, especially that made from sheep milk and/or goat milk, is particularly healthful and has a thick, rich, creamy texture. Many people who are intolerant of cow's milk find the sheep- or goat-milk yogurts ideal.

BEANS (LEGUME FAMILY)

- *Best bets:* Chana dal (aka Bengal gram dal or cholar dal), lentils, chickpeas
    Note: Chana gram dal comes from a distinct variety of the same plant that gives us chickpeas (*Cicer arietinum*), but the chana dal bean is much smaller and darker and is higher in fiber and phytoceuticals. In India, these two types of chickpea are called *desi* (chana dal) and *kabuli* (chickpeas). This distinction is important because chickpeas have a much higher glycemic index (albeit still low, in relative terms) than chana dal.

- *Good choices:* Mung beans, hummus (chickpea purée), kidney beans, navy beans, pinto beans, black beans
- *Anti-aging benefits:* Rich in soluble fibers and (colorful varieties only) anti-inflammatory antioxidants that discourage the degenerative processes leading to common health disorders (e.g., cardiovascular disease, diabetes, cancer)

HERITAGE WHOLE GRAINS: OATS, HULL-LESS BARLEY, BUCKWHEAT

- *Anti-aging benefits:* Oats and barley are high in fibers that enhance weight control and discourage cardiovascular disease; the beta-glucan fiber in oats and barley exerts beneficial antiglycemic effects as well, helping to stabilize blood sugar.

  Buckwheat is a seed rather than a grain and has many healthful anti-aging properties. Buckwheat is by far the richest food source of rare carbohydrate compounds called fagopyritols—especially D-*chiro*-inositol—which, in diabetic rats, reduces blood sugar levels very substantially. It is also rich in anti-inflammatory antioxidants.

SPICY SUGAR-FIGHTERS: CINNAMON, FENUGREEK, CLOVES

Those with diabetes should consult a physician before relying on any food or supplement to help control blood sugar.

- *Anti-aging benefits:* Rich in phytonutrients (fenugreek) and anti-inflammatory antioxidants (cinnamon and cloves) that enhance weight control and discourage common degenerative conditions (e.g., cardiovascular disease, diabetes, cancer). Cinnamon is also an outstanding blood sugar stabilizer, as discussed in Chapter Two ("Lean for Life").

ANTI-AGING "RAINBOW" VEGGIES

- *Best bets:* Spinach, kale, chard, collards, escarole, broccoli rabe, root vegetable greens (turnip, mustard, beet), sea vegetables (seaweed)

- *Good choices:* Brussels sprouts, broccoli florets, broccoli sprouts, bell peppers, onion and garlic (allium) family, eggplant, green or red cabbage (red has the higher antioxidant potential), lettuces (various types; multicolored are best)
- *Anti-aging benefits:* Rich in fiber, anti-inflammatory antioxidants, and other phytonutrients that enhance weight control and discourage common degenerative conditions (e.g., cardiovascular disease, diabetes, cancer)

ANTI-INFLAMMATORY SPICES AND HERBS: GINGER, TURMERIC, GALANGAL, LEMON GRASS, AROMATIC CULINARY HERBS

Culinary herbs are parsley, mint, dill, marjoram, oregano, rosemary, thyme, and basil.

- *Anti-aging benefits:* Extremely high in anti-inflammatory antioxidants and other anti-inflammatory phytonutrients. The yellow pigment in turmeric (curcumin) is rich in antioxidants (curcuminoids) that exert potent anti-Alzheimer's effects in animals. Turmeric (like cinnamon) also has powerful blood sugar–stabilizing effects and can halt the changes caused by excessive alcohol consumption that lead to liver damage.

  In clinical trials, ginger and turmeric have shown the ability to ease arthritis symptoms, since they act on the same inflammation/pain pathways as prescription COX-2 inhibitor drugs (e.g., Vioxx and Celebrex), but without any of the significant adverse side effects associated with those drugs.

EXTRA VIRGIN OLIVE OIL, MACADAMIA NUT OIL, AND HIGH-OLEIC SAFFLOWER OR SUNFLOWER OIL

- *Anti-aging benefits:* These oils are high in heart-healthy monounsaturated fatty acids and low in the inflammatory omega-6 fatty acids that

DR. PERRICONE'S 7 SECRETS TO BEAUTY, HEALTH, AND LONGEVITY

dominate most common cooking oils (e.g., canola, corn, regular saf-flower and sunflower, soy). EVOO is also uniquely rich in extremely potent antioxidants called hydroxytyrosols. (Lesser grades are not.)

Make Smart Cookware Selections

Cooking should be a pleasure unsullied by concerns about cookware. While many of the most popular types may pose serious health risks, fortunately there are excellent alternatives that will protect your family. An added benefit is that they will usually yield superior culinary outcomes.

COOKWARE TO AVOID

Two types of cookware should be avoided because of health concerns.

- *Nonstick plastic pan coatings:* Controversy rages over the safety of non-stick surfaces, which are applied to pans made of aluminum and steel. According to the Cookware Manufacturers Association, some 90% of all aluminum cookware sold in the United States in 2001 was coated with nonstick synthetic surfaces.

  Nonstick synthetic surfaces are easily damaged, causing the plastic to flake and get in food. And when heated, cookware coated with Teflon and other nonstick materials emits fumes proven to kill pet birds. These unfortunate avian victims raised the alarm by acting as canaries in the kitchen rather than the coal mine.

  According to a study by the 3M company, a chemical used in the manufacture of Teflon—called perfluorooctanoic acid, or PFOA—can be found in the blood of 90% of Americans. Of the 600 children tested, 90% had PFOA in their blood. And because PFOA does not break down, it persists in the environment indefinitely.

  While it is not clear how much of this PFOA comes from nonstick pans—it is also used to coat microwave popcorn bags and paper plates, among other food-related applications—cookware is likely to be a major source. And as toxicologist Tim Kropp of the Environmental Working Group told the *New York Times* in 2005, "Any amount of PFOA you are ingesting may be a problem because we don't know what levels are safe."

Teflon maker DuPont reached a $16.5 million settlement with the Environmental Protection Agency over the company's failure to report health risks from PFOA. The Environmental Working Group reported that their tests showed that Teflon emits fumes at only 325° Fahrenheit, while DuPont claims that it resists breakdown at temperatures lower than 660° Fahrenheit.

Speaking for myself, the evidence of possible harm is clear enough to make me stick to (no pun intended) more traditional surfaces. I recommend that you heed the warning provided by the DuPont settlement with the Environmental Protection Agency and replace your nonstick cookware as soon as possible.

- *Aluminum (regular, nonanodized)*: Evidence from some studies indicates that Alzheimer's patients have abnormally high levels of aluminum in the amyloid protein plaques that characterize the disease, although it remains unclear whether this accumulation is a contributing factor to or an effect of the disease process.

The soft aluminum used to make standard aluminum pans transfers to foods readily, which poses possible neurological risks and imparts a metallic taste to foods. These drawbacks lead me to recommend against using standard aluminum pans. Anodized aluminum pans are likely to be safer, and these are discussed below.

PREFERRED COOKWARE

While the available alternatives may be a tad less convenient in certain circumstances, they will perform better in the kitchen and certainly won't harm your health.

- *Porcelain-enameled cast iron, my top choice:* Famed *New York Times* food writer Marian Burros recommends enameled cast-iron pans because they yield superb cooking results and long-lasting performance on all heat sources. Once it gets hot, enameled cast iron requires only a low heat setting to keep food cooking. And excepting pieces with wooden handles, most enameled cast iron cookware can be used on burners, in the oven, and under the broiler.

  In addition, the vitreous (glass-containing) enamel cooking surface is impervious to acids and other chemicals, so it can hold raw or cooked foods that are marinating or being stored in the refrigerator or freezer.

  One of my favorite brands for this type of cookware is Le Creuset. It is initially more expensive than other types of cookware but will provide many years of faithful service. It also comes in a variety of beautiful colors.

  Chef's Classic Ceramic Bakeware by Cuisinart is heavy, commercial-quality stoneware that gracefully moves from oven to broiler to table to freezer. The nonporous glaze will not absorb moisture or odors, so foods cooled and served in this ceramic bakeware maintain their natural flavor and juices.

- *Stainless steel:* When *Cook's Illustrated* magazine reviewed sauté pans in 2001, they chose a stainless-steel pan over otherwise identical nonstick models and found that stainless-steel pan roasters performed better than nonstick pans. This terrific choice also browns foods better than nonstick surfaces. And, tests by a leading consumer magazine indicate that stainless steel and steel–aluminum alloy pans are the easiest to clean.

  You can season stainless-steel pans to make them virtually nonstick:

  - Put about 2 tablespoons of olive oil or high-oleic safflower oil and 2 tablespoons of salt in the pan.
  - Heat the pan to the point where the oil is almost beginning to emit smoke, and then let it start cooling down.

- Scrub the salt into the pan using a clean, lint-free cloth or paper towel.
- Wipe the pan out, re-oil it, wipe it out again, and you will have created a nonstick layer.

Perform this process when the pan is new, and repeat the process periodically. As with a seasoned cast-iron pan, clean the pan by wiping it out with (or without) a bit of warm water, without using soap or detergent. Should food bits become stuck to the pan, you may need to scrub it with detergent and reseason the pan.

COOKWARE RUNNERS-UP

While these cookware choices have their drawbacks, they appear to be safer than pans with standard nonstick surfaces.

- *Cast iron:* This old standby can be preheated to temperatures that will brown meat and will withstand oven temperatures well above those considered safe for nonstick pans. Cast iron is extremely durable and can be seasoned to provide a smooth, stick-resistant surface or can be purchased preseasoned.

  However, I recommend minimizing its use—and avoiding it altogether if you have a personal or family history of heart trouble. Cast-iron cookware leaches iron into foods, and an excess of dietary iron acts as a pro-oxidant agent proven to promote dangerous oxidation of cholesterol.
- *Ceramic titanium:* This type of pan is made by permanently bonding a ceramic–titanium surface that contains a synthetic nonstick substance to a dense, high-pressure–cast aluminum pan. The ceramic–titanium compound is anchored to the pan base and then impregnated with a proprietary nonstick formula that is free of PFOA, the toxic chemical used to make Teflon. Since the nonstick formula is proprietary, it is hard to know whether it is as safe as claimed. And the leading manufacturer—Scanpan—admits that the

nonstick surface will begin to break down and emit fumes at temperatures of 500° Fahrenheit or higher.

- *Anodized aluminum:* Anodized aluminum pans—such as the ubiquitous Calphalon line—are made by electrochemically treating their cooking surfaces to increase their hardness and reduce the normal rate at which aluminum transfers to foods. Anodized aluminum is not, however, highly scratch resistant, so the hard surface layer may wear away over time, exposing the plain, soft aluminum underneath. *Note:* According to tests by a leading consumer magazine, "infused" anodized aluminum holds up to wear no better than standard anodized aluminum pans.

MENUS

&

RECIPES

For the recipe section of your anti-aging kitchen I have created special menus to celebrate the four seasons of the year: spring, summer, autumn, and winter. Each menu contains recipes keyed to nature's bounty at these special times of the year.

When shopping for the finest, freshest ingredients, always purchase organic meats, vegetables, and condiments when possible, and choose locally grown organic food when you can. It is not just your own precious life and health that will benefit but also that of the planet—its rivers, lakes, oceans, the land, the plant life, and beneficial insects and animals, both large and small. A simple choice made in the supermarket aisle has far-reaching effects.

Our first menu celebrates springtime's bounty of fresh asparagus served with a baked fillet of wild salmon. An added bonus: Each of these salmon recipes works equally well with boneless breast of chicken (remember to choose organic, free-range chicken) or firm tofu.

One of the wonderful harbingers of spring, along with the return of the robin and the appearance of spring flowers, is fresh asparagus. This delicious, nutritious vegetable is a rich source of folic acid, also known as folate or folacin.

When taken in sufficient quantities by pregnant women, folic acid can effectively reduce the risk of neural tube birth defects such as spina bifida. This explains why, in 1998, the FDA mandated that grain products must be enriched with folic acid. The U.S. Public Health Service recommends that all women of childbearing age who are capable of becoming pregnant should consume 0.4 milligrams (400 micrograms) of folacin per day to reduce their babies' risk of suffering neural tube birth defects. Folic acid is also essential to blood cell formation and growth, and in the prevention of liver disease.

This underappreciated B vitamin also appears to help prevent strokes. The results of a new study reveal that stroke mortality rates in both the United States and Canada dropped substantially after the FDA's grain-fortification mandate took effect.

But why eat heavily processed, synthetically fortified foods when you can enjoy fresh fruits and vegetables that also provide anti-inflammatory antioxidants and a wealth of anti-aging phytonutrients? The best sources of folic acid are asparagus and leafy dark-green vegetables such as spinach and collards. A 4-ounce serving of asparagus (8 medium-thick spears) provides 178 micrograms of folic acid, which is 45% of the recommended daily allowance (400 micrograms).

Its wealth of nutrients, fiber, and very low sodium and calorie content make asparagus a nutritionally wise (and delicious) choice.

Key Attributes of Asparagus

- Is low in calories, with only 26 per 4-ounce serving, or less than 4 calories per spear
- Contains no fat or cholesterol
- Is very low in sodium
- Is an excellent source of folic acid (178 micrograms per 4-ounce serving)
- Is a good source of potassium
- Is a significant source of thiamin
- Is a significant source of vitamin B$_6$
- Is a source of fiber (2.4 grams per 4-ounce serving)
- Is one of the richest sources of rutin. This antioxidant bioflavonoid compound strengthens and may help prevent unsightly breaks in small capillaries in the skin.
- Is abundant in glutathione, an essential tripeptide antioxidant found within our cells. This is one of the body's most effective fighters of cell-damaging free radicals, and it constitutes a critical part of our antioxidant defense system. Glutathione also detoxifies certain carcinogens and protects against chemicals that promote cell transformation or cell death.

A significant source of an essential nutrient provides 10% or more of the RDA, a good source provides 25% or more, and an excellent source provides 40% or more. A source of fiber provides 2 grams or more per serving, a good source contains 5 grams or more, and an excellent source contains 8 grams or more.

Celebrating Springtime's Bounty

· M E N U ·

Baked Fillet of Salmon with Asparagus and Caper-Enriched
Lemon Sauce

Spinach Salad with Fresh Raspberries

Feta, Toasted Walnut, and Fresh Pear Platter

Pinot Noir

Pinot noir is a delightful wine to accompany salmon because pinot noirs have enough acidity in them to mitigate the fatty content in Alaska's oil-rich salmon species. They are also generally low in tannins, preventing the somewhat bitter aftertaste of some red wines. Pinot noir (and Pinot gris, its white wine cousin) is a great balance for salmon.

BAKED FILLET OF SALMON WITH ASPARAGUS AND CAPER-ENRICHED LEMON SAUCE

Serves 4

2 tablespoons fresh lemon juice

2 tablespoons minced shallots (may substitute red onion)

1 tablespoon drained capers, chopped

1 teaspoon minced fresh thyme

½ teaspoon grated lemon zest (use organic only or omit from recipe)

 Sea salt and freshly ground black pepper to taste

24 ounces wild salmon fillet (1¼ to 1½ inches thick; skinless if available)

1 pound asparagus, trimmed

1 tablespoon extra virgin olive oil

 Lemon slices

• Preheat oven to 450°F. Briskly stir first 5 ingredients in small bowl to blend. Add sea salt and freshly ground black pepper to taste.

• Slice three ½-inch-deep slits crosswise in top of salmon (as if dividing into 4 equal pieces), but do not cut through.

• Arrange asparagus in an even layer on a rimmed baking sheet. Drizzle with oil and turn to coat. Sprinkle with salt and pepper.

• Place salmon atop asparagus; sprinkle with salt and pepper. Roast until salmon is just opaque in center, about 20 minutes.

• Transfer asparagus and salmon to platter. Spoon sauce over salmon. Cut into 4 pieces along slits, garnish with lemon slices, and serve.

This delightful entrée recipe is easy enough for everyday enjoyment but elegant enough for a dinner party. The piquant flavor of the capers enhances the delicate yet distinctive flavors of the wild salmon and fresh asparagus. Capers are an outstanding way to turn a super dish into the sublime—without adding unwanted calories or fat.

SPINACH SALAD WITH FRESH RASPBERRIES

Serves 4

The addition of the fresh raspberries transforms this salad from the delightful to the divine.

DRESSING INGREDIENTS

  2 tablespoons raspberry vinegar (available at specialty foods shops and some supermarkets)

  1 tablespoon balsamic vinegar

  1 tablespoon low-sodium tamari (soy sauce)

  ¾ teaspoon Dijon mustard

  1½ teaspoons minced, peeled fresh ginger root

  1 garlic clove, minced and mashed to a paste with ¼ teaspoon salt

  ¼ teaspoon chili powder

  ¼ teaspoon freshly ground black pepper, or to taste

  ⅓ cup extra virgin olive oil

SALAD INGREDIENTS

  1 pound baby spinach, coarse stems discarded and leaves washed well and spun dry

  16 cherry tomatoes

  ⅔ cup fresh raspberries (rinsed and dried)

  4 scallions, chopped fine

  ¼ cup walnuts, toasted and chopped coarsely

To make dressing: In a bowl, whisk together all dressing ingredients except oil. Add oil in a stream, whisking, and whisk until emulsified. (Dressing may be made 2 days ahead and chilled, covered.)

• Combine salad ingredients except for walnuts in a bowl and toss with dressing. Sprinkle with walnuts for a garnish.

FETA, TOASTED WALNUT, AND FRESH PEAR PLATTER

½ pound feta cheese, cut into ¼-inch slices
3 pears, peeled, cored and cut into ¼-inch slices
 Fresh black pepper
1 cup toasted walnuts

- Arrange the feta slices down the center of a large platter.
- Arrange the pear slices around the feta.
- Grate fresh black pepper over the feta; sprinkle with toasted walnuts and serve.

Feta cheese is a rich and creamy soft cheese of Greece, authentically made of whole sheep's milk, although many cheeses are now made with goat's milk or a mixture of the two. When possible, purchase feta cheese made from goat's milk and/or sheep's milk. This is far superior to feta made from cow's milk.

Celebrating Summer's Bounty with Our

BACKYARD HEALTHY HOLIDAY BARBECUE

· MENU ·

Salmon, Chicken, or Tofu Kabobs with a Marinade of Fresh
Lime and Rosemary

Grilled Veggie Kabobs

Rainbow Parfait

Amarone della Valpolicella Classico Riserva

Iced Green Tea with Sprigs of Fresh Mint and
Lemon Wedges

When it comes to barbecue, the experts recommend a rich red wine that can stand up to the powerful flavors of barbecue sauces and marinades. One of my favorites is amarone, an exceptional wine from Veneto, the same northeastern area of Italy that produces valpolicella. Well balanced, this complex wine is smooth and elegant on the palate and delivers cherry and raisinlike flavors. Delightful with food, including salmon, amarone is often enjoyed alone, sipped outside of mealtimes with good conversation and good friends.

If your idea of a summer barbecue is grilled fat- and chemical-laden hot dogs and greasy burgers, this menu is the ideal antidote. Grilled veggie kabobs make the perfect accompaniment to savory skewered salmon, chicken, or tofu.

Wild salmon is superb when cooked on the grill and offers a far healthier nutritional profile than does farm-raised salmon. Wild salmon is high in the anti-inflammatory omega-3 fatty acids sorely lacking in Western diets. It is these omega-3s that enhance mood, mental function, weight control, and heart health—is it any wonder so many of us are depressed and overweight? The savory salmon kabobs will deliver a healthy dose of the omega-3s as well as superior taste and flavor. Here's another reason to "go wild" when it comes to salmon: Farmed salmon is high in the inflammatory omega-6 fatty acids found in extreme excess in the standard American diet.

For wild salmon of superior taste and quality—especially sockeye, which is the kind highest in omega-3s—I recommend Vital Choice Seafood (http://www.vitalchoice.com). See the "Resources" section for more details.

This recipe also works wonders with shrimp, scallops, boneless chicken breast, and firm tofu.

SALMON, CHICKEN, OR TOFU KABOBS WITH A MARINADE OF FRESH LIME AND ROSEMARY

Serves 4

KABOB INGREDIENTS

>   4 (6 ounces each) skinless and boneless wild Alaskan salmon
>   fillets, boneless chicken breasts, or bricks of firm tofu
>   Salt and freshly ground black pepper

MARINADE INGREDIENTS

>   2 garlic cloves, pressed
>   2 rosemary sprigs, leaves removed and finely chopped
>   7 tablespoons extra virgin olive oil
>   2 tablespoons freshly squeezed lime juice (use organic limes to
>   avoid the pesticide residue that accumulate in citrus rinds)
>   Lime slices
>   Rosemary sprigs

- Rinse the salmon, chicken, or tofu and pat dry. Cut into large cubes suitable for skewering.

- Place the salmon, chicken, or tofu cubes in a shallow baking dish and sprinkle them with freshly grated sea salt and pepper.

- Place the marinade ingredients in a small bowl and whisk them together until blended.

- Pour the marinade over the salmon, chicken, or tofu and allow to marinate for at least 10 minutes.

- Preheat the broiler (or preheat grill to medium-high).

- Lace the salmon, chicken, or tofu onto the skewers and broil (or grill) for 5 minutes, turning them once.

- While the salmon (or chicken or tofu) is cooking, pour the marinade in a small saucepan and heat it over medium heat.

- To serve: Divide among 4 serving plates and spoon some of the heated marinade over each. Garnish each plate with a few lime slices and a sprig of fresh rosemary and serve.

Note: if using wooden skewers, presoak in water for about 20 minutes.

GRILLED VEGGIE KABOBS

Serves 4 to 6

½ pound whole small mushrooms
2 large green or red bell peppers
1½ pounds small zucchini, cut into 1-inch slices
12 to 16 cherry tomatoes
1 large yellow onion cut into 1-inch slices

MARINADE AND BASTING SAUCE

⅓ cup chopped shallots
⅓ cup extra virgin olive oil
3 tablespoons Dijon mustard
3 tablespoons fresh lemon juice
2 tablespoons chopped fresh thyme
1 tablespoon grated lemon zest (use organic lemons to avoid the pesticide residue that accumulate in citrus rinds)
Freshly ground sea salt and black pepper to taste

- Place the marinade ingredients in a bowl and whisk them together until blended.

- Wash mushrooms; remove and discard stems. Wash peppers, remove seeds and veins and cut into 1-inch slices. Pat dry and place mushrooms, sliced zucchini, peppers, onion, and cherry tomatoes in marinade.

- Optional: Let vegetables marinate in refrigerator for at least 4 hours. If this is not possible, just baste them liberally during cooking.

- Drain vegetables, reserving marinade. Thread vegetables alternately onto skewers. Cook on grill over medium heat for about 10 minutes, turning occasionally and basting with reserved marinade. Grilled veggie kabobs make the perfect accompaniment to the savory skewered salmon, chicken, or tofu.

Rainbow Parfait

Serves 4 to 6

2 cups ¾-inch honeydew melon balls (from about a 3-pound
    piece, seeded)
2 cups ¾-inch cantaloupe balls (from about a 3-pound piece,
    seeded)
1 cup wild organic blueberries (see "Resources" section)
¼ cup fresh lime juice
    Fresh mint sprigs

• Gently layer melon, cantaloupe, and berries into tall parfait glasses.

• Drizzle equal amounts of the lime juice over each glass of fruit.

• Top with sprig of fresh mint.

Celebrating Autumn's Harvest

A CORNUCOPIA OF CULINARY DELIGHTS

Many of us make our biggest dietary mistakes during the holidays. In fact statistics show that Thanksgiving is when we are most apt to put on unwanted weight. Here is a Thanksgiving menu that offers healthy alternatives to fat- and carb-heavy fare. The RS in the chick peas (garbanzo beans) used to make the hummus will ensure that your blood sugar is not raised to unhealthy levels—as will the cinnamon in the pies.

THE PERRICONE THANKSGIVING

• MENU •

Appetizer: Hummus and Basil Kefir Dips with Crudités

Main Course: Turkey and Side Dishes

Dessert: Pumpkin and Apple Pies

Châteauneuf-du-Pape

Châteauneuf-du-Pape is a beautiful wine made in the southern Rhône region of France. This is a robust wine that goes particularly well with the classic country autumn and winter fare. Although poultry and seafood are customarily linked with a white wine, a "big" red wine, such as Châteauneuf-du-Pape, is a delightful, full-bodied accompaniment to a traditional Thanksgiving dinner.

APPETIZER: HUMMUS AND BASIL KEFIR DIPS WITH CRUDITÉS

HUMMUS

    4 garlic cloves, crushed

    1 teaspoon salt

    Two 19-ounce cans of chickpeas, drained and rinsed

    ⅔ cup well-stirred tahini

    ¼ cup fresh lemon juice, or to taste

    ½ cup extra virgin olive oil, or to taste

    ¼ cup fresh parsley leaves

    2 tablespoons pine nuts, toasted lightly

Mix all of the ingredients in a food processor until creamy.

BASIL KEFIR DIP

    ½ pound of fresh basil, blanched

    1 pint of plain or low-fat kefir (or yogurt)

    2 tablespoons fresh lemon juice

    Sea salt and pepper to taste

Blend ingredients thoroughly and refrigerate.

CRUDITÉS

    Julienned cucumber

    Zucchini

    Broccoli florets

    Red peppers

    Cauliflower florets

    Grape tomatoes

    Sliced apples

    Sliced pears

Fresh berries

Assorted olives

Flaxseed crackers

Bowl of almonds, hazelnuts, and walnuts

Serve all items arranged on a large platter with bowls of hummus and basil kefir dip.

Main Course: Turkey and Side Dishes

The Turkey

15-pound whole turkey, preferably fresh (and organic free range)
¾ cup extra virgin olive oil
⅓ cup freshly squeezed lemon juice
6 to 8 cloves fresh garlic, peeled
1 tablespoon lemon zest
1 teaspoon salt
1 teaspoon freshly ground black pepper
Parsley and other fresh herbs
Lemon wedges

- Remove giblets and neck from turkey; reserve. Rinse turkey with cold running water and drain well.

- In blender, combine olive oil and lemon juice. While blending, drop in garlic cloves one at a time. Gradually add lemon zest. Continue to blend until mixture is puréed.

- Using an injector, inject marinade into all parts of the turkey. (Strain marinade if it is too thick to pass through the injector.)

- Gently massage turkey to distribute marinade.

- Place turkey in a large plastic bag (cooking bag or food service–grade plastic bag). Close bag and refrigerate overnight.

- Preheat oven to 325°F.

- Remove turkey and drain and discard excess marinade. Do not reuse marinade to baste the turkey.

- Fold the neck skin and fasten to the back with 1 or 2 skewers. Fold the wings under the back of the turkey. Return the legs to tucked position.

- Place turkey, breast side up, on a rack in a large, shallow (about 2½ inches deep) roasting pan. Rub turkey with salt and pepper.

- Insert oven-safe meat thermometer into the thickest part of the turkey's thigh, being careful that the pointed end of the thermometer does not touch the bone.

- Roast the turkey in preheated oven for about 3¾ hours. During the last hour of roasting time, baste with pan drippings. If necessary, loosely cover with foil to prevent excessive browning.

- Continue roasting until the thermometer registers 180° in the thigh or 170° in the breast. Remove turkey from the oven and allow it to rest for 15 to 20 minutes before carving.

- Place turkey on a warm large platter and garnish with fresh herbs and lemon wedges.

GRAVY *(Yield: 1.5 cups)*
    ½ cup finely chopped onion
    2 tablespoons chopped fresh parsley
    2½ cups low-fat chicken broth
    1 tablespoon cornstarch
    Pepper to taste

- Cook onions and parsley in ¼ cup of broth until onions are translucent.

- In separate mixing bowl, combine cornstarch, pepper, and 1 cup broth and stir until smooth.

- Add mixture to pan with the remaining broth, stirring continuously. Boil for 2 minutes.

BUCKWHEAT STUFFING
    1 cup kasha (medium or coarse)
    1 egg, slightly beaten

¼ cup butter

1 cup each chopped onion and celery

2 cups chopped unpeeled apples

½ teaspoon ground sage

2 cups boiling chicken or turkey broth

Salt and pepper to taste

- Combine kasha and egg.

- Heat heavy skillet or pan lightly coated with oil (with tightly fitting lid); sear kasha until egg is cooked (2 to 3 minutes); remove from pan.

- Add butter to same pan; sauté onion, celery, and apples; season with sage.

- Return kasha to pan and carefully add boiling broth; reduce heat and simmer, covered, until liquid is absorbed (8 to 11 minutes). Adjust seasonings to taste.

- Bake separately in covered casserole at 350° Fahrenheit for 45 minutes.

CRANBERRY SAUCE *(Yield: 1¼ cups)*

2 cups fresh cranberries, washed

½ cup water

¼ cup agave nectar (or stevia, as desired)

1 orange, peeled and sectioned, discarding seeds and membranes, and puréed

- Place berries and water in saucepan and cook over high heat until berries begin to pop. Stir continuously to prevent sticking.

- Add desired amount of stevia or agave to sweeten as berries gel.

- When everything is completely dissolved, add orange and mix.

- Refrigerate to chill.

MASHED CAULIFLOWER

    1 head cauliflower
    ⅛ cup skim milk
    ½ cup Gruyère cheese, grated
      Salt and pepper
      Paprika

- Preheat oven to 350°F.
- Cook cauliflower until fork tender.
- Place cauliflower (in pieces), skim milk, cheese, salt, and pepper in blender. Whip until smooth.
- Pour cauliflower mixture into small baking dish. Sprinkle with paprika and bake until bubbly.

OVEN-ROASTED BRUSSELS SPROUTS WITH APPLES

Serves 2

    1 pint Brussels sprouts, cleaned and left whole
    1 apple peeled, cored, and cut into eighths
    1 teaspoon extra virgin olive oil

- Preheat oven to 375°F. In large bowl, toss Brussels sprouts, apple, and oil together.
- Cover a cookie sheet with aluminum foil; spread apple–Brussels sprout mixture evenly. Roast until lightly browned.

SPICED WINTER SQUASH WITH FENNEL

Serves 4

    1½ pounds butternut squash, peeled, halved lengthwise, seeded, halved crosswise, then cut lengthwise into ¾-inch-wide wedges

1 fennel bulb, trimmed, cut lengthwise into 1-inch-wide wedges

1 large onion, root end left intact, then cut lengthwise into ½-inch-wide wedges

3 tablespoons extra virgin olive oil

1 teaspoon ground cumin

1 teaspoon ground cinnamon

1 teaspoon chili powder

½ teaspoon turmeric

Salt and pepper to taste

- Position rack in bottom third of oven and preheat oven to 450°F.

- Combine squash, fennel, and onion on heavy, large, rimmed baking sheet. Add oil and toss vegetables to coat.

- Mix all spices in small bowl to blend. Sprinkle spice mixture over vegetables and toss them to coat. Sprinkle with salt and generous amount of pepper.

- Roast vegetables, turning once, about 45 minutes, until they are tender and browned. Transfer them to shallow dish and serve.

Desserts: Pumpkin and Apple Pies

Serves 8 (per pie)

Pumpkin Pie

PIE CRUST

> 1 cup rolled oats
> 10 almonds
> 1 cup brown rice flour
> ¼ teaspoon salt
> 2 tablespoons sesame oil
> ⅔ cup ice water

- Preheat oven to 350°F.
- Blend oats and almonds in dry blender to flour consistency.
- Combine in a bowl with rice flour and salt; add oil and stir; add water and mix to soft dough consistency.
- Press mixture into lightly oiled and sprayed pie pan, pressing from center outward; crimp edges with fork or dampened fingertips.
- Prebake for 10–15 minutes at 350°F and cool before adding filling.

PIE FILLING

> One 15-ounce can pumpkin (about 1¾ cups)
> 8 ounces skim milk
> 3 eggs
> ½ cup agave nectar
> Pumpkin pie spice to taste
> Cinnamon to taste

- Preheat oven to 425°F.
- Mix pumpkin, milk, and eggs until smooth.

- Gradually stir in agave nectar (¼ cup at a time).
- Add the pumpkin pie spice, taste; add more if needed.
- Pour mixture into crust and spread evenly.
- Bake in the oven for 15 minutes, then reduce the temperature to 350°F and bake for another 45 minutes (time may vary depending on oven).
- Lightly sprinkle cinnamon on top of pie and let cool.

Apple Pie

UNBAKED PIE CRUST: SEE RECIPE ON P. 224.

PIE FILLING

    2 firm, tart apples, peeled, cored, and sliced
    ⅓ cup raisins (optional)
    4 large eggs
    ½ cup agave nectar
    1 cup plain yogurt
    1 teaspoon pure vanilla extract
    ½ teaspoon cinnamon
    ¼ teaspoon salt

- Preheat oven to 375°F.
- Spread apples and raisins evenly in unbaked pie shell.
- In a blender, combine the eggs, agave syrup, yogurt, vanilla extract, cinnamon, and salt, and blend until creamy.
- Pour this custard over the apples and bake for about 1 hour, or until set. Allow to cool before serving.

Celebrating a Winter Wonderland with a

ROMANTIC VALENTINE DINNER

for TWO

Valentine's Day is another holiday in which our usual dietary decorum flies out the window as we indulge in rich desserts and fine champagne. Here is a romantic Valentine dinner for two that will satisfy the senses without sacrifice.

I chose these recipes for two reasons: because both feature heart-healthy foods that will nourish body and spirit, and to help set the mood for a lovely evening. In addition to superior nutrition, these recipes also feature foods that possess powerful anti-inflammatory properties that can help protect body and brain alike from the harmful effects of aging.

· MENU ·

Almond-Encrusted Wild Salmon Fillets on a Bed of
Wilted Greens

Parsley and Saffron-Scented Oat Pilaf

Cabernet Sauvignon

Extra-Dark Organic Chocolate with Blueberries

Green Tea

Cabernet Sauvignon is the dominant grape in the famed Bordeaux region of France and the premier red wine grape in the world. It is usually blended with other varieties, such as Merlot, to make wines with increased complexity. When you think of the finest red wines in the world, you often are thinking of wines made with Cabernet Sauvignon. In addition to Cabernet's taste characteristics, which are dark cherry, cedar, tobacco, and black currant, this red grape has a higher concentration of antioxidants than any other grape. To learn more about this and other fine wines, visit www.cellarnotes.net.

ALMOND-ENCRUSTED WILD SALMON FILLETS ON A BED OF WILTED GREENS

Hazelnuts, walnuts, or sunflower seeds may be used in place of almonds.

Serves 2

½ cup coarsely ground almonds
¼ cup chopped fresh parsley
1 tablespoon grated organic lemon zest (use organic lemons; nonorganic lemon rind is treated with fungicide)
  Dash of sea salt and fresh pepper
  Two 6-ounce wild salmon skinless fillets
2 tablespoons extra virgin olive oil
4 cups mixed organic baby greens (arugula, mesclun, spinach, etc.)
  Lemon wedges

• Grind the almonds in a coffee grinder or food processor—do not overgrind and turn them into a paste.

• Mix ground almonds, parsley, grated lemon zest, salt, and pepper on plate.

• Dry the salmon; dredge salmon on both sides in the almond mixture.

• Heat the oil in a large skillet over medium heat.

• Add the salmon and cook about 5 minutes on each side, making sure that the salmon is cooked through.

• Arrange 1 cup of greens—such as spinach, or a mix of greens such as baby lettuce, arugula, turnip or mustard greens, herbs, endive, and escarole—on each of 2 plates.

• Transfer the hot salmon fillets to plates.

• Garnish with lemon wedges and serve immediately.

PARSLEY AND SAFFRON-SCENTED OAT PILAF

Serves 4

2 cups water or soup stock

⅛ teaspoon saffron, crushed

2 tablespoons extra virgin olive oil

1 large clove of garlic, minced

1 medium yellow onion, diced

1 cup whole oat groats, rinsed (they look like brown rice and are available at natural-food stores)

½ cup fresh parsley

2 stalks fresh rosemary (or 1 teaspoon dried rosemary)

4 tablespoons Parmesan or Romano cheese (if possible, use imported cheese and grate it yourself for superior flavor)

Freshly grated black pepper to taste

- Boil ½ cup of the water or stock and pour over the saffron. Set aside.

- Heat the oil in a large saucepan. Sauté the garlic and onion over medium heat for about 5 minutes.

- Add the oats and stir to coat all the grains. Cook over medium heat for about 5 minutes, stirring frequently.

- Add the remaining 1½ cups of water or stock to the oats; add the saffron mixture and bring to a boil. Reduce the heat to a simmer and cook, covered, for about 45 minutes, or until all the water is absorbed.

- Remove rosemary leaves from stalk and coarsely chop. Discard stalk. Coarsely chop parsley leaves.

- Remove the pot cover, fluff the oats with a fork, fold in the rosemary and the parsley, and serve immediately.

- Top each serving with 1 tablespoon grated Parmesan or Romano cheese and with black pepper. I prefer imported Parmigiano-Reggiano for superior flavor.

Foods for Lovers . . . and a Longer, Healthier Life

A closer look at their key ingredients reveals why I chose these recipes for your Valentine's Day dinner.

WILD SALMON is probably the world's most heart healthy source of protein. It is rich in long-chain omega-3 EFAs—the most beneficial kind—which protect heart health, inhibit inflammation, act as natural antidepressants, increase feelings of well-being, and help keep skin young, supple, and radiant.

NUTS AND SEEDS such as hazelnuts, walnuts, and almonds are rich in short-chain omega-3 EFAs, which inhibit the accumulation of fats in artery walls that promote angina, strokes, and heart attacks. Nuts are also high in the amino acid arginine, which prompts the body to release vital hormones, stimulates sexuality, increases lean muscle mass, burns fat, lowers cholesterol, and boosts the immune system.

OAT PILAF is a delightful way to enjoy the benefits of the complex carbohydrates in an extraordinarily healthful whole grain, which provide sustained energy and also stimulate release of serotonin, a key neurotransmitter that can lift mood and cut carbohydrate cravings. Oats are also rich in vitamins, minerals, fibrous lignans, and phytochemicals that protect against heart disease, cancers, diabetes, and a whole host of diseases.

DARK LEAFY GREENS are rich in the antioxidant plant pigments known as carotenoids, which enhance immune response, protect skin cells against UV radiation, and spare liver enzymes that neutralize carcinogens and other toxins. Their important antioxidant, anti-inflammatory effects reduce the risk of heart disease, block sunlight-induced inflammation in the skin—which leads to wrinkles and skin cancer—and protect the eyes (especially the lutein found in spinach and kale), and may prevent cataracts and macular degeneration.

CABERNET SAUVIGNON: Red wine contains a powerful heart-healthy, anticancer, anti-aging antioxidant called resveratrol. It also appears that resveratrol helps protect the skin against the sun's UV radiation. Many studies have suggested that moderate alcohol drinking helps to reduce the likelihood of heart disease. But it seems that wine—particularly red wines such as Cabernet Sauvignon—interferes with the production of a body chemical vital to the process that leads to clogged arteries and an increased risk of heart attack. White wine and rosé do not offer the same protection.

EXTRA-DARK CHOCOLATE, especially that containing 80 percent cocoa solids or more, is uniquely high in potent, heart-healthy flavon-3-ol antioxidants. In fact, cocoa contains double the flavon-3-ol antioxidant content of red wine and five times that of green tea. Chocolate also contains arginine, whose benefits we addressed under "Nuts and Seeds" above. Chocolate is also a source of several mood-elevating constituents, including tryptophan (precursor to serotonin), anandamide (a natural brain chemical very similar to the cannabinoids in marijuana), theobromine (far milder cousin to caffeine), phenylethylamine, and magnesium. While the amounts of each of these potentially mood-elevating components appear too small to affect most people's mood significantly, the combination can and does produce feelings of elation, even ecstasy, in some sensitive individuals.

GREEN TEA: Enjoy a cup of green tea after your meal and don't worry about the caffeine, since a compound in green tea called theonine blocks the negative effects of caffeine while acting as a natural mood elevator and promoting feelings of well-being. Because green tea is rich in polyphenol antioxidants, it can help fight inflammation and age-accelerating free radicals, protect against heart disease and cancer, boost the body's natural defenses, and exert antiviral and antibacterial effects.

MAGNESIUM MAGIC: Many of the foods in our recipes are excellent sources of magnesium, a vital mineral that many of us do not get enough of. Thanks to its calming effects on the nervous system, magnesium can help ease anxiety, relax muscles, promote stress relief, decrease levels of the stress hormone cortisol, and promote a good night's sleep.

A Final Note on the Anti-aging Kitchen

If you are angry or upset, it is better to avoid cooking or preparing a meal, if possible. It's a well-known fact that many of us use food to influence our feelings. That means that if you're angry while you're cooking, you're likely to snack while you prepare the meal, make more than you or your family needs, go for foods that contain more sugar and/or starch than is good for you, and possibly even spark an eating binge. A study conducted at Ohio State University in 2000 revealed that anger increases the levels of homocysteine in the blood, an amino acid that has been linked to cardiovascular disease and hardening of the arteries. The good news is that adding folate to your diet (by trying the delicious asparagus recipe above, for example) can help alleviate homocysteine's harmful effects.

Creating health and longevity is as much a mental and spiritual discipline as it is physical—perhaps even more so. When we bring a positive and thankful attitude to even the simplest or most tedious of tasks, we quickly find that it becomes much more enjoyable. Remember that in many ways the kitchen is the heart and soul of the home, the perfect place for all of your positive energy. And as important as pure water, healthy food choices, and safe cookware are, perhaps the most critical ingredient we can bring into the anti-aging kitchen is a spirit of love and joy.

Here is a small sampling of the best foods to choose when stocking your anti-aging kitchen. *A special note:* Save very sweet fresh fruit for the end of the meal to keep blood sugar levels normal.

Adzuki beans
Alaskan halibut
Alaskan salmon
Almond butter
Almonds
Anasazi
Appaloosa
Apples
Artichokes
Arugula
Asparagus
Bamboo shoots
Barley
Basil
Bean sprouts
Berries (blackberries, blueberries, strawberries, etc.)
Black-eyed peas
Bok choy
Brazil nuts
Broccoli
Broccoli rabe
Broccoli sprouts
Brussels sprouts
Buckwheat
Butter (use in moderation)
Buttermilk
Cabbage
Cannellini
Cantaloupe and muskmelon
Cauliflower
Celeriac
Celery
Celery root

Cheese (especially Parmigiano-Reggiano and sheep's milk and goat's milk cheeses such as feta and Pecorino Romano)
Cherries
Chervil
Chestnuts
Chicken (choose free range, raised without added hormones and antibiotics and never fed animal by-products)
Chickory
Chickpeas
Chinese cabbage
Chives
Cilantro
Cinnamon
Cloves
Cod
Collards
Coriander
Cottage cheese
Cranberry
Crawfish
Cucumbers
Culinary herbs and spices
Cumin
Daikon radish
Dairy products (choose organic and low-fat unless from grass-fed animals)
Dandelion greens

Dill

Dungeness crab

Eggplant

Eggs (choose omega-3 eggs
    from free-range chicken)

Endive

Escarole

European soldier beans

Farmed clams and mussels
    (Unlike farmed fish, farmed
    clams and mussels require
    no feeding. The culture of
    these mollusks is very
    friendly to the surrounding
    environment, unlike many
    of the wild mussel and
    clam fisheries that drag the
    sea floor to harvest them
    or destroy their habitat
    through raking. These
    mollusks filter-feed on the
    crystal-clear water,
    eliminating the need
    to feed them, and they
    clean the water in the
    process.)

Farmer's cheese

Fava

Fennel

Flageolets

Ginger root

Grapefruit

Grass-fed beef, lamb, etc.

Great Northern beans

Green beans

Green tea

Green, red, yellow, and orange
    bell peppers

Hazelnuts

Honeydew melon

Hot peppers (cherry, serrano,
    jalepeño, etc.)

Kale

Kefir

Kidney beans

Kohlrabi

Lemons

Lentils (all varieties)

Lettuce (dark-red and dark-
    green varieties)

Lima (butter) beans

Limes

Lupini beans

Macadamia nuts

Marjoram

Milk

Mint

Mung beans

Mushrooms

Natto (fermented soy product
    high in bone-building
    vitamin K_2)

Navy beans

Nutmeg

Nuts and seed butter (avoid
    commercial peanut butter)

Oatmeal (slow-cooking)

Oats (whole or steel-cut)

Olive oil (extra virgin olive oil is
the recommended variety)

Olives (black and green)

Oranges (temple, mandarin,
blood, navel, etc.)

Oregano

Oysters

Parsley

Pea pods

Peanuts

Pears

Peas (split), dried

Pecans

Pine nuts

Pineapple

Pinto beans

Pistachios

Plums

Pomegranate

Pumpkin seeds

Quinoa

Radicchio

Radish

Red beans

Red kidney beans

Rhubarb

Ricotta

Romaine lettuce

Rosemary

Rutabaga

Sage

Scallops

Sea vegetables (nori, kelp,
arame, dulse, etc.)

Seafood

Sesame seeds

Sesame tahini

Shallot

Shellfish

Shrimp

Snow peas

Soba (buckwheat noodles)

Sorrel

Soybeans

Spinach

Sprouts

Squash

String beans

Sunflower seeds

Swiss chard

Tangelos

Tangerines

Thyme

Tofu

Tomatoes

Trout beans

Turkey

Turmeric

Turnips

Walnuts

Water chestnuts

Watercress

Watermelon

Yogurt

And here is a brief sampling of foods that can cause inflammation, thereby accelerating aging. This is because they are either high glycemic (that is, they cause a rise in blood sugar and insulin) or high in saturated fats, which can be pro-inflammatory.

Bacon (except turkey bacon)
Bagels
Beer
Breads, rolls, baked goods
Cake
Candy
Cereals (except slow-cooking oatmeal)
Chocolate (except extra-dark)
Cookies
Corn syrup
Cornbread, corn muffins
Cornstarch
Crackers
Fast food
Flour
French fries
Fried food
Fruit juice
Granola
Honey
Hot dogs
Ice cream, frozen yogurt, Italian ices
Jam, jelly, preserves

Mangoes
Margarine
Molasses
Muffins
Noodles
Pancakes
Pasta
Pastry
Pie (commercial)
Pita bread
Pizza
Popcorn
Potatoes
Pudding
Relish
Rice
Sherbet
Snack foods (e.g., potato chips, pretzels, corn chips, rice and corn cakes)
Soda
Sugar (white and brown)
Tacos
Tortillas
Waffles

Caralluma fimbriata
Safety Profile

HARRY G. PREUSS, M.D., MACN, CNS
Professor of Physiology, Medicine, and Pathology
Georgetown University Medical Center

Source of Information

Much background material on *Caralluma fimbriata* was supplied by Gencor Pacific. This information proved useful, especially the company's safety reports on *Caralluma fimbriata*. Additional information was obtained from PubMed (http://ncbi.nlm.nih.gov/entrez/query.fcgi) and from Web searches.

Safety of *Caralluma fimbriata* and Its Extract

In addition to the long history of safe ingestion of the cactus as a food, further proof of safety of its extract is evident through an acute oral toxicity study on rats and two clinical studies. The former was carried out by the Department of Pharmacology of St. John's Medical College in Bangalore, India. Doses of 2 grams per kilogram of body weight and 5 grams per kilogram of body weight were gavaged to rats. All animals survived until the scheduled necropsy at the end of the study period of 14 days. Histology revealed no abnormalities in the various organs.

Overall View of *Caralluma fimbriata* and Its Extract

I have reviewed the Gencor Pacific report on *Caralluma fimbriata* and believe the information is correct and accurate. Accordingly, all current evidence points to the safety of *Caralluma fimbriata* extract at the recommended doses.

I believe, on the basis of the following, that *Caralluma fimbriata* is safe to consume at recommended doses:

1. The cactus has been in the food chain of India for years and has not been associated with any significant adverse side effects.
2. *Caralluma fimbriata* is listed in the Wealth of India as a famine food and by various individuals on the Internet as a safe-to-consume food.
3. Various testimonials by doctors and scientists confirm its safety.
4. Testimonials by individuals who regularly consume the product describe its safety.
5. The daily dose of the extract contains the same concentration of ingredients as commonly eaten daily in the raw vegetable.

6. A study to determine LD$_{50}$ (the amount of a substance that is toxic to half of the experimental animals exposed to it) did not disclose toxicity, and it was reported that the LD$_{50}$ exceeded 5 grams per kilogram of body weight.

7. Two clinical studies composed of 44 individuals consuming the extract failed to reveal any significant adverse effects.

For a complete bibliography, see "References," the section for Chapter Two.

Abbreviations and Acronyms

2"-O-GIV:	2"-*O*-glycosylisovitexin
AI:	adequate intake
AIDS:	acquired immuno-deficiency syndrome
ALA:	alpha lipoic acid
ALC:	acetyl-L-carnitine
AP-1:	activator protein 1
ATP:	adenosine triphosphate
BMD:	bone mineral density
ch-OSA:	choline-stabilized orthosilicic acid
CLA:	conjugated linoleic acid
Co-Q$_{10}$:	coenzyme Q$_{10}$
COX-2:	cyclooxygenase-2

DHA:	docosahexaenoic acid
DHEA:	dehydroepiandrosterone
DHLA:	dihydrolipoic acid
DMAE:	dimethylaminoethanol
DNA:	deoxyribonucleic acid
EFA:	essential fatty acid
EMS:	electronic muscle stimulation
EPA:	eicosapentaenoic acid
EVOO:	extra virgin olive oil
GC:	glucocorticoid
GLA:	gamma linoleic acid
GSH:	glutathione
GSSG:	glutathione disulfide

HFCS:	high-fructose corn syrup	PFOA:	perfluorooctanoic acid
HGH:	human growth hormone	PS:	phosphatidylserine
HPA axis:	hypothalamic-pituitary-adrenal axis	PTH:	parathyroid hormone
HRT:	hormone-replacement therapy	RDA:	recommended daily allowance
		R-DHLA:	R-dihydrolipoic acid
LDL-C:	low-density lipoprotein cholesterol	RLA:	R-lipoic acid
		RNA:	ribonucleic acid
		ROS:	reactive oxygen species
MHC:	major histocompatibility complex	RS:	resistant starch
MRSA:	methicillin-resistant *Staphylococcus aureus*	SARS:	severe acute respiratory syndrome
		SOD:	superoxide dismutase
NFkB:	nuclear factor kappa B	SP:	substance P
NIH:	National Institutes of Health		
		UV:	ultraviolet
ORAC:	Oxygen Radical Absorbance Capacity	VNO:	vomeronasal organ

Resources

To receive updates on the latest health, beauty, and anti-aging news (and more) featured in *Dr. Perricone's 7 Secrets to Health, Beauty, and Longevity*, visit *www.perriconesecrets.com*.

TOPICAL ANTIOXIDANT, ANTI-AGING, ANTI-INFLAMMATORY SKIN PRODUCTS

- N.V. Perricone, M.D., Ltd., at 888-823-7837 or *www.nvperriconemd.com*
- N.V. Perricone, M.D., Ltd. flagship store, at 791 Madison Avenue (at 67th Street), New York, New York
- Nordstrom
- Sephora
- Select Saks stores
- Select Neiman Marcus stores
- Henri Bendel
- Clyde's, at 926 Madison Avenue at 74th Street, New York, New York
- Select Bloomingdale's stores

Light-Therapy Mask
- N.V. Perricone, M.D., Therapeutics, at 888-823-7837 or *www.nvperriconemd.com*

- N.V. Perricone, M.D., Ltd. flagship store, at 791 Madison Avenue (at 67th Street), New York, New York

Electronic Muscle Stimulation Glove
- N.V. Perricone, M.D., Therapeutics, at 888-823-7837 or www.nvperriconemd.com
- N.V. Perricone, M.D., Ltd. flagship store, at 791 Madison Avenue (at 67th Street), New York, New York

PRODUCTS FOR INFLAMMATORY SKIN CONDITIONS, INCLUDING ACNE

Light-Therapy Mask
- N.V. Perricone, M.D., Therapeutics, at 888-823-7837 or www.nvperriconemd.com
- N.V. Perricone, M.D., Ltd. flagship store, at 791 Madison Avenue (at 67th Street), New York, New York

Skin Clear Nutritional Support System
- N.V. Perricone, M.D., Therapeutics, at 888-823-7837 or www.nvperriconemd.com
- N.V. Perricone, M.D., Ltd. flagship store, at 791 Madison Avenue (at 67th Street), New York, New York

Nonchemical Sunscreen for Face and Body: Active Tinted Moisturizer with SPF 15
- N.V. Perricone, M.D., Therapeutics, at 888-823-7837 or www.nvperriconemd.com
- N.V. Perricone, M.D., Ltd. flagship store, at 791 Madison Avenue (at 67th Street), New York, New York
- Nordstrom
- Sephora
- Select Saks stores
- Select Neiman Marcus stores
- Henri Bendel
- Clyde's, at 926 Madison Avenue at 74th Street, New York, New York
- Select Bloomingdale's stores

LIBIDO, ENERGY, AND WELL-BEING ENHANCERS

Neuropeptide and Pheromone Therapeutic Anti-aging Fragrance
This unique, patented formula combines pheromones with a fragrance rich in therapeutic botanical essences. This results in a therapeutic mood enhancer and libido booster that also can greatly enhance memory and mental clarity, lift depression, increase self-confidence, and increase one's attractiveness to the opposite sex.

Additionally, because the limbic portion of the brain controls autonomous body functions, these fragrances can also lower blood pressure, increase blood flow to the brain (eliminating the confusion that sometimes plagues older people), increase problem-solving skills, reduce levels of the stress hormones cortisol and adrenaline, and actually slow the aging process.

- N.V. Perricone, M.D., Therapeutics, at 888-823-7837 or www.nvperriconemd.com
- N.V. Perricone, M.D., Ltd. flagship store, at 791 Madison Avenue (at 67th Street), New York, New York

Botanicals to Promote Sexual Health and Libido Enhancement
MacaPure rhodiola, tongkat ali, and other key botanicals have been specially formulated for both men and women under the brand names Hot Plants for Her and Hot Plants for Him by Enzymatic Therapy (www.enzy.com).

MacaPure extract is also available as Better World MacaTru, by Enzymatic Therapy (www.enzy.com).

Tongkat ali is also available in a stand-alone extract as LJ100, available at www.herbalpowers.com.

Rhodiola rosea is also available in a stand-alone extract as Rhodiola Energy, by Enzymatic Therapy (www.enzy.com).

WEIGHT MANAGEMENT SUPPLEMENTS AND BLOOD SUGAR STABILIZERS

Weight Management Supplements
- *Caralluma fimbriata*
- Chromate brand of chromium
- Maitake D-Fraction and SX Fraction Extract
- Conjugated linoleic acid
- Coenzyme Q_{10}
- Carnitine and acetyl-L-carnitine
- Alpha-lipoic acid
- Gamma linoleic acid
- L-glutamine powder

All of the above are available at N.V. Perricone, M.D., Ltd., at 888-823-7837 or www.nvperriconemd.com, and at N.V. Perricone, M.D., Ltd. flagship store, at 791 Madison Avenue (at 67th Street), New York, New York.

High-Quality Fish Oil Capsules
- N.V. Perricone, M.D., Ltd., at 888-823-7837 or www.nvperriconemd.com
- N.V. Perricone, M.D., Ltd. flagship store, at 791 Madison Avenue (at 67th Street), New York, New York
- Vital Choice Seafood, at 800-608-4825 or www.vitalchoice.com
- Optimum Health International at 800-228-1507 or www.opthealth.com

NUTRITIONAL SUPPLEMENTS, MITOCHONDRIAL REJUVENATORS, AND ANTI-AGING, ANTI-INFLAMMATORY SUPPLEMENTS

Skin and total body nutritional supplements, formulated by N.V. Perricone, M.D., are available from

- N.V. Perricone, M.D., Ltd., at 888-823-7837 or www.nvperriconemd.com
- N.V. Perricone, M.D., Ltd. flagship store, at 791 Madison Avenue (at 67th Street), New York, New York
- Nordstrom
- Sephora
- Select Saks stores
- Select Neiman Marcus stores
- Henri Bendel
- Clyde's, at 926 Madison Avenue at 74th Street, New York, New York
- Select Bloomingdale's stores

AstaREAL Astaxanthin Supplements
AstaREAL is available from N.V. Perricone, M.D., Ltd., at 888-823-7837 or www.nvperriconemd.com.

Supplements for Bone Health and Cardiovascular Support
Vitamin K_2 and bone solutions are available from

- Advanced Biosolutions, 1-888-887-7498 or www.drsinatra.com
- Jarrow Formulas, www.jarrow.com: Choline-stabilized orthosilicic acid (ch-OSA) and BioSil

Oreganol P73 and Related Products
Oil of oregano is an herbal product that has been used since biblical times. It was widely used in ancient Greece for many medical purposes. Oil of oregano is a potent antiseptic, meaning that it kills germs. Research proves that it is highly effective for killing a wide range of fungi, yeast, and bacteria, including methicillin-resistant *Staphylococcus aureus* and avian flu, as well as parasites and viruses. It is available from North American Herb & Spice, 800-243-5242 or www.oreganol.com.

Recommended Reading
Natural Cures for Killer Germs and *The Cure Is in the Cupboard*
by Dr. Cass Ingram
Available from www.amazon.com

RECOMMENDED FOODS

Wild Salmon and Seafood
You can get wild Alaskan salmon and seafood delivered to your door—Alaskan salmon, scallops, halibut, sablefish, and low-mercury Pacific tuna,

Alaskan salmon sausage and burgers, smoked wild salmon and sablefish, and canned wild salmon, tuna, and sardines—from Vital Choice Seafood. Wild Alaskan salmon has a far healthier fatty acid profile than does farmed salmon. It has much lower levels of saturated and inflammatory omega-6 fats, and a much higher ratio of anti-inflammatory omega-3 fatty acids to omega-6 and saturated fats. Vital Choice Seafood fish are caught at sea, flash-frozen immediately, packed in dry ice, and delivered via air courier at affordable prices. Most Vital Choice Seafood products are certified kosher.

Note: The wild Alaskan salmon and Pacific halibut fisheries are certified sustainable by the Marine Stewardship Council; Alaska's Weathervane Scallop Fishery is governed by state and federal plans that enforce sustainability measures. Vital Choice offers only small, troll-caught, low-mercury albacore tuna.

Contact Vital Choice Seafood at www.vitalchoice.com or 800-608-4825.

Acai—Amazonian Fruit High in Antioxidants
Acai fruit has more antioxidants than wild blueberries, pomegranate, or red wine; it also contains essential omegas (healthy fats), amino acids, calcium, and fiber.

Super Berry Powder with Acai is a berry powder drink containing high amounts of antioxidants and anti-inflammatories. Both qualities maintain cell health, protect from free-radical damage, and provide support to the major organ functions in the body.

- N.V. Perricone, M.D., Ltd., at 888-823-7837 or www.nvperriconemd.com
- N.V. Perricone, M.D., Ltd. flagship store, 791 Madison Avenue (at 67th Street), New York, New York
- Nationwide at Whole Foods Market and Wild Oats stores, and at www.sambazon.com: Sambazon brand acai beverages

Avocado
For recipes and health information, visit the website of the California Avocado Board, at www.avocado.org.

Beans and Lentils
Westbrae Natural markets certified-organic beans, including rare heirloom varieties, nationwide. www.westbrae.com/products/index.html or call 800-434-4246.

Coconut Oil
Spectrum Organic Products offers coconut oil at www.spectrumorganics.com.

Foods Alive Organic Golden Flax Crackers (Grain Free)
Foods Alive offers organic flax crackers at www.foodsalive.com.

Goji Berry
All goji berry supply worldwide is processed through the Office of the Tibetan Goji Berry Company (866-328-4654 or www.gojiberry.com). This single-source

supply office is an ecological control put in place for botanical conservation purposes and to protect against overharvesting of the limited crop of wild-crafted goji berry.

Grass-Fed Beef
Eatwild.com is your source for safe, healthy, natural, and nutritious grass-fed beef, lamb, goats, bison, poultry, pork, and dairy products. The website has three goals:

- To link consumers with reliable suppliers of all-natural, delicious, grass-fed products
- To provide comprehensive, accurate information about the benefits of raising animals on pasture
- To provide a marketplace for farmers who raise their livestock on pasture from birth to market and who actively promote the welfare of their animals and the health of the land

Neff Family Ranch (www.nfrnaturalbeef.com) offers 100% grass-fed beef grazed on organic pasture.

Recommended Reading
Pasture Perfect: The Far-Reaching Benefits of Choosing Meat, Eggs, and Dairy Products from Grass-Fed Animals
By Jo Robinson
Available from www.eatwild.com

The Omnivore's Dilemma
By Michael Pollen
Available at bookstores, www.amazon.com, and www.eatwild.com

Green Foods
Certified organic barley grass and Green Magma powder and supplements are available at natural-food stores, including Whole Foods and Wild Oats. For additional retailers and online retailers, visit www.greenfoods.com.

Green Tea
For high-quality teas (green, white, and black) and tea buds with the highest polyphenol content, contact the Red Blossom Tea Company at 415-395-0868 or www.redblossomtea.com.

Kefir and Yogurt
- Helios Nutrition is a small organic dairy in Sauk Centre, Minnesota, that makes several flavors of organic kefir with added FOS (prebiotic polysaccharide). Locate retail outlets at 888-3-HELIOS or www.heliosnutrition.com/html/where_to_buy.html.
- Stonyfield Farm yogurt is available at many food markets. See the store locator at www.stonyfield.com/storelocator/.

- Horizon Organic yogurt is available at many food markets. See the store locator at www.horizonorganic.com/stores/index.html.
- Diamond Organics sells organic yogurt direct to consumers at www.diamondorganics.com/prod_detail_list/41 161 or 1-888-ORGANIC (888-674-2642).

Organic Berries, Chocolates, Seasonings, Oils, and Teas Delivered to Your Door
Vital Choice Seafood, a purveyor of premium-quality seafood, also offers top-quality certified-organic foods. Go to www.vitalchoice.com or call 800-608-4825.

Organic Fruits and Vegetables Delivered to Your Home
Diamond Organics sells certified-organic berries (in season, May through October) direct to consumers. Go to www.diamondorganics.com or call 888-ORGANIC (888-674-2642).

Organic Markets Nationwide
For fish, meat, poultry, eggs, fruits and vegetables, barley, oats, buckwheat, beans and lentils, hot peppers, nuts, seeds, extra virgin olive oil, herbs, spices, spring water, tea (green, white, and black), nutritional supplements, kefir, yogurt, and more:

- Whole Foods Market has an outstanding choice of natural and organic foods. Go to the company's website to find a store near you: www.wholefoods.com.
- Wild Oats is another national chain offering an excellent selection of organic and natural food. To find a store near you, visit www.wildoats.com.

Polysaccharide Peptide Food Products (Anti-inflammatory and Antiaging)
- N.V. Perricone, M.D., Ltd., at 888-823-7837 or www.nvperriconemd.com
- N.V. Perricone, M.D., Ltd., flagship store, at 791 Madison Avenue (at 67th Street), New York, New York

Pistachio Nuts
You can find information about California pistachio nuts at www.everybodysnuts.com and can buy them in grocery stores nationwide.

Pomegranate Juice and Concentrate (Extremely High in Antioxidants)
You can find stores that carry POM Wonderful by calling 310-966-5800 or going to www.pomwonderful.com. The juice and concentrate are also available at supermarkets and natural-food stores.

Pure Spring Water
- Poland Spring brand spring water can be found in grocery stores nationwide.

- FIJI Water, natural artesian water bottled at its source in the Fiji Islands, is available at leading grocery and convenience store chains. FIJI Water is also available for home delivery in the continental United States at www.fijiwater.com.

Sea Vegetables
- Maine Coast Sea Vegetables (www.seaveg.com)
- Eden Foods (www.edenfoods.com)

Sprouts
The International Sprout Growers Association at www.isga-sprouts.org is the professional association of sprout growers and companies that supplies products and services to the sprout industry. Visit the association's website for outstanding information, recipes, and health notes.

Turmeric
- New Chapter markets high-potency turmeric extract under the brand name Turmericforce. Go to www.new-chapter.com or call 800-543-7279.
- Most natural-food stores and grocers also carry fresh turmeric root.

RECOMMENDED COOK- AND BAKEWARE

It should come as no surprise that my favorite cook- and bakeware hail from France, one of the countries most famed for superior cuisine. The cookware that you choose is very important to your health as well as to the flavor of your food. Porcelain and enameled cookware will not interact with your food, which is important to know when you are dealing with acidic foods such as vinegar and lemon. As mentioned, avoid nonstick cook- and bakeware. Although the recommended items cost a bit more, proper care will ensure that they last a lifetime—a wise investment that you have to make only once.

Emile Henry Cookware
The Burgundy region in the heart of France is the home of Emile Henry cookware. Since 1850 five generations of the Henry family have been handcrafting this famous line of oven-to-tableware. Emile Henry is the largest manufacturer of pottery in France. Since its cookware was first produced, the major benefits of cooking in oven-to-tableware has been the ability to allow gradual, even heat distribution through the food so that the fibers soften slowly, without toughening. The cookware is available at fine stores such as Williams-Sonoma. For a complete listing of retail and online sellers, visit www.emilehenry.com.

Le Creuset
Le Creuset is the world's leading manufacturer of enameled cast-iron cookware. Like Emile Henry, Le Creuset is as beautiful as it is functional. The only challenge when it comes to shopping for Le Creuset is choosing the color. All

Le Creuset cookware is made from enameled cast iron. Cast iron has been used for cooking utensils since the Middle Ages. The Le Creuset factory is at Fresnoy-le-Grand in northern France.

In 1925, the foundry began producing cast iron by hand-casting molten iron in sand molds—still the most delicate stage of the production process. Even today, after casting, each mold is destroyed and the cookware is polished and sanded by hand, then scrutinized for imperfections. Once declared good for enameling, the items are sprayed with two separate coats of enamel and fired after each process at a temperature of 800° Centigrade. The enamel then becomes extremely hard and durable, making it almost completely resistant to damage during normal use. Since much of the finishing is done by hand, each Le Creuset cast-iron cookware piece is unique.

RECOMMENDED HOUSEHOLD PRODUCTS

Sun & Earth www.sunandearth.com

Seventh Generation
There is an alternative to toxic cleansers and environmentally unfriendly paper and plastic. I recommend Seventh Generation, which offers a complete line of nontoxic household products. All of its products are designed to work as well as their traditional counterparts but use renewable, nontoxic, phosphate-free, and biodegradable ingredients and are never tested on animals. They are as gentle on the planet as they are on people, and they don't create fumes or leave residues that may affect the health of your family or your pets. Seventh Generation products are widely available nationwide. To learn more and find a local or online retailer, visit www.seventhgeneration.com.

HEALTH EDUCATION INFORMATION

These websites offer interesting information on the topics of nutrition, natural healing, food, and holistic health:

- For up-to-the-minute scientific news and information on food and nutritional supplements, see www.lef.org.
- For science-based information on food and food-related topics to the media, health and nutrition professionals, educators, and opinion leaders, visit the website of the European Food Information Council, a nonprofit organization, at www.eufic.org.
- For information on the glycemic index, see www.glycemicindex.com.
- For excellent information on general health and nutrition, including different types of meat and sugars, see www.mercola.com.
- For information on the cancer-preventing phytonutrients found in fruits and vegetables, visit the website of the American Institute for Cancer Research, at www.aicr.org.

- For outstanding information on the benefits of various types of exercise, including detailed information with drawings, visit, the websites of the President's Council on Physical Fitness (www.fitness.gov) and the National Institute on Aging (www.niapublications.org).

Health Benefits of Olive Oil
Information about the health benefits of olive oil can be found at www.internationaloliveoil.org/oliveworld_mediet.asp.

Nonglycemic Sweeteners
- To learn more about the pros and cons of sweeteners, both natural and chemical, visit www.holisticmed.com/sweet/.
- For information on stevia, visit www.stevia.net.
- For information on ZSweet natural sugar substitute, visit www.zsweet.com.

Soy Foods
For comprehensive information on soy foods, visit www.soyfoods.com.

Seafood Safety
- Union of Concerned Scientists: www.ucsusa.org
- U.S. Food and Drug Administration fish safety website: www.cfsan.fda.gov/~frf/sea-mehg.html
- Environmental Protection Agency: www.epa.gov/ost/fish, www.epa.gov/mercury

Anti-aging Exercise for Both Mind and Body
For information and instruction, read *Chi Kung: The Chinese Art of Mastering Energy*, by Yves Réquéna, published by Healing Arts Press. It is available from www.innertraditions.com.

T-Tapp
Learn more about T-Tapp, an innovative wellness workout that incorporates many different elements to build balanced muscle tissue along with strength and flexibility, at www.t-tapp.com or read *Fit and Fabulous in 15 Minutes*, by Teresa Tapp, published by Ballantine Books and available at most bookstores.

References

CHAPTER 1

Aggarwal BB, Kumar A, Bharti AC. Anticancer potential of curcumin: preclinical and clinical studies. *Anticancer Research* 2003; 23(1A):363–98. Review.

Aggarwal BB, Shishodia S. Suppression of the nuclear factor-kappaB activation pathway by spice-derived phytochemicals: reasoning for seasoning. *Annals of the New York Academy of Sciences* 2004; 1030:434–41. Review.

Aggarwal S, Ichikawa H, Takada Y, Sandur SK, Shishodia S, Aggarwal BB. Curcumin (diferuloylmethane) down-regulates expression of cell proliferation and anti-apoptotic and metastatic gene products through suppression of IkappaBalpha kinase and Akt activation. *Molecular Pharmacology* 2006;69(1):195–206. Epub 2005 Oct 11.

Agmon Y, Khandheria BK, Meissner I, Petterson TM, O'Fallon WM, Wiebers DO, Christianson TJ, McConnell JP, Whisnant JP, Seward JB, Tajik AJ. C-reactive protein and atherosclerosis of the thoracic aorta: a population-based trans-esophageal echocardiographic study. *Archives of Internal Medicine* 2004;164(16): 1781–87.

Allen RG, Tresini M. Oxidative stress and gene regulation. *Free Radical Biology & Medicine* 2000 1;28(3):463–99. Review.

Amato P, Morales AJ, Yen SS. Effects of chromium picolinate supplementation on insulin sensitivity, serum lipids, and body composition in healthy, nonobese, older men and women. *The Journals of Gerontology—Series A, Biological Sciences and Medical Sciences* 2000;55(5):M260–63.

Ames BN. Delaying the mitochondrial decay of aging. *Annals of the New York Academy of Sciences* 2004; 1019:406–11. Review.

Ames BN, Liu J. Delaying the mitochondrial decay of aging with acetylcarnitine. *Annals of the New York Academy of Sciences* 2004;1033:108–16. Review.

Anderson RA. Effects of chromium on body composition and weight loss. *Nutrition Reviews* 1998;56:266–70.

Anti-inflammatory effect may help explain fish benefit: best results seen among people who ate more than half a pound of fish each week. Accessed July 8, 2005 at http://www.acc.org/media/releases/highlights/2005/july05/fish.htm.

Aquaxan™ HD algal meal use in aquaculture diets: enhancing nutritional performance and pigmentation. Technical report 2102.001. Available at http://www.fda.gov/ohrms/dockets/dailys/00/jun00/061900/rpt0065_tab6.pdf

Arab L, Steck S. Lycopene and cardiovascular disease. *American Journal of Clinical Nutrition* 2000;71:1691S–5S.

Arafa HM. Curcumin attenuates diet-induced hypercholesterolemia in rats. *Medical Science Monitor* 2005;11(7):BR228–34. Epub 2005 Jun 29.

Arimoto T, Ichinose T, Yoshikawa T, Shibamoto T. Effect of the natural antioxidant 2"-O-glycosylisovitexin on superoxide and hydroxyl radical generation. *Food and Chemical Toxicology* 2000;38(9):849–52.

Arita M, Bianchini F, Aliberti J, Sher A, Chiang N, Hong S, Yang R, Petasis NA, Serhan CN. Sterochemical assignment, antiinflammatory properties, and receptor for the omega-3 lipid mediator resolvin E1. *Journal of Experimental Medicine* 2005;201: 713–22.

Arroyo-Espliguero R, Avanzas P, Cosin-Sales J, Aldama G, Pizzi C, Kaski JC. C-reactive protein elevation and disease activity in patients with coronary artery disease. *European Heart Journal* 2004;25(5):401–8.

Atalay M, Gordillo G, Roy S, Rovin B, Bagchi D, Bagchi M, Sen CK. Anti-angiogenic property of edible berry in a model of hemangioma. *FEBS Letters* 2003;544(1–3): 252–57.

Aviram M. 11th biennial meeting of the Society for Free Radical Research International, Paris, 2002.

Aviram M, Dornfeld L. Pomegranate juice consumption inhibits serum angiotensin converting enzyme activity and reduces systolic blood pressure. *Atherosclerosis* 2001;158(1):195–98.

Aviram M, Dornfeld L, Kaplan M, Coleman R, Gaitini D, Nitecki S, Hofman A, Rosenblat M, Volkova N, Presser D, Attias J, Hayek T, Fuhrman B. Pomegranate juice flavonoids inhibit low-density lipoprotein oxidation and cardiovascular diseases: studies in atherosclerotic mice and in humans. *Drugs Under Experimental and Clinical Research* 2002;28(2–3):49–62. Review.

Aviram M, Dornfeld L, Rosenblat M, Volkova N, Kaplan M, Coleman R, Hayek T,

Presser D, Fuhrman B. Pomegranate juice consumption reduces oxidative stress, atherogenic modifications to LDL, and platelet aggregation: studies in humans and in atherosclerotic apolipoprotein E-deficient mice. *American Journal of Clinical Nutrition* 2000;71(5):1062–76.

Bagchi D, Bagchi M, Balmoori J, Ye X, Stohs SJ. Comparative induction of oxidative stress in cultured J774A.1 macrophage cells by chromium picolinate and chromium nicotinate. *Research Communications in Molecular Pathology and Pharmacology* 1997;97(3):335–46. Erratum in: *Research Communications in Molecular Pathology and Pharmacology* 1998;99(2):240.

Bagchi D, Bagchi M, Stohs SJ, Das DK, Ray SD, Kuszynski CA, Joshi SS, Pruess HG. Free radicals and grape seed proanthocyanidin extract: importance in human health and disease prevention. *Toxicology.* 2000;148(2–3):187–97.

Bagchi D, Bagchi M, Stohs S, Ray SD, Sen CK, Preuss HG. Cellular protection with proanthocyanidins derived from grape seeds. *Annals of the New York Academy of Sciences* 2002;957:260–70. Review.

Bagchi D, Sen CK, Bagchi M, Atalay M. Anti-angiogenic, antioxidant, and anti-carcinogenic properties of a novel anthocyanin-rich berry extract formula. *Biochemistry Biokhimila* 2004;69(1):75–80.

Bagga D, Wang L, Farias-Eisner R, Glaspy JA, Reddy ST. Differential effects of prostaglandin derived from omega-6 and omega-3 polyunsaturated fatty acids on COX-2 expression and IL-6 secretion. *Proceedings of the National Academy of Sciences of the United States of America* 2003;100:1751–56.

Bahadori B, Wallner S, Schneider H, Wascher TC, Toplak H. [Effect of chromium yeast and chromium picolinate on body composition of obese, non-diabetic patients during and after a formula diet]. *Acta Med Austriaca* 1997;24(5):185–57. German.

Bassuk SS, Rifai N, Ridker PM. High-sensitivity C-reactive protein: clinical importance. *Current Problems in Cardiology* 2004;29(8):439–93. Review.

Bast A, Haenen GR. Interplay between lipoic acid and glutathione in the protection against microsomal lipid peroxidation. *Biochimica et Biophysica Acta.* 1988;963(3):558–61.

Baynes JW. The role of AGEs in aging: causation or correlation. *Experimental Gerontology* 2001;36(9):1527–37. Review.

Baynes JW, Thorpe SR. Glycoxidation and lipoxidation in atherogenesis. *Free Radical Biology and Medicine* 2000;28(12):1708–16. Review.

Beal MF. Bioenergetic approaches for neuroprotection in Parkinson's disease. *Annals of Neurology* 2003;53(suppl 3):S39–47; discussion S47–48. Review.

Beal MF. Mitochondria, oxidative damage, and inflammation in Parkinson's disease. *Annals of the New York Academy of Sciences* 2003;991:120–31. Review.

Beal MF. Mitochondrial dysfunction and oxidative damage in Alzheimer's and Parkinson's diseases and coenzyme Q_{10} as a potential treatment. *Journal of Bioenergetics and Biomembranes* 2004;36(4):381–86. Review.

Becker EW, Jakober B, Luft D, et al. Clinical and biochemical evaluations of the alga Spirulina with regard to its application in the treatment of obesity. A double-blind cross-over study. *Nutrition Reports International* 1986;33:565–574.

Bell JG, Henderson RJ, Tocher DR, Sargent JR. Replacement of dietary fish oil with increasing levels of linseed oil: modification of flesh fatty acid compositions in Atlantic salmon (*Salmo salar*) using a fish oil finishing diet. *Lipids* 2004;39(3): 223–32.

Bell JG, Tocher DR, Henderson RJ, Dick JR, Crampton VO. Altered fatty acid compositions in Atlantic salmon (*Salmo salar*) fed diets containing linseed and rapeseed oils can be partially restored by a subsequent fish oil finishing diet. *Journal of Nutrition* 2003;133(9):2793–801.

Bertram JS, Vine AL. Cancer prevention by retinoids and carotenoids: independent action on a common target. *Biochimica et Biophysica Acta* 2005;1740(2):170–8. Epub 2005 Jan 25. Review.

Beyer RE. An analysis of the role of coenzyme Q in free radical generation and as an antioxidant. *Biochemistry and Cell Biology* 1992;70(6):390–403. Review.

Bharti AC, Donato N, Singh S, Aggarwal BB. Curcumin (diferuloylmethane) down-regulates the constitutive activation of nuclear factor-kappa B and Ikappa-Balpha kinase in human multiple myeloma cells, leading to suppression of proliferation and induction of apoptosis. *Blood* 2003;101(3):1053–62. Epub 2002 Sep 5.

Bhattacharya A, Lawrence RA, Krishnan A, Zaman K, Sun D, Fernandes G. Effect of dietary n-3 and n-6 oils with and without food restriction on activity of antioxidant enzymes and lipid peroxidation in livers of cyclophosphamide treated autoimmune-prone NZB/W female mice. *Journal of the American College of Nutrition* 2003;22(5):388–99.

Bhosale P, Bernstein PS. Microbial xanthophylls. *Applied Microbiology and Biotechnology* 2005;68(4):445–55. Epub 2005 Oct 26. Review.

Bianchini F, Vainio H. Wine and resveratrol: mechanisms of cancer prevention? *European Journal of Cancer Prevention* 2003;12(5):417–25. Review.

Bierhaus A, Chevion S, Chevion M, Hofmann M, Quehenberger P, Illmer T, Luther T, Berentshtein E, Tritschler H, Muller M, Wahl P, Ziegler R, Nawroth PP. Advanced glycation end product-induced activation of NF-kappaB is suppressed by alpha-lipoic acid in cultured endothelial cells. *Diabetes* 1997;46(9):1481–90.

Biewenga GP, Haenen GR, Bast A. The pharmacology of the antioxidant lipoic acid. *General Pharmacology* 1997;29(3):315–31.

Biewenga GP, Veening-Griffioen DH, Nicastia AJ, Haenen GR, Bast A. Effects of dihydro-lipoic acid on peptide methionine sulfoxide reductase. Implications for antioxidant drugs. *Arzneimittelforschung* 1998;48(2):144–48.

Blankenberg S, Rupprecht HJ, Bickel C, Peetz D, Hafner G, Tiret L, Meyer J. Circulating cell adhesion molecules and death in patients with coronary artery disease. *Circulation* 2001;104(12):1336–42.

Blankenberg S, Tiret L, Bickel C, Peetz D, Cambien F, Meyer J, Rupprecht HJ; Athero-Gene Investigators. Interleukin-18 is a strong predictor of cardiovascular death in stable and unstable angina. *Circulation* 2002;106(1):24–30.

Blinkova LP, Gorobets OB, Baturo AP. [Biological activity of Spirulina]. *Zhurnal mikrobiologii, epidemiologii, immunobiologii* 2001;(2):114–18. Russian.

Block G, Patterson B, Subar A. Fruit, vegetables, and cancer prevention: a review of the epidemiological evidence. *Nutrition and Cancer* 1992;18(1):1–29. Review.

Bordin L, Prianti G, Musacchio E, Giunco S, Tibaldi E, Clari G, Baggio B. Arachidonic acid-induced IL-6 expression is mediated by PKC-α activation in osteoblastic cells. *Biochemistry* 2003;42:4485–91.

Bourre JM. Where to find omega-3 fatty acids and feeding animals with diet enriched in omega-3 fatty acids to increase nutritional value of derived products for human: what is actually useful? *Journal of Nutrition, Health & Aging* 2005;9(4):232–42. Review.

Breinholt V, Arbogast D, Loveland P, Pereira C, Dashwood R, Hendricks J, Bailey G. Chlorophyllin chemoprevention: an evaluation of reduced bioavailability vs. target organ protective mechanisms. *Toxicology and Applied Pharmacology* 1999; 158:141–51.

Breinholt V, Hendricks J, Pereira C, Arbogast D, Bailey G. Dietary chlorophyllin is a potent inhibitor of aflatoxin B1 hepatocarcinogenesis in rainbow trout. *Cancer Research* 1995;55:57–62.

Brouet I, Ohshima H. Curcumin, an anti-tumour promoter and anti-inflammatory agent, inhibits induction of nitric oxide synthase in activated macrophages. *Biochemical and Biophysical Research Communications* 1995;206(2):533–40.

Burke JD, Curran-Celentano J, Wenzel AJ. Diet and serum carotenoid concentrations affect macular pigment optical density in adults 45 years and older. *Journal of Nutrition* 2005;135(5):1208–14.

Burros M. Farmed salmon looking less rosy. *New York Times*, May 28, 2003.

Bustamante J, Lodge JK, Marcocci L, Tritschler HJ, Packer L, Rihn BH. Alpha-lipoic acid in liver metabolism and disease. *Free Radical Biology & Medicine* 1998;24(6): 1023–39. Review.

Caballero-George C, Vanderheyden PM, De Bruyne T, Shahat AA, Van den Heuvel H, Solis PN, Gupta MP, Claeys M, Pieters L, Vauquelin G, Vlietinck AJ. In vitro inhibition of [3H]-angiotensin II binding on the human AT1 receptor by proanthocyanidins from *Guazuma ulmifolia* bark. *Planta Medica* 2002;68(12):1066–71.

Cakatay U, Telci A, Kayali R, Sivas A, Akcay T. Effect of alpha-lipoic acid supplementation on oxidative protein damage in the streptozotocin-diabetic rat. *Research in Experimental Medicine* 2000;199(4):243–51.

Cal C, Garban H, Jazirehi A, Yeh C, Mizutani Y, Bonavida B. Resveratrol and cancer: chemoprevention, apoptosis, and chemo-immunosensitizing activities. *Current Medicinal Chemistry Anti-cancer Agents* 2003;3(2):77–93. Review.

Calabrese V, Scapagnini G, Colombrita C, Ravagna A, Pennisi G, Giuffrida Stella AM,

Galli F, Butterfield DA. Redox regulation of heat shock protein expression in aging and neurodegenerative disorders associated with oxidative stress: a nutritional approach. *Amino Acids* 2003;25(3–4):437–44. Epub 2003 Nov 07.

Calder PC. N-3 fatty acids and cardiovascular disease: evidence explained and mechanisms explored. *Clinical Science (London)*. 2004;107(1):1–11. Review.

Calder PC. N-3 polyunsaturated fatty acids and inflammation: from molecular biology to the clinic. *Lipids* 2003;38:342–52.

Calixto JB, Yunes RA. Natural bradykinin antagonists. *Memorias do Instituto Oswaldo Cruz* 1991;86(suppl 2):195–202. Review.

Camandola S, Leonarduzzi G, Musso T, Varesio L, Carini R, Scavazza A, Chiarpotto E, Baeuerle PA, Poli G. Nuclear factor κB is activated by arachidonic acid but not by eicosapentenoic acid. *Biochemical and Biophysical Research Communications* 1996; 229:643–47.

Campbell WW, Joseph LJ, Anderson RA, Davey SL, Hinton J, Evans WJ. Effects of resistive training and chromium picolinate on body composition and skeletal muscle size in older women. *International Journal of Sport Nutrition and Exercise Metabolism* 2002;12(2):125–35.

Campbell WW, Joseph LJ, Davey SL, Cyr-Campbell D, Anderson RA, Evans WJ. Effects of resistance training and chromium picolinate on body composition and skeletal muscle in older men. *Journal of Applied Physiology* 1999;86(1):29–39.

Cao G, Russell RM, Lischner N, Prior RL. Serum antioxidant capacity is increased by consumption of strawberries, spinach, red wine or vitamin C in elderly women. *Journal of Nutrition* 1998;128(12):2383–90.

Cao G, Shukitt-Hale B, Bickford PC, Joseph JA, McEwen J, Prior RL. Hyperoxia-induced changes in antioxidant capacity and the effect of dietary antioxidants. *Journal of Applied Physiology* 1999;86(6):1817–22.

Carson C, Lee S, De Paola C, et al. Antioxidant intake and cataract in the Melbourne Visual Impairment Project [abstract]. *American Journal of Epidemiology* 1994;139 (suppl 11):A65.

Cefalu WT, Bell-Farrow AD, Wang ZQ, Sonntag WE, Fu MX, Baynes JW, Thorpe SR. Caloric restriction decreases age-dependent accumulation of the glycoxidation products, N epsilon-(carboxymethyl)lysine and pentosidine, in rat skin collagen. *Journals of Gerontology; Series A, Biological Sciences and Medical Sciences* 1995; 50(6):B337–41.

Chainani-Wu N. Safety and anti-inflammatory activity of curcumin: a component of turmeric (*Curcuma longa*). *Journal of Alternative and Complementary Medicine* 2003; 9(1):161–68. Review.

Chan KY, Boucher ES, Gandhi PJ, Silva MA. HMG-CoA reductase inhibitors for lowering elevated levels of C-reactive protein. *American Journal of Health-System Pharmacy* 2004;61(16):1676–81. Review.

Chan MM. Inhibition of tumor necrosis factor by curcumin, a phytochemical. *Biochemical Pharmacology* 1995;49(11):1551–56.

Chan MM, Huang HI, Fenton MR, Fong D. In vivo inhibition of nitric oxide synthase gene expression by curcumin, a cancer preventive natural product with anti-inflammatory properties. *Biochemical Pharmacology* 1998;55(12):1955–62.

Chauhan DP. Chemotherapeutic potential of curcumin for colorectal cancer. *Current Pharmaceutical Design* 2002;8(19):1695–706. Review.

Chernomorsky S, Segelman A, Poretz RD. Effect of dietary chlorophyll derivatives on mutagenesis and tumor cell growth. *Teratogenesis, Carcinogenesis, and Mutagenesis* 1999;19(5):313–22.

Chew GT, Watts GF. Coenzyme Q_{10} and diabetic endotheliopathy: oxidative stress and the 'recoupling hypothesis.' *QJM.* 2004;97(8):537–48. Review.

Chitchumroonchokchai C, Bomser JA, Glamm JE, Failla ML. Xanthophylls and alpha-tocopherol decrease UVB-induced lipid peroxidation and stress signaling in human lens epithelial cells. *Journal of Nutrition* 2004;134(12):3225–32.

Clancy SP, Clarkson PM, DeCheke ME, Nosaka K, Freedson PS, Cunningham JJ, Valentine B. Effects of chromium picolinate supplementation on body composition, strength, and urinary chromium loss in football players. *International Journal of Sport Nutrition* 1994;4(2):142–53.

Conney AH, Lysz T, Ferraro T, Abidi TF, Manchand PS, Laskin JD, Huang MT. Inhibitory effect of curcumin and some related dietary compounds on tumor promotion and arachidonic acid metabolism in mouse skin. *Advances in Enzyme Regulation* 1991;31:385–96.

Crane FL. Biochemical functions of coenzyme Q_{10}. *Journal of the American College of Nutrition* 2001;20(6):591–98. Review.

Curran-Celentano J, Hammond BR Jr., Ciulla TA, Cooper DA, Pratt LM, Danis RB. Relation between dietary intake, serum concentrations, and retinal concentrations of lutein and zeaxanthin in adults in a Midwest population. *American Journal of Clinical Nutrition* 2001;74(6):796–802.

Curtis CL, Hughes CD, Flannery CR, Little CB, Harwood JL, Caterson B. N-3 fatty acids specifically modulate catabolic factors involved in articular cartilage degradation. *Journal of Biological Chemistry* 2000;275:721–24.

Curtis CL, Rees SG, Little CB, Flannery CR, Hughes CE, Wilson C, Dent CM, Otterness IG, Harwood JL, Caterson B. Pathologic indicators of degradation and inflammation in human osteoarthritic cartilage are abrogated by exposure to n-3 fatty acids. *Arthritis and Rheumatism* 2002;46:1544–53.

D'Anci KE, Rosenberg IH. Folate and brain function in the elderly. *Current Opinion in Clinical Nutrition and Metabolic Care* 2004;7(6):659–64. Review.

Dashwood RH, Breinholt V, Bailey GS. Chemopreventive properties of chlorophyllin: inhibition of aflatoxin B1 (AFB1)-DNA binding in vivo and antimutagenic activity against AFB1 and two heterocyclic amines in the *Salmonella* mutagenicity assay. *Carcinogenesis* 1991;12:939–42.

Dauer A, Hensel A, Lhoste E, Knasmuller S, Mersch-Sundermann V. Genotoxic and antigenotoxic effects of catechin and tannins from the bark of *Hamamelis virginiana L.* in metabolically competent, human hepatoma cells (Hep G2) using single cell gel electrophoresis. *Phytochemistry* 2003;63(2):199–207.

Deodhar SD, Sethi R, Srimal RC. Preliminary study on antirheumatic activity of curcumin (diferuloyl methane). *Indian Journal of Medical Research* 71:632–34.

Divecha H, Sattar N, Rumley A, Cherry L, Lowe GD, Sturrock R. Cardiovascular risk parameters in men with ankylosing spondylitis in comparison to non-inflammatory control subjects: relevance of systemic inflammation. *Clinical Science (London)* 2005;109(2):171–76. [Epub ahead of print]

Dooper MM, Wassink L, M'Rabet L, Graus YM. The modulatory effects of prostaglandin-E on cytokine production by human peripheral blood mononuclear cells are independent of the prostaglandin subtype. Immunology 2002; 107:152–59.

Dorai T, Cao YC, Dorai B, Buttyan R, Katz AE. Therapeutic potential of curcumin in human prostate cancer. III. Curcumin inhibits proliferation, induces apoptosis, and inhibits angiogenesis of LNCaP prostate cancer cells in vivo. *Prostate* 2001; 47(4):293–303.

Duan CL, Qiao SY, Wang NL, Zhao YM, Qi CH, Yao XS. [Studies on the active polysaccharides from *Lycium barbarum* L.] *Yao Xue Xue Bao.* 2001;36(3):196–99. Chinese.

Durak I, Avci A, Kacmaz M, Buyukkocak S, Cimen MY, Elgun S, Ozturk HS. Comparison of antioxidant potentials of red wine, white wine, grape juice and alcohol. *Current Medical Research and Opinion* 1999;15(4):316–20.

Duvoix A, Blasius R, Delhalle S, Schnekenburger M, Morceau F, Henry E, Dicato M, Diederich M. Chemopreventive and therapeutic effects of curcumin. *Cancer Letters* 2005;223(2):181–90. Epub 2004 Nov 11. Review.

Duvoix A, Morceau F, Delhalle S, Schmitz M, Schnekenburger M, Galteau MM, Dicato M, Diederich M. Induction of apoptosis by curcumin: mediation by glutathione S-transferase P1-1 inhibition. *Biochemical Pharmacology* 2003;66(8): 1475–83.

Elias MF, Robbins MA, Budge MM, Elias PK, Brennan SL, Johnston C, Nagy Z, Bates CJ. Homocysteine, folate, and vitamins B_6 and B_{12} blood levels in relation to cognitive performance: the Maine-Syracuse study. *Psychosomatic Medicine* 2006; 68(4):547–54.

Engler MM, Engler MB, Malloy M, Chiu E, Besio D, Paul S, Stuehlinger M, Morrow J, Ridker P, Rifai N, Mietus-Snyder M. Docosahexaenoic acid restores endothelial function in children with hyperlipidemia: results from the EARLY study. *International Journal of Clinical Pharmacology and Therapeutics* 2004;42(12):672–79.

Erkkila AT, Lichtenstein AH, Mozaffarian D, Herrington DM. Fish intake is associated with a reduced progression of coronary artery atherosclerosis in postmenopausal women with coronary artery disease. *American Journal of Clinical Nutrition* 2004;80(3):626–32.

Evans JL, Goldfine ID. Alpha-lipoic acid: a multifunctional antioxidant that improves insulin sensitivity in patients with type 2 diabetes. *Diabetes Technology & Therapeutics* 2000;2(3):401–13. Review.

Fahey JW, Zhang Y, Talalay P. Broccoli sprouts: an exceptionally rich source of inducers of enzymes that protect against chemical carcinogens. *Proceedings of the National Academy of the Sciences of the United States of America* 1997;94(19):10367–72.

Fisher ND, Hughes M, Gerhard-Herman M, Hollenberg NK. Flavanol-rich cocoa induces nitric-oxide-dependent vasodilation in healthy humans. *Journal of Hypertension* 2003;21(12):2281–86.

Frances FJ. Pigments and other colorants. In OR Fennema (ed.): *Food Chemistry*, 2nd ed. Marcel Dekker, Inc, New York, 1985.

Flagg EW, Coates RJ, Greenberg RS. Epidemiologic studies of antioxidants and cancer in humans. *Journal of the American College of Nutrition* 1995;14:419–27.

Flower RJ, Perretti M. Controlling inflammation: a fat chance? [editorial] *Journal of Experimental Medicine* 2005;201:671–74.

Freedman JE, Parker C III, Li L, Perlman JA, Frei B, Ivanov V, Deak LR, Iafrati MD, Folts JD. Select flavonoids and whole juice from purple grapes inhibit platelet function and enhance nitric oxide release. *Circulation* 2001;103:2792–98.

Frieling UM, Schaumberg DA, Kupper TS, Muntwyler J, Hennekens CH. A randomized, 12-year primary-prevention trial of beta carotene supplementation for nonmelanoma skin cancer in the physician's health study. *Archives of Dermatology* 2000;136:179–84.

Fu M-X, Réquéna JR, Jenkins AJ, Lyons TJ, Baynes JW, Thorpe SR. The advanced glycation end-product, Ne-(carboxymethyl)lysine, is a product of both lipid peroxidation and glycoxidation reactions. *Journal of Biological Chemistry* 1996;271: 9982–86.

Fu MX, Wells-Knecht KJ, Blackledge JA, Lyons TJ, Thorpe SR, Baynes JW. Glycation, glycoxidation, and cross-linking of collagen by glucose. Kinetics, mechanisms, and inhibition of late stages of the Maillard reaction, *Diabetes* 1994;43(5):676–83.

Fuchs J, Milbradt R. Antioxidant inhibition of skin inflammation induced by reactive oxidants: evaluation of the redox couple dihydrolipoate/lipoate. *Skin Pharmacology* 1994;7(5):278–84.

Galli RL, Shukitt-Hale B, Youdim KA, Joseph JA. Fruit polyphenolics and brain aging: nutritional interventions targeting age-related neuronal and behavioral deficits. *Annals of the New York Academy of Sciences* 2002;959:128–32. Review.

Genser D, Prachar H, Hauer R, Halbmayer WM, Mlczoch J, Elmadfa I. Homocysteine, folate and vitamin B(12) in patients with coronary heart disease. *Annals of Nutrition & Metabolism* 2006;50(5):413–19. [Epub ahead of print]

Gil MI, Tomas-Barberan FA, Hess-Pierce B, Holcroft DM, Kader AA. Antioxidant activity of pomegranate juice and its relationship with phenolic composition and processing. *Journal of Agricultural and Food Chemistry* 2000;48(10):4581–89.

Gilroy DJ, Kauffman KW, Hall RA, Huang X, Chu FS. Assessing potential health risks from microcystin toxins in blue-green algae dietary supplements. *Environmental Health Perspectives* 2000;108(5):435–39.

Giovannucci E. Tomatoes, tomato-based products, lycopene, and cancer: review of the epidemiologic literature. *Journal of the National Cancer Institute* 1999;91:317–31.

Goldberg J, Flowerdew G, Smith E, Brody JA, Tso MO. Factors associated with age-related macular degeneration. An analysis of data from the first National Health and Nutrition Examination Survey. *American Journal of Epidemiology* 1988; 128:700–10.

Gorman C, Park A. The fires within. *Time.* Monday, February 23, 2004.

Grant KE, Chandler RM, Castle AL, Ivy JL. Chromium and exercise training: effect on obese women. *Medicine and Science in Sports and Exercise* 1997;29(8):992–98.

Haag M. Essential fatty acids and the brain. *Canadian Journal of Psychiatry* 2003;48: 195–203.

Hackett AM. In Cody V, Middleton EJ Jr., Harborne JB (eds.): *Plant Flavonoids in Biology and Medicine: Biochemical, Pharmacological, and Structure-activity Relationships.* New York: Liss 1986, pp. 177–94.

Hagen TM, Liu J, Lykkesfeldt J, Wehr CM, Ingersoll RT, Vinarsky V, Bartholomew JC, Ames BN. Feeding acetyl-L-carnitine and lipoic acid to old rats significantly improves metabolic function while decreasing oxidative stress. *Proceedings of the National Academy of the Sciences of the United States of America* 2000;99(4):1870–75. Erratum in *Proceedings of the National Academy of the Sciences in the United States of America* 2002;99(10):7184.

Hagen TM, Moreau R, Suh JH, Visioli F. Mitochondrial decay in the aging rat heart: evidence for improvement by dietary supplementation with acetyl-L-carnitine and/or lipoic acid. *Annals of the New York Academy of Sciences* 2002;959:491–507. Review.

Hager K, Marahrens A, Kenklies M, Riederer P, Munch G. Alpha-lipoic acid as a new treatment option for Alzheimer type dementia. *Archives of Gerontology and Geriatrics* 2001;32(3):275–82.

Han B, Jaurequi J, Tang BW, Nimni ME. Proanthocyanidin: a natural crosslinking reagent for stabilizing collagen matrices. *Journal of Biomedical Materials Research, Part A* 2003;65(1):118–24.

Han D, Handelman G, Marcocci L, Sen CK, Roy S, Kobuchi H, Tritschler HJ, Flohe L, Packer L. Lipoic acid increases de novo synthesis of cellular glutathione by improving cystine utilization. *Biofactors* 1997;6(3):321–38.

Han G, Duan Y. [Advances in pharmacological study of natural active polysaccharides in China]. *Zhong Yao Cai* 2003;26(2):138–41. Review. Chinese.

Han SS, Keum YS, Seo HJ, Surh YJ. Curcumin suppresses activation of NF-kappaB and AP-1 induced by phorbol ester in cultured human promyelocytic leukemia cells. *Journal of Biochemistry and Molecular Biology* 2002;35(3):337–42.

Haramaki N, Assadnazari H, Zimmer G, Schepkin V, Packer L. The influence of vitamin E and dihydro-lipoic acid on cardiac energy and glutathione status under hypoxia-reoxygenation. *Biochemistry and Molecular Biology International* 1995;37(3): 591–97.

Haramaki N, Packer L, Assadnazari H, Zimmer G. Cardiac recovery during post-ischemic reperfusion is improved by combination of vitamin E with dihydro-lipoic acid. *Biochemical and Biophysical Research Communications* 1993;196(3):1101–7.

Harman D. Nutritional implications of the free-radical theory of aging. *Journal of the American College of Nutrition* 1982;1(1):27–34.

Hasegawa T, Matsuguchi T, Noda K, Tanaka K, Kumamoto S, Shoyama Y, Yoshikai Y. Toll-like receptor 2 is at least partly involved in the antitumor activity of glyco-protein from *Chlorella vulgaris*. *International Immunopharmacology* 2002;2(4):579–89.

Hasegawa T, Okuda M, Makino M, Hiromatsu K, Nomoto K, Yoshikai Y. Hot water ex-tracts of *Chlorella vulgaris* reduce opportunistic infection with *Listeria* monocyto-genes in C57BL/6 mice infected with LP-BM5 murine leukemia viruses. *International Journal of Immunopharmacology* 1995;17(6):505–12.

Hayashi K, Hayashi T, Morita N, Kajima I. An extract from *Spirulina platensis* is a selec-tive inhibitor of herpes simplex virus type 1 penetration into HeLa cells. *Phytotherapy Research* 1993;7:76–80.

Hayashi O, Katoh T, Okuwaki Y. Enhancement of antibody production in mice by di-etary *Spirulina platensis*. *Journal of Nutritional Science and Vitaminology* 1994;40:431–41.

Hayashi T, Hayashi K. Calcium spirulan, an inhibitor of enveloped virus replication, from a blue-green alga *Spirulina platensis*. *Journal of Natural Products* 1996;59:83–87.

Heeschen C, Dimmeler S, Hamm CW, Fichtlscherer S, Boersma E, Simoons ML, Zei-her AM; CAPTURE Study Investigators. Serum level of the antiinflammatory cytokine interleukin-10 is an important prognostic determinant in patients with acute coronary syndromes. *Circulation* 2003;107(16):2109–14. Epub 2003 Mar 31.

Hennekens CH, Buring JE, Manson JE, et al. Lack of effect of long-term supplemen-tation with beta carotene on the incidence of malignant neoplasms and car-diovascular disease. *New England Journal of Medicine* 1996;334:1145–49.

Hensley K, Robinson KA, Gabbita SP, Salsman S, Floyd RA. Reactive oxygen species, cell signaling, and cell injury. *Free Radical Biology & Medicine* 2000;28(10):1456–62. Review.

Herbal/plant therapies: turmeric (*Curcuma longa* Linn.) and curcumin. University of Texas MD Anderson Cancer Center, 2002 (updated May 2004). Accessed Febru-ary 18, 2006, at http://www.mdanderson.org/departments/cimer/display.cfm?id=fa324b1c-b0ca-4e93-903082f85808558f&method=displayfull&pn=6eb86a59-ebd9-11d4-810100508b603a14.

Hernandez-Corona A, Nieves I, Meckes M, Chamorro G, Barron BL. Antiviral activity of *Spirulina maxima* against herpes simplex virus type 2. *Antiviral Research* 2002;56(3):279–85.

Higuera-Ciapara I, Felix-Valenzuela L, Goycoolea FM. Astaxanthin: a review of its chemistry and applications. *Critical Reviews in Food Science and Nutrition* 2006;46(2):185–96.

Hix LM, Lockwood SF, Bertram JS. Bioactive carotenoids: potent antioxidants and regulators of gene expression. *Redox Report: Communications in Free Radical Research* 2004;9(4):181–91.

Hoffmeister A, Rothenbacher D, Kunze M, Brenner H, Koenig W. Prognostic value of inflammatory markers alone and in combination with blood lipids in patients with stable coronary artery disease. *European Journal of Internal Medicine* 2005; 16(1):47–52.

Hofmann M, Mainka P, Tritschler H, Fuchs J, Zimmer G. Decrease of red cell membrane fluidity and -SH groups due to hyperglycemic conditions is counteracted by alpha-lipoic acid. *Archives of Biochemistry and Biophysics* 1995;324(1): 85–92.

Holick CN, Michaud DS, Stolzenberg-Solomon R, Mayne ST, Pietinen P, Taylor PR, Virtamo J, Albanes D. Dietary carotenoids, serum beta-carotene, and retinol and risk of lung cancer in the alpha-tocopherol, beta-carotene cohort study. *American Journal of Epidemiology* 2002;156(6):536–47.

Hollenberg NK. Flavanols and cardiovascular health: what is the evidence for chocolate and red wine? American Heart Association Scientific Sessions, Unofficial Satellite Symposium, Nov. 11, 2001, Anaheim, CA.

Hou DX. Potential mechanisms of cancer chemoprevention by anthocyanins. *Current Molecular Medicine* 2003;3(2):149–59. Review.

Hou DX, Kai K, Li JJ, Lin S, Terahara N, Wakamatsu M, Fujii M, Young MR, Colburn N. Anthocyanidins inhibit activator protein 1 activity and cell transformation: structure-activity relationship and molecular mechanisms. *Carcinogenesis* 2004; 25(1):29–36. Epub 2003 Sep 26.

Howell AB. Cranberry proanthocyanidins and the maintenance of urinary tract health. *Critical Reviews in Food Science and Nutrition* 2002;42(suppl 3):273–78. Review.

Howell AB, Foxman B. Cranberry juice and adhesion of antibiotic-resistant uropathogens. *JAMA* 2002;287(23):3082–83. No abstract available.

Hussein G, Sankawa U, Goto H, Matsumoto K, Watanabe H. Astaxanthin, a carotenoid with potential in human health and nutrition. *Journal of Natural Products* 2006;69(3):443–49. Review.

Ito H, Kobayashi E, Takamatsu Y, Li SH, Hatano T, Sakagami H, Kusama K, Satoh K, Sugita D, Shimura S, Itoh Y, Yoshida T. Polyphenols from *Eriobotrya japonica* and their cytotoxicity against human oral tumor cell lines. *Chemical & Pharmaceutical Bulletin (Tokyo)*. 2000;48(5):687–93.

Ito Y, Gajalakshmi KC, Sasaki R, Suzuki K, Shanta V. A study on serum carotenoid levels in breast cancer patients of Indian women in Chennai (Madras), India. *Journal of Epidemiology* 1999;9(5):306–14.

Iwata K, Inayama T, Kato T. Effects of *Spirulina platensis* on plasma lipoprotein lipase activity in fructose-induced hyperlipidemic rats. *Journal of Nutritional Science and Vitaminology* 1990;36:165–71.

Jacob S, Henriksen EJ, Tritschler HJ, Augustin HJ, Dietze GJ. Improvement of insulin-stimulated glucose-disposal in type 2 diabetes after repeated parenteral administration of thioctic acid. *Experimental and Clinical Endocrinology & Diabetes*. 1996;104(3):284–88.

Jang M, Pezzuto JM. Cancer chemopreventive activity of resveratrol. *Drugs Under Experimental and Clinical Research* 1999;25(2–3):65–77.

Jeppesen J, Hein HO, Suadicani P, Gyntelberg F. Relation of high TG-low HDL choles-terol and LDL cholesterol to the incidence of ischemic heart disease. An 8-year follow-up in the Copenhagen Male Study. *Arteriosclerosis Thrombosis, and Vascular Biology* 1997;17(6):1114–20.

Jobin C, Bradham CA, Russo MP, Juma B, Narula AS, Brenner DA, Sartor RB. Cur-cumin blocks cytokine-mediated NF-kappa B activation and proinflammatory gene expression by inhibiting inhibitory factor I-kappa B kinase activity. *Journal of Immunology* 1999;163(6):3474–83.

Kaats GR, Blum K, Fisher JA, Adelman JA. Effects of chromium picolinate supple-mentation on body composition: a randomized, double-masked, placebo-controlled study. *Current Therapeutic Research* 1996;57:747–56.

Kaats GR, Blum K, Pullin D, Keith SC, Wood R. A randomized, double-masked, placebo-controlled study of the effects of chromium picolinate supplementa-tion on body composition: a replication and extension of a previous study. *Current Therapeutic Research* 1998;59:379–88.

Kagan VE, Shvedova A, Serbinova E, Khan S, Swanson C, Powell R, Packer L. Dihy-drolipoic acid—a universal antioxidant both in the membrane and in the aqueous phase. Reduction of peroxyl, ascorbyl and chromanoxyl radicals. *Bio-chemical Pharmacology* 1992;44(8):1637–49.

Kahler W, Kuklinski B, Ruhlmann C, Plotz C. Diabetes mellitus—a free radical–asso-ciated disease. Results of adjuvant antioxidant supplementation. *Zeitschrift für die gesamte innere Medizin und ihre Grenzgebiete* 1993;48(5):223–32.

Kakegawa H, Matsumoto H, Endo K, Satoh T, Nonaka G, Nishioka I. Inhibitory ef-fects of tannins on hyaluronidase activation and on the degranulation from rat mesentry mast cells. *Chemical & Pharmaceutical Bulletin* 1985;33(11):5079–82.

Kalmijn S. Fatty acid intake and the risk of dementia and cognitive decline: a review of clinical and epidemiological studies. *Journal of Nutrition, Health & Aging* 2000;4: 202–7.

Kang G, Kong PJ, Yuh YJ, Lim SY, Yim SV, Chun W, Kim SS. Curcumin suppresses lipopolysaccharide-induced cyclooxygenase-2 expression by inhibiting activa-tor protein 1 and nuclear factor kappaB bindings in BV2 microglial cells. *Journal of Pharmacological Sciences* 2004;94(3):325–28.

Kaplan M, Hayek T, Raz A, Coleman R, Dornfeld L, Vaya J, Aviram M. Pomegranate juice supplementation to atherosclerotic mice reduces macrophage lipid per-oxidation, cellular cholesterol accumulation and development of atheroscle-rosis. *Journal of Nutrition* 2001;131(8):2082–89.

Karunagaran D, Rashmi R, Kumar TR. Induction of apoptosis by curcumin and its implications for cancer therapy. *Current Cancer Drug Targets.* 2005;5(2):117–29. Review.

Keck AS, Finley JW. Cruciferous vegetables: cancer protective mechanisms of glu-cosinolate hydrolysis products and selenium. *Integrative Cancer Therapies* 2004; 3(1):5–12.

Kempaiah RK, Srinivasan K. Beneficial influence of dietary curcumin, capsaicin and garlic on erythrocyte integrity in high-fat fed rats. *Journal of Nutritional Biochemistry* 2006;17(7):471–78. [Epub ahead of print]

Kempaiah RK, Srinivasan K. Influence of dietary spices on the fluidity of erythrocytes in hypercholesterolaemic rats. *British Journal of Nutrition* 2005;93(1):81–91.

Khor TO, Keum YS, Lin W, Kim JH, Hu R, Shen G, Xu C, Gopalakrishnan A, Reddy B, Zheng X, Conney AH, Kong AN. Combined inhibitory effects of curcumin and phenethyl isothiocyanate on the growth of human PC-3 prostate xenografts in immunodeficient mice. *Cancer Research* 2006;66(2):613–21.

Kilic F, Handelman GJ, Serbinova E, Packer L, Trevithick JR. Modelling cortical cataractogenesis 17: in vitro effect of a-lipoic acid on glucose-induced lens membrane damage, a model of diabetic cataractogenesis. *Biochemistry and Molecular Biology International* 1995;37(2):361–70.

Kilic F, Handelman GJ, Traber K, Tsang K, Packer L, Trevithick JR. Modelling cortical cataractogenesis XX. In vitro effect of alpha-lipoic acid on glutathione concentrations in lens in model diabetic cataractogenesis. *Biochemistry and Molecular Biology International* 1998;46(3):585–95.

Kim HM, Lee EH, Cho HH, Moon YH. Inhibitory effect of mast cell-mediated immediate-type allergic reactions in rats by spirulina. *Biochemical Pharmacology* 1998; 55(7):1071–76.

Kim ND, Mehta R, Yu W, Neeman I, Livney T, Amichay A, Poirier D, Nicholls P, Kirby A, Jiang W, Mansel R, Ramachandran C, Rabi T, Kaplan B, Lansky E. Chemopreventive and adjuvant therapeutic potential of pomegranate (*Punica granatum*) for human breast cancer. *Breast Cancer Research and Treatment* 2002;71(3):203–17.

Kim YJ, Kim HJ, No JK, Chung HY, Fernandes G. Anti-inflammatory action of dietary fish oil and calorie restriction. *Life Sciences* 2006;78(21):2523–32. Epub 2006 Jan 24.

Kim YJ, Yokozawa T, Chung HY. Effects of energy restriction and fish oil supplementation on renal guanidino levels and antioxidant defences in aged lupus-prone B/W mice. *British Journal of Nutrition* 2005;93(6):835–44.

Kim YJ, Yokozawa T, Chung HY. Suppression of oxidative stress in aging NZB/NZW mice: effect of fish oil feeding on hepatic antioxidant status and guanidino compounds. *Free Radical Research* 2005;39(10):1101–10.

Kim YS, Milner JA. Targets for indole-3-carbinol in cancer prevention. *Journal of Nutritional Biochemistry* 2005;16(2):65–73. Review.

Knight JA. The biochemistry of aging. *Advances in Clinical Chemistry* 2000;35:1–62. Review.

Kocak G, Aktan F, Canbolat O, Ozogul C, Elbeg S, Yildizoglu-Ari N, Karasu C. Alpha-lipoic acid treatment ameliorates metabolic parameters, blood pressure, vascular reactivity and morphology of vessels already damaged by streptozotocin-diabetes. *Diabetes, Nutrition & Metabolism* 2000;13(6):308–18.

Kodentsova VM, Gmoshinskii IV, Vrzhesinskaia OA, Beketova NA, Kharitonchik LA,

Nizov AA, Mazo VK. [Use of the microalgae *Spirulina platensis* and its selenium-containing form in nutrition of patients with nonspecific ulcerative colitis]. *Voprosy Pitaniia* 2001;70(5):17–21. Russian.

Kohlmeier L, Weterings KGC, Steck S, Kok FJ. Tea and cancer prevention: an evaluation of the epidemiologic literature. *Nutrition and Cancer* 1997;27:1–13.

Kollar P, Hotolova H. [Biological effects of resveratrol and other constituents of wine]. *Ceskaa Slovenska farmacie* 2003;52(6):272–81. Review. Czech.

Konishi F, Mitsuyama M, Okuda M, Tanaka K, Hasegawa T, Nomoto K. Protective effect of an acidic glycoprotein obtained from culture of *Chlorella vulgaris* against myelosuppression by 5-fluorouracil. *Cancer Immunology, Immunotherapy* 1996;42:268–74.

Konishi F, Tanaka K, Kumamoto S, et al. Enhanced resistance against *Escherichia coli* infection by subcutaneous administration of the hot-water extract of *Chlorella vulgaris* in cyclophosphamide-treated mice. *Cancer Immunology and Immunotherapy* 1990;32:1–7.

Kotrbacek V, Halouzka R, Jurajda V, Knotkova Z, Filka J. [Increased immune response in broilers after administration of natural food supplements. *Veterinární medicína* 1994;39(6):321–28. Czech.

Kozlov AV, Gille L, Staniek K, Nohl H. Dihydro-lipoic acid maintains ubiquinone in the antioxidant active form by two-electron reduction of ubiquinone and one-electron reduction of ubisemiquinone. *Archives of Biochemistry and Biophysics* 1999;363(1):148–54.

Krinsky NI. Micronutrients and their influence on mutagenicity and malignant transformation. *Annals of the New York Academy of Sciences* 1993;686:229–42. Review.

Krinsky NI, Landrum JT, Bone RA. Biologic mechanisms of the protective role of lutein and zeaxanthin in the eye. *Annual Review of Nutrition* 2003;23:171–201. Epub Feb 27, 2003.

Kris-Etherton PM, Keen CL. Evidence that the antioxidant flavonoids in tea and cocoa are beneficial for cardiovascular health. *Current Opinion in Lipidology* 2002;13(1):41–49. Review.

Krishnaswamy K, Polasa K. Diet, nutrition & cancer—the Indian scenario. *Indian Journal of Medical Research* 1995;102:200–9. Review.

Kumar AP, Garcia GE, Ghosh R, Rajnarayanan RV, Alworth WL, Slaga TJ. 4-Hydroxy-3-methoxybenzoic acid methyl ester: a curcumin derivative targets Akt/NF kappa B cell survival signaling pathway: potential for prostate cancer management. *Neoplasia* 2003;5(3):255–66.

Kunt T, Forst I, Wilhelm A, Tritschler H, Pfuetzner A, Harzer O, Engelbach M, Zschaebitz A, Stoft E, Beyer J. Alpha-lipoic acid reduces expression of vascular cell adhesion molecule-1 and endothelial adhesion of human monocytes after stimulation with advanced glycation end products. *Clinical Science* (London) 1999;96(1):75–82.

Kuttan R, Donnelly PV, Di Ferrante N. Collagen treated with (+)-catechin becomes resistant to the action of mammalian collagenases. *Experientia* 1981;37(3):221–23.

La Vecchia C, Tavani A. Fruit and vegetables, and human cancer. *European Journal of Cancer Prevention* 1998;7(1):3–8. Review.

Lai C-N. Chlorophyll: the active factor in wheat sprout extract inhibiting the metabolic activation of carcinogens in vitro. *Nutrition and Cancer* 1979;1:19–21.

Lai C-N, Dabney BJ, Shaw CR. Inhibition of in vitro metabolic activation of carcinogens by wheat sprout extracts. *Nutrition and Cancer.* 1978;1:27–30.

Lambert JD, Hong J, Yang GY, Liao J, Yang CS. Inhibition of carcinogenesis by polyphenols: evidence from laboratory investigations. *American Journal of Clinical Nutrition* 2005;81(suppl 1):284S–91S. Review.

Lamson DW, Brignall MS. Antioxidants and cancer, part 3: quercetin. *Alternative Medicine Review* 2000;5(3):196–208. Review.

Lamson DW, Plaza SM. Mitochondrial factors in the pathogenesis of diabetes: a hypothesis for treatment. *Alternative Medicine Review* 2002;7(2):94–111. Review.

Lapenna D, Ciofani G, Pierdomenico SD, Giamberardino MA, Cuccurullo F. Dihydrolipoic acid inhibits 15-lipoxygenase-dependent lipid peroxidation. *Free Radical Biology & Medicine* 2003;35(10):1203–9.

Lavrovsky Y, Chatterjee B, Clark RA, Roy AK. Role of redox-regulated transcription factors in inflammation, aging and age-related diseases. *Experimental Gerontology* 2000;35(5):521–32. Review.

Lee EH, Faulhaber D, Hanson KM, Ding W, Peters S, Kodali S, Granstein RD. Dietary lutein reduces ultraviolet radiation-induced inflammation and immunosuppression. *Journal of Investigative Dermatology* 2004;122(2):510–17.

Lee IM, Cook NR, Manson JE, et al. Beta-carotene supplementation and incidence of cancer and cardiovascular disease: the Women's Health Study. *Journal of the National Cancer Institute* 1999;91:2102–6.

Lee KW, Kim YJ, Kim DO, Lee HJ, Lee CY. Major phenolics in apple and their contribution to the total antioxidant capacity. *Journal of Agricultural and Food Chemistry* 2003;51(22):6516–20.

Lee KW, Kim YJ, Lee HJ, Lee CY. Cocoa has more phenolic phytochemicals and a higher antioxidant capacity than teas and red wine. *Journal of Agricultural and Food Chemistry* 2003;51(25):7292–95.

Lenaz G, D'Aurelio M, Merlo Pich M, Genova ML, Ventura B, Bovina C, Formiggini G, Parenti Castelli G. Mitochondrial bioenergetics in aging. *Biochimica et Biophysica Acta.* 2000;1459(2–3):397–404. Review.

Leu TH, Maa MC. The molecular mechanisms for the antitumorigenic effect of curcumin. *Current Medical Chemistry Anticancer Agents* 2002;2(3):357–70. Review.

Levy BD, Clish CB, Schmidt B, Gronert K, Serhan CN. Lipid mediator class switching during acute inflammation: signals in resolution. *Nature Immunology* 2001;2: 612–19.

Li L, Aggarwal BB, Shishodia S, Abbruzzese J, Kurzrock R. Nuclear factor-kappaB and

IkappaB kinase are constitutively active in human pancreatic cells, and their down-regulation by curcumin (diferuloylmethane) is associated with the suppression of proliferation and the induction of apoptosis. *Cancer* 2004;101(10): 2351–62.

Li WG, Zhang XY, Wu YJ, Tian X. Anti-inflammatory effect and mechanism of proanthocyanidins from grape seeds. *Acta pharmacologica Sinica* 2001;22(12):1117–20.

Liacini A, Sylvester J, Li WQ, Huang W, Dehnade F, Ahmad M, Zafarullah M. Induction of matrix metalloproteinase-13 gene expression by TNF-alpha is mediated by MAP kinases, AP-1, and NF-kappaB transcription factors in articular chondrocytes. *Experimental Cell Research* 2003;288(1):208–17.

Lim GP, Chu T, Yang F, Beech W, Frautschy SA, Cole GM. The curry spice curcumin reduces oxidative damage and amyloid pathology in an Alzheimer transgenic mouse. *Journal of Neuroscience* 2001;21(21):8370–77.

Lin JK, Lin-Shiau SY. Mechanisms of cancer chemoprevention by curcumin. *Proceedings of the National Science Council, Republic of China: Part B, Life Sciences* 2001;25(2): 59–66. Review.

Lin JK, Pan MH, Lin-Shiau SY. Recent studies on the biofunctions and biotransformations of curcumin. *Biofactors* 2000;13(1–4):153–58. Review.

Lin Y, Rajala MW, Berger JP, Moller DE, Barzilai N, Scherer PE. Hyperglycemia-induced production of acute phase reactants in adipose tissue. *Journal of Biological Chemistry* 2001;276(45):42077–83.

Linetsky M, James HL, Ortwerth BJ. Spontaneous generation of superoxide anion by human lens proteins and by calf lens proteins ascorbylated in vitro. *Experimental Eye Research* 1999;69(2):239–48.

Liu J, Atamna H, Kuratsune H, Ames BN. Delaying brain mitochondrial decay and aging with mitochondrial antioxidants and metabolites. *Annals of the New York Academy of Sciences* 2002;959:133–66. Review.

Liu J, Head E, Gharib AM, Yuan W, Ingersoll RT, Hagen TM, Cotman CW, Ames BN. Memory loss in old rats is associated with brain mitochondrial decay and RNA/DNA oxidation: partial reversal by feeding acetyl-L-carnitine and/or R-alpha-lipoic acid. *Proceedings of the National Academy of Sciences of the United States of America* 2002;99(4):2356–61.

Liu J, Killilea DW, Ames BN. Age-associated mitochondrial oxidative decay: improvement of carnitine acetyltransferase substrate-binding affinity and activity in brain by feeding old rats acetyl-L-carnitine and/or R-alpha-lipoic acid. *Proceedings of the National Academy of Sciences of the United States of America* 2002;99(4): 1876–81.

Liu XL, Sun JY, Li HY, Zhang L, Qian BC. [Extraction and isolation of active component for inhibiting PC3 cell proliferation in vitro from the fruit of *Lycium barbarum* L.]. Zhongguo Zhong Yao Za Zhi. 2000;25(8):481–83. Chinese.

Livolsi JM, Adams GM, Laguna PL. The effect of chromium picolinate on muscular strength and body composition in women athletes. *Journal of Strength and Conditioning Research* 2001;15(2):161–66.

Lockwood SF, Gross GJ. Disodium disuccinate astaxanthin (Cardax): antioxidant and antiinflammatory cardioprotection. *Cardiovascular Drug Reviews* 2005;23(3): 199–216. Review.

Lopez-Garcia E, Schulze MB, Manson JE, Meigs JB, Albert CM, Rifai N, Willett WC, Hu FB. Consumption of (n-3) fatty acids is related to plasma biomarkers of inflammation and endothelial activation in women. *Journal of Nutrition* 2004;134(7): 1806–11.

Lopez-Garcia E, Schulze MB, Meigs JB, Manson JE, Rifai N, Stampfer MJ, Willett WC, Hu FB. Consumption of trans fatty acids is related to plasma biomarkers of inflammation and endothelial dysfunction. *Journal of Nutrition* 2005;135(3):562–66.

Lopez-Velez M, Martinez-Martinez F, Del Valle-Ribes C. The study of phenolic compounds as natural antioxidants in wine. *Critical Reviews in Food Science and Nutrition* 2003;43(3):233–44. Review.

Lovell MA, Xie C, Xiong S, Markesbery WR. Protection against amyloid beta peptide and iron/hydrogen peroxide toxicity by alpha lipoic acid. *Journal of Alzheimer's Disease* 2003;5(3):229–39.

Lugasi A, Hovari J. Antioxidant properties of commercial alcoholic and nonalcoholic beverages. *Die Nahrung.* 2003;47(2):79–86.

Luo Q, Yan J, Zhang S. [Effects of pure and crude *Lycium barbarum* polysaccharides on immunopharmacology]. *Zhong Yao Cai* 1999;22(5):246–49. Chinese.

Luo Q, Yan J, Zhang S. [Isolation and purification of *Lycium barbarum* polysaccharides and its antifatigue effect]. *Wei Sheng Yan Jiu* 2000;29(2):115–17. Chinese.

Madhusudan S, Smart F, Shrimpton P, Parsons JL, Gardiner L, Houlbrook S, Talbot DC, Hammonds T, Freemont PA, Sternberg MJ, Dianov GL, Hickson ID. Isolation of a small molecule inhibitor of DNA base excision repair. *Nucleic Acids Research* 2005;33(15):4711–24.

Madsen T, Christensen JH, Blom M, Schmidt EB. The effect of dietary n-3 fatty acids on serum concentrations of C-reactive protein: a dose-response study. *British Journal of Nutrition* 2003;89(4):517–22.

Madsen T, Skou HA, Hansen VE, Fog L, Christensen JH, Toft E, Schmidt EB. C-reactive protein, dietary n-3 fatty acids, and the extent of coronary artery disease. *American Journal of Cardiology* 2001;88(10):1139–42.

Malik M, Zhao C, Schoene N, Guisti MM, Moyer MP, Magnuson BA. Anthocyanin-rich extract from *Aronia meloncarpa E* induces a cell cycle block in colon cancer but not normal colonic cells. *Nutrition and Cancer* 2003;46(2):186–96.

Marcheselli VL, Hong S, Lukiw WJ, Tian XH, Gronert K, Musto A, Hardy M, Gimenez JM, Chiang N, Serhan CN, Bazan NG. Novel docosanoids inhibit brain ischemia-reperfusion-mediated leukocyte infiltration and pro-inflammatory gene expression. *Journal of Biological Chemistry* 2003;278:43807–17.

Matsuyama W, Mitsuyama H, Watanabe M, Oonakahara K, Higashimoto I, Osame M, Arimura K. Effects of omega-3 polyunsaturated fatty acids on inflammatory markers in COPD. *Chest* 2005;128(6):3817–27.

Mazza G, Kay CD, Cottrell T, Holub BJ. Absorption of anthocyanins from blueberries and serum antioxidant status in human subjects. *Journal of Agricultural and Food Chemistry* 2002;50(26):7731–37.

Mazza G, Miniati E. Small fruits. In: *Anthocyanins in Fruits, Vegetables, and Grains.* CRC Press, Boca Raton, FL, 1993, pp. 85–130.

McAlindon TE, Jacques P, Zhang Y, Hannan MT, Aliabadi P, Weissman B, Rush D, Levy D, Felson DT. Do antioxidant micronutrients protect against the development and progression of knee osteoarthritis? *Arthritis and Rheumatism* 1996;39:648–56.

McBride J. High-ORAC foods may slow aging. USDA Agricultural Research Service website: http://www.ars.usda.gov/is/pr/1999/990208.htm.

McCowen KC, Bistrian BR. Essential fatty acids and their derivatives. *Current Opinion in Gastroenterology* 2005;21(2):207–15.

McCullough JL, Kelly KM. Prevention and treatment of skin aging. *Annals of the New York Academy of Sciences* 2006;1067:323–31. Review.

Melhem MF, Craven PA, Derubertis FR. Effects of dietary supplementation of alpha-lipoic acid on early glomerular injury in diabetes mellitus. *Journal of the American Society of Nephrology* 2001;12(1):124–33.

Melhem MF, Craven PA, Liachenko J, DeRubertis FR. Alpha-lipoic acid attenuates hyperglycemia and prevents glomerular mesangial matrix expansion in diabetes. *Journal of the American Society of Nephrology* 2002;13(1):108–16.

Merchant RE, Andre CA. A review of recent clinical trials of the nutritional supplement *Chlorella pyrenoidosa* in the treatment of fibromyalgia, hypertension, and ulcerative colitis. *Alternative Therapies in Health and Medicine* 2001;7:79–80, 82–91.

Merchant RE, Carmack CA, Wise CM. Nutritional supplementation with *Chlorella pyrenoidosa* for patients with fibromyalgia syndrome: a pilot study. *Phytotherapy Research* 2000;14:167–173.

Merin JP, Matsuyama M, Kira T, Baba M, Okamoto T. Alpha-lipoic acid blocks HIV-1 LTR-dependent expression of hygromycin resistance in THP-1 stable transformants. *FEBS Letters* 1996;394(1):9–13.

Meyer M, Pahl HL, Baeuerle PA. Regulation of the transcription factors NF-kappa B and AP-1 by redox changes. *Chemico-Biological Interactions* 1994;91(2–3):91–100.

Meyer M, Schreck R, Baeuerle PA. H_2O_2 and antioxidants have opposite effects on activation of NF-kappa B and AP-1 in intact cells: AP-1 as secondary antioxidant-responsive factor. *EMBO Journal* 1993;12(5):2005–15.

Micozzi MS, Beecher GR, Taylor PR, Khachik F. Carotenoid analyses of selected raw and cooked foods associated with a lower risk for cancer. *Journal of the National Cancer Institute* 1990;82(4):282–85. Erratum in: *Journal of the National Cancer Institute* 1990;82(8):715.

Midaoui AE, Elimadi A, Wu L, Haddad PS, de Champlain J. Lipoic acid prevents hypertension, hyperglycemia, and the increase in heart mitochondrial superoxide production. *American Journal of Hypertension* 2003;16(3):173–79.

Miles EA, Allen E, Calder PC. In vitro effects of eicosanoids derived from different

20-carbon fatty acids on production of monocyte-derived cytokines in human whole blood cultures. *Cytokine* 2002;20:215–23.

Miller MJ, Vergnolle N, McKnight W, Musah RA, Davison CA, Trentacosti AM, Thompson JH, Sandoval M, Wallace JL. Inhibition of neurogenic inflammation by the Amazonian herbal medicine sangre de grado. *Journal of Investigative Dermatology* 2001;117(3):725–30.

Mingrone G. Carnitine in type 2 diabetes. *Annals of the New York Academy of Science* 2004;1033:99–107. Review.

Miranda MS, Cintra RG, Barros SB, Mancini Filho J. Antioxidant activity of the microalga *Spirulina maxima*. *Brazilian Journal of Medical and Biological Research* 1998; 31(8):1075–79.

Miranda MS, Sato S, Mancini-Filho J. Antioxidant activity of the microalga *Chlorella vulgaris* cultured on special conditions. *Bollettino Chimico Farmaceutico* 2001;140(3): 165–68.

Mittal A, Elmets CA, Katiyar SK. Dietary feeding of proanthocyanidins from grape seeds prevents photocarcinogenesis in SKH-1 hairless mice: relationship to decreased fat and lipid peroxidation. *Carcinogenesis* 2003;24(8):1379–88. Epub 2003 Jun 05.

Moeller SM, Jacques PF, Blumberg JB. The potential role of dietary xanthophylls in cataract and age-related macular degeneration. *Journal of the American College of Nutrition* 2000;19(suppl 5):522S–27S. Review.

Mohandas KM, Desai DC. Epidemiology of digestive tract cancers in India. V. Large and small bowel. *Indian Journal of Gastroenterology* 1999;18(3):118–21. Review.

Mohandas KM, Jagannath P. Epidemiology of digestive tract cancers in India. VI. Projected burden in the new millennium and the need for primary prevention. *Indian Journal of Gastroenterology* 2000;19(2):74–78.

Morita K, Matsueda T, Iida T, Hasegawa T. Chlorella accelerates dioxin excretion in rats. *Journal of Nutrition* 1999;129:1731–36.

Moyer RA, Hummer KE, Finn CE, Frei B, Wrolstad RE. Anthocyanins, phenolics, and antioxidant capacity in diverse small fruits: vaccinium, rubus, and ribes. *Journal of Agricultural and Food Chemistry* 2002;50(3):519–25.

Murphy KJ, Chronopoulos AK, Singh I, Francis MA, Moriarty H, Pike MJ, Turner AH, Mann NJ, Sinclair AJ. Dietary flavanols and procyanidin oligomers from cocoa (*Theobroma cacao*) inhibit platelet function. *American Journal of Clinical Nutrition* 2003;77(6):1466–73.

Nahata MC, Slencsak, CA, Kamp J. Effect of chlorophyllin on urinary odor in incontinent geriatric patients. *Drug Intelligence & Clinical Pharmacy* 1983;17:732–34.

Nakaya N, Homma Y, Goto Y. Cholesterol lowering effect of spirulina. *Nutrition Reports International* 1988;37:1329–37.

Narayan S. Curcumin, a multi-functional chemopreventive agent, blocks growth of colon cancer cells by targeting beta-catenin-mediated transactivation and cell-cell adhesion pathways. *Journal of Molecular Histology* 2004;35(3):301–7. Review.

Ni H, Qing D, Kaisa S, Lu J. [The study on the effect of LBP on cleaning hydroxygen free radical by EPR technique]. *Zhong Yao Cai* 2004;27(8):599–600. Chinese.

Nishiyama T, Hagiwara Y, Hagiwara H, Shibamoto T. Inhibitory effect of 2″-O-glycosyl isovitexin and alpha-tocopherol on genotoxic glyoxal formation in a lipid peroxidation system. *Food and Chemical Toxicology* 1994;32(11):1047–51.

Noda K, Ohno N, Tanaka K, Kamiya N, Okuda M, Yadomae T, Nomoto K, Shoyama Y. A water-soluble antitumor glycoprotein from *Chlorella vulgaris*. *Planta Medica* 1996;62:423–26.

Novak TE, Babcock TA, Jho DH, Helton WS, Espat NJ. NF-kappaB inhibition by omega-3 fatty acids modulates LPS-stimulated macrophage TNF-alpha transcription. *American Journal of Physiology* 2003;284:L84–L89.

Obrenovich ME, Monnier VM. Vitamin B_1 blocks damage caused by hyperglycemia. *Science of Aging Knowledge Environment* 2003;2003(10):PE6.

O'Byrne DJ, Devaraj S, Grundy SM, Jialal I. Comparison of the antioxidant effects of Concord grape juice flavonoids alpha-tocopherol on markers of oxidative stress in healthy adults. *American Journal of Clinical Nutrition* 2002;76(6):1367–74. [Cosponsored by Welch's Foods Inc. (Concord, MA) and the National Institutes of Health].

Omenn GS, Goodman GE, Thornquist MD, Balmes J, Cullen MR, Glass A, Keogh JP, Meyskins FL, Valanis B, Williams JH, Barnhart S, Hammar S. Effects of a combination of beta carotene and vitamin A on lung cancer and cardiovascular disease. *New England Journal of Medicine* 1996;334:1150–55.

Ong TM, Whong WZ, Stewart J, Brockman HE. Chlorophyllin: a potent antimutagen against environmental and dietary complex mixtures. *Mutation Research* 1986; 173:111–15.

Onoda M, Inano H. Effect of curcumin on the production of nitric oxide by cultured rat mammary gland. *Nitric Oxide: Biology and Chemistry* 2000;4(5):505–15.

Ookawara T, Kawamura N, Kitagawa Y, Taniguchi N. Site-specific and random fragmentation of Cu,Zn-superoxide dismutase by glycation reaction. Implication of reactive oxygen species. *Journal of Biological Chemistry* 1992;267(26):18505–10.

Orsini F, Pelizzoni F, Verotta L, Aburjai T, Rogers CB. Isolation, synthesis, and antiplatelet aggregation activity of resveratrol 3-O-beta-D-glucopyranoside and related compounds. *Journal of Natural Products* 1997;60(11):1082–87.

Otles S, Pire R. Fatty acid composition of *Chlorella* and *Spirulina* microalgae species. *Journal of AOAC International* 2001;84(6):1708–14.

Packer L, Kraemer K, Rimbach G. Molecular aspects of lipoic acid in the prevention of diabetes complications. *Nutrition* 2001;17(10):888–95. Review.

Packer L, Roy S, Sen CK. Alpha-lipoic acid: a metabolic antioxidant and potential redox modulator of transcription. *Advances in Pharmacology* 1996;38:79–101.

Packer L, Tritschler HJ, Wessel K. Neuroprotection by the metabolic antioxidant alpha-lipoic acid. *Free Radical Biology & Medicine* 1997;22(1–2):359–78. Review.

Packer L, Witt EH, Tritschler HJ. Alpha-lipoic acid as a biological antioxidant. *Free Radical Biology & Medicine* 1995;19(2):227–50. Review.

Pan MH, Lin-Shiau SY, Lin JK. Comparative studies on the suppression of nitric oxide synthase by curcumin and its hydrogenated metabolites through down-regulation of IkappaB kinase and NFkappaB activation in macrophages. *Biochemical Pharmacology* 2000;60(11):1665–76.

Pani G, Colavitti R, Bedogni B, Fusco S, Ferraro D, Borrello S, Galeotti T. Mitochondrial superoxide dismutase: a promising target for new anticancer therapies. *Current Medicinal Chemistry* 2004;11(10):1299–308.

Park JM, Adam RM, Peters CA, Guthrie PD, Sun Z, Klagsbrun M, Freeman MR. AP-1 mediates stretch-induced expression of HB-EGF in bladder smooth muscle cells. *American Journal of Physiology* 1999;277(2 Pt 1):C294–301.

Patrick L, Uzick M. Cardiovascular disease: C-reactive protein and the inflammatory disease paradigm: HMG-CoA reductase inhibitors, alpha-tocopherol, red yeast rice, and olive oil polyphenols. A review of the literature. *Alternative Medicine Review* 2001;6(3):248–71. Review.

Perricone N, Nagy K, Horvath F, Dajko G, Uray I, Zs-Nagy I. Alpha lipoic acid (ALA) protects proteins against the hydroxyl free radical-induced alterations: rationale for its geriatric application. *Archives of Gerontology and Geriatrics* 1999;29(1):45–56.

Perricone NV. Topical 5% alpha lipoic acid cream in the treatment of cutaneous rhytids. *Aesthetic Surgery Journal* 2000;20(3):218–22.

Peryt B, Miloszewska J, Tudek B, Zielenska M, Szymczyk T. Antimutagenic effects of several subfractions of extract from wheat sprout toward benzo[a]pyrene-induced mutagenicity in strain TA98 of *Salmonella typhimurium*. *Mutation Research* 1988;206:221–25.

Peryt B, Szymczyk T, Lesca P. Mechanism of antimutagenicity of wheat sprout extracts. *Mutation Research* 1992;269:201–15.

Phan TT, See P, Lee ST, Chan SY. Protective effects of curcumin against oxidative damage on skin cells in vitro: its implication for wound healing. *Journal of Trauma* 2001;51(5):927–31.

Pischon T, Hankinson SE, Hotamisligil GS, Rifai N, Willett WC, Rimm EB. Habitual dietary intake of n-3 and n-6 fatty acids in relation to inflammatory markers among US men and women. *Circulation* 2003;108(2):155–60. Epub 2003 Jun 23.

Pittler MH, Stevinson C, Ernst E. Chromium picolinate for reducing body weight: meta-analysis of randomized trials. *International Journal of Obesity and Related Metabolic Disorders* 2003;27(4):522–29.

Plummer SM, Holloway KA, Manson MM, Munks RJ, Kaptein A, Farrow S, Howells L. Inhibition of cyclo-oxygenase 2 expression in colon cells by the chemopreventive agent curcumin involves inhibition of NF-kappaB activation via the NIK/IKK signalling complex. *Oncogene* 1999;18(44):6013–20.

Pobezhimova TP, Voinikov VK. Biochemical and physiological aspects of ubiquinone function. *Membrane & Cell Biology* 2000;13(5):595–602. Review.

Podda M, Rallis M, Traber MG, Packer L, Maibach HI. Kinetic study of cutaneous and subcutaneous distribution following topical application of [7,8-14C]rac-alpha-lipoic acid onto hairless mice. *Biochemical Pharmacology* 1996;52(4):627–33.

Podda M, Tritschler HJ, Ulrich H, Packer L. Alpha-lipoic acid supplementation prevents symptoms of vitamin E deficiency. *Biochemical and Biophysical Research Communications* 1994;204(1):98–104.

Podda M, Zollner TM, Grundmann-Kollmann M, Thiele JJ, Packer L, Kaufmann R. Activity of alpha-lipoic acid in the protection against oxidative stress in skin. *Current Problems in Dermatology* 2001;29:43–51.

The polyphenol flavonoids content and anti-oxidant activities of various juices: a comparative study. Lipid Research Laboratory, Technion Faculty of Medicine, Rappaport Family Institute for Research in the Medical Sciences and Rambam Medical Center, Haifa, Israel.

Premkumar K, Pachiappan A, Abraham SK, Santhiya ST, Gopinath PM, Ramesh A. Effect of *Spirulina fusiformis* on cyclophosphamide and mitomycin-C induced genotoxicity and oxidative stress in mice. *Fitoterapia* 2001;72(8):906–11.

Preuss HG, Grojec PL, Lieberman S, Anderson RA. Effects of different chromium compounds on blood pressure and lipid peroxidation in spontaneously hypertensive rats. *Clinical Nephrology* 1997;47(5):325–30.

Priante G, Bordin L, Musacchio E, Clari G, Baggio B. Fatty acids and cytokine mRNA expression in human osteoblastic cells: a specific effect of arachidonic acid. *Clinical Science (London)* 2002;102:403–9.

Price JA 3rd, Sanny C, Shevlin D. Inhibition of mast cells by algae. *Journal of Medicinal Food* 2002;5(4):205–10.

Pugh N, Pasco DS. Characterization of human monocyte activation by a water soluble preparation of *Aphanizomenon flos-aquae*. *Phytomedicine*. 2001;8(6):445–53.

Pugh N, Ross SA, ElSohly HN, ElSohly MA, Pasco DS. Isolation of three high molecular weight polysaccharide preparations with potent immunostimulatory activity from *Spirulina platensis*, *Aphanizomenon flos-aquae* and *Chlorella pyrenoidosa*. *Planta Medica* 2001;67(8):737–42.

Queiroz ML, Rodrigues AP, Bincoletto C, Figueiredo CA, Malacrida S. Protective effects of *Chlorella vulgaris* in lead-exposed mice infected with *Listeria monocytogenes*. *International Immunopharmacology* 2003;3(6):889–900.

Qureshi MA, Ali RA. *Spirulina platensis* exposure enhances macrophage phagocytic function in cats. *Immunopharmacology and Immunotoxicology* 1996;18:457–63.

Qureshi MA, Garlich JD, Kidd MT. Dietary *Spirulina platensis* enhances humoral and cell-mediated immune functions in chickens. *Immunopharmacology and Immunotoxicology* 1996;18:465–76.

Ram VJ. Herbal preparations as a source of hepatoprotective agents. *Drug News & Perspectives* 2001;14(6):353–63.

Ramirez-Tortosa MC, Mesa MD, Aguilera MC, Quiles JL, Baro L, Ramirez-Tortosa CL, Martinez-Victoria E, Gil A. Oral administration of a turmeric extract inhibits LDL oxidation and has hypocholesterolemic effects in rabbits with experimental atherosclerosis. *Atherosclerosis* 1999;147(2):371–78.

Rao CV, et al. Antioxidant activity of curcumin and related compounds. Lipid peroxide formation in experimental inflammation. *Cancer Research* 1993;55:259.

Rao PV, Gupta N, Bhaskar AS, Jayaraj R. Toxins and bioactive compounds from cyanobacteria and their implications on human health. *Journal of Environmental Biology* 2002;23(3):215–24. Review.

Reber F, Geffarth R, Kasper M, Reichenbach A, Schleicher ED, Siegner A, Funk RH. Graded sensitiveness of the various retinal neuron populations on the glyoxal-mediated formation of advanced glycation end products and ways of protection. *Graefe's Archive for Clinical and Experimental Ophthalmology* 2003;241(3): 213–25.

Reddy AP, Harttig U, Barth MC, Baird WM, Schimerlik M, Hendricks JD, Bailey GS. Inhibition of dibenzo[a,l]pyrene-induced multi-organ carcinogenesis by dietary chlorophyllin in rainbow trout. *Carcinogenesis* 1999;20:1919–26.

Reed LJ, DeBusk BG, Gunsalus IC, Hornberger CS Jr. Crystalline alpha-lipoic acid; a catalytic agent associated with pyruvate dehydrogenase. *Science* 1951;27; 114(2952):93–4.

Ridker PM, Hennekens CH, Buring JE, Rifai N. C-reactive protein and other markers of inflammation in the prediction of cardiovascular disease in women. *New England Journal of Medicine* 2000;342(12):836–43.

Ridker PM. Inflammation in atherothrombosis: how to use high-sensitivity C-reactive protein (hsCRP) in clinical practice. *American Heart Hospital Journal* 2004; 2(4 suppl 1):4–9. Review.

Ritenbaugh C. Diet and prevention of colorectal cancer. *Current Oncology Reports* 2000;2(3):225–33. Review.

Robert AM, Tixier JM, Robert L, Legeais JM, Renard G. Effect of procyanidolic oligomers on the permeability of the blood-brain barrier. *Pathologie-Biologie (Paris)*. 2001;49(4):298–304.

Robins EW, Nelson RL. Inhibition of 1,2-dimethylhydrazine-induced nuclear damage in rat colonic epithelium by chlorophyllin. *Anticancer Research* 1989;9:981–85.

Rock CL, Saxe GA, Ruffin MT 4th, August DA, Schottenfeld D. Carotenoids, vitamin A, and estrogen receptor status in breast cancer. *Nutrition and Cancer* 1996;25: 281–96.

Rogan EG. The natural chemopreventive compound indole-3-carbinol: state of the science. *In Vivo* 2006;20(2):221–28. Review.

Rosenfeldt F, Hilton D, Pepe S, Krum H. Systematic review of effect of coenzyme Q_{10} in physical exercise, hypertension and heart failure. *Biofactors* 2003;18(1–4): 91–100. Review.

Ross JA, Moses AG, Fearon KC. The anti-catabolic effects of n-3 fatty acids. *Current Opinion in Clinical Nutrition and Metabolic Care* 1999;2:219–26.

Roy S, Khanna S, Alessio HM, Vider J, Bagchi D, Bagchi M, Sen CK. Anti-angiogenic property of edible berries. *Free Radical Research* 2002;36(9):1023–31.

Roy S, Sen CK, Tritschler HJ, Packer L. Modulation of cellular reducing equivalent homeostasis by alpha-lipoic acid. Mechanisms and implications for diabetes and ischemic injury. *Biochemical Pharmacology.* 1997;53(3):393–99.

Rudich A, Tirosh A, Potashnik R, Khamaisi M, Bashan N. Lipoic acid protects against oxidative stress induced impairment in insulin stimulation of protein kinase B and glucose transport in 3T3-L1 adipocytes. *Diabetologia* 1999;42(8):949–57.

Rukkumani R, Aruna K, Varma PS, Rajasekaran KN, Menon VP. Comparative effects of curcumin and its analog on alcohol- and polyunsaturated fatty acid–induced alterations in circulatory lipid profiles. *Journal of Medicinal Food* 2005; 8(2):256–60.

Saliou C, Kitazawa M, McLaughlin L, Yang JP, Lodge JK, Tetsuka T, Iwasaki K, Cillard J, Okamoto T, Packer L. Antioxidants modulate acute solar ultraviolet radiation-induced NF-kappa-B activation in a human keratinocyte cell line. *Free Radical Biology & Medicine* 1999;26(1–2):174–83.

Sano T, Kumamoto Y, Kamiya N, Okuda M, Tanaka Y. Effect of lipophilic extract of *Chlorella vulgaris* on alimentary hyperlipidemia in cholesterol-fed rats. *Artery* 1988;15:217–24.

Sano T, Tanaka Y. Effect of dried, powdered *Chlorella vulgaris* on experimental atherosclerosis and alimentary hypercholesterolemia in cholesterol-fed rabbits. *Artery* 1987;14:76–84.

Satoskar RR, Shah SJ, Shenoy SG. Evaluation of anti-inflammatory property of curcumin (diferuloyl methane) in patients with postoperative inflammation. *International Journal of Clinical Pharmacology, Therapy, and Toxicology* 1986;24(12):651–54.

Schmidt K. Antioxidant vitamins and beta-carotene: effects on immunocompetence. *American Journal of Clinical Nutrition* 1991;53(suppl 1):383S–85S.

Schubert SY, Lansky EP, Neeman I. Antioxidant and eicosanoid enzyme inhibition properties of pomegranate seed oil and fermented juice flavonoids. *Journal of Ethnopharmacology* 1999;66(1):11–17.

Seddon JM, Ajani UA, Sperduto RD, Hiller R, Blair N, Burton TC, Farber MD, Gragoudas ES, Haller J, Miller DT, et al. Dietary carotenoids, vitamins A, C, and E, and advanced age-related macular degeneration. Eye Disease Case-Control Study Group. *JAMA* 1994;272:1413–20. Erratum in: *JAMA* 1995;273(8):622.

Seeram NP, Zhang Y, Nair MG. Inhibition of proliferation of human cancer cells and cyclooxygenase enzymes by anthocyanidins and catechins. *Nutrition and Cancer* 2003;46(1):101–6.

Seierstad SL, Seljeflot I, Johansen O, Hansen R, Haugen M, Rosenlund G, Froyland L, Arnesen H. Dietary intake of differently fed salmon; the influence on markers of human atherosclerosis. *European Journal of Clinical Investigation* 2005;35(1):52–9.

Sen CK, Packer L. Antioxidant and redox regulation of gene transcription. FASEB *Journal* 1996;10:709–20.

Serhan CN, Clish CB, Brannon J, Colgan SP, Chiang N, Gronert K. Novel functional sets of lipid-derived mediators with antiinflammatory actions generated from omega-3 fatty acids via cyclooxygenase 2-nonsteroidal antiinflammatory drugs and transcellular processing. *Journal of Experimental Medicine* 2000;192: 1197–1204.

Serhan CN, Jain A, Marleau S, Clish C, Kantarci A, Behbehani B, Colgan SP, Stahl GL, Merched A, Petasis NA, Chan L, Van Dyke TE. Reduced inflammation and tissue damage in transgenic rabbits overexpressing 15-lipoxygenase and endogenous anti-inflammatory lipid mediators. *Journal of Immunology* 2003;171:6856–65.

Shah BH, Nawaz Z, Pertani SA, Roomi A, Mahmood H, Saeed SA, Gilani AH. Inhibitory effect of curcumin, a food spice from turmeric, on platelet-activating factor– and arachidonic acid–mediated platelet aggregation through inhibition of thromboxane formation and Ca2+ signaling. *Biochemical Pharmacology* 1999; 58(7):1167–72.

Shapiro TA, Fahey JW, Wade KL, Stephenson KK, Talalay P. Chemoprotective glucosinolates and isothiocyanates of broccoli sprouts: metabolism and excretion in humans. *Cancer Epidemiology, Biomarkers & Prevention* 2001;10(5):501–8.

Sharma RA, Gescher AJ, Steward WP. Curcumin: the story so far. *European Journal of Cancer* 2005;41(13):1955–68. Review.

Sharma SC, Mukhtar H, Sharma SK, Krishna Murt CR. Lipid peroxide formation in experimental inflammation. *Biochemical Pharmacology* 1972;21:1210.

Shi J, Yu J, Pohorly JE, Kakuda Y. Polyphenolics in grape seeds—biochemistry and functionality. *Journal of Medicinal Food* 2003;6(4):291–99.

Shigenaga MK, Hagen TM, Ames BN. Oxidative damage and mitochondrial decay in aging. *Proceedings of the National Academy of Sciences of the United States of America* 1994; 91(23):10771–78. Review.

Shih SR, Tsai KN, Li YS, Chueh CC, Chan EC. Inhibition of enterovirus 71-induced apoptosis by allophycocyanin isolated from a blue-green alga *Spirulina platensis*. *Journal of Medical Virology* 2003;70(1):119–25.

Singh S, Aggarwal BB. Activation of transcription factor NF-kappa B is suppressed by curcumin (diferuloylmethane) [corrected]. *Journal of Biological Chemistry* 1995;270 (42):24995–5000. Erratum in: *Journal of Biological Chemistry* 1995;270(50):30235.

Singletary KW, Meline B. Effect of grape seed proanthocyanidins on colon aberrant crypts and breast tumors in a rat dual-organ tumor model. *Nutrition and Cancer* 2001;39(2):252–58.

Singletary KW, Stansbury MJ, Giusti M, Van Breemen RB, Wallig M, Rimando A. Inhibition of rat mammary tumorigenesis by concord grape juice constituents. *Journal of Agricultural and Food Chemistry* 2003;51(25):7280–86.

Sinha R, Anderson DE, McDonald SS, Greenwald P. Cancer risk and diet in India. *Journal of Postgraduate Medicine* 2003;49(3):222–28. Review.

Siwak DR, Shishodia S, Aggarwal BB, Kurzrock R. Curcumin-induced antiproliferative and proapoptotic effects in melanoma cells are associated with suppression of IkappaB kinase and nuclear factor kappaB activity and are independent of the B-Raf/mitogen-activated/extracellular signal-regulated protein kinase pathway and the Akt pathway. *Cancer* 2005;104(4):879–90.

Slomski G. Lycopene. In Krapp, JL, Lange (eds.): *Gale Encyclopedia of Alternative Medicine*. Gale Group, Detroit, 2001.

Soliman KF, Mazzio EA. In vitro attenuation of nitric oxide production in C6 astrocyte cell culture by various dietary compounds. *Proceedings of the Society for Experimental Biology and Medicine* 1998;218(4):390–97.

Soni KB, Kuttan R. Effect of oral curcumin administration on serum peroxides and cholesterol levels in human volunteers. *Indian Journal of Physiology and Pharmacology* 1992;(36):273–75.

Spencer JP, Schroeter H, Rechner AR, Rice-Evans C. Bioavailability of flavan-3-ols and procyanidins: gastrointestinal tract influences and their relevance to bioactive forms in vivo. *Antioxidants & Redox Signaling* 2001;3(6):1023–39. Review.

Spiteller G. Peroxidation of linoleic acid and its relation to ageing and age dependent diseases. *Mechanisms of Ageing and Development* 2001;122(7):617–57. Review.

Sreekanth KS, Sabu MC, Varghese L, Manesh C, Kuttan G, Kuttan R. Antioxidant activity of Smoke Shield in-vitro and in-vivo. *Journal of Pharmacy and Pharmacology* 2003;55(6):847–53.

Srimal R, Dhawan B. Pharmacology of diferuloyl methane (curcumin), a nonsteroidal anti-inflammatory agent. *Journal of Pharmacy and Pharmacology* 1973;(25)447–52.

Srinivas L, Shalini VK, Shylaja M. Turmerin: a water-soluble antioxidant peptide from turmeric [*Curcuma longa*]. *Archives of Biochemistry and Biophysics* 1992;292(2):617–23.

Srivasta R, Srimal RC. Modification of certain inflammation-induced biochemical changes by curcumin. *Indian Journal of Medical Research* 1985;(81):215–23.

Steele PE, Tang PH, DeGrauw AJ, Miles MV. Clinical laboratory monitoring of coenzyme Q_{10} use in neurologic and muscular diseases. *American Journal of Clinical Pathology* 2004;121(suppl):S113–20. Review.

Steinmetz KA, Potter JD. Vegetables, fruit, and cancer prevention: a review. *Journal of the American Dietetic Association* 1996;96(10):1027–39. Review.

Stoclet JC, Kleschyov A, Andriambeloson E, Diebolt M, Andriantsitohaina R. Endothelial no release caused by red wine polyphenols. *Journal of Physiology and Pharmacology* 1999;50(4):535–40.

Subarnas A, Wagner H. Analgesic and anti-inflammatory activity of the proanthocyanidin shellegueain A from *Polypodium feei* METT. *Phytomedicine* 2000;7(5):401–5.

Sugawara T, Miyazawa T. Beneficial effect of dietary wheat glycolipids on cecum short-chain fatty acid and secondary bile acid profiles in mice. *Journal of Nutritional Science and Vitaminology* (Tokyo) 2001;47(4):299–305.

Suh JH, Shigeno ET, Morrow JD, Cox B, Rocha AE, Frei B, Hagen TM. Oxidative stress in the aging rat heart is reversed by dietary supplementation with (R)-(alpha)-lipoic acid. *FASEB Journal* 2001;15(3):700–6.

Surh YJ. Anti-tumor promoting potential of selected spice ingredients with antioxidative and anti-inflammatory activities: a short review. *Food and Chemical Toxicology* 2002;40(8):1091–97. Review.

Surh YJ, Chun KS, Cha HH, Han SS, Keum YS, Park KK, Lee SS. Molecular mechanisms underlying chemopreventive activities of anti-inflammatory phytochemicals: down-regulation of COX-2 and iNOS through suppression of NF-kappa B activation. *Mutation Research* 2001;480–481:243–68. Review.

Surh YJ, Han SS, Keum YS, Seo HJ, Lee SS. Inhibitory effects of curcumin and capsaicin on phorbol ester-induced activation of eukaryotic transcription factors, NF-kappaB and AP-1. *Biofactors* 2000;12(1–4):107–12.

Susan M, Rao MNA. Induction of glutathione S-transferase activity by curcumin in mice. *Arzneimmittelforschung* 1992;42:962.

Suzuki Y, Ohgami K, Shiratori K, Jin XH, Ilieva I, Koyama Y, Yazawa K, Yoshida K, Kase S, Ohno S. Suppressive effects of astaxanthin against rat endotoxin-induced uveitis by inhibiting the NF-kappaB signaling pathway. *Experimental Eye Research* 2006;82(2):275–81. Epub 2005 Aug 26.

Suzuki YJ, Aggarwal BB, Packer L. Alpha-lipoic acid is a potent inhibitor of NF-kappa B activation in human T cells. *Biochemical and Biophysical Research Communications* 1992;189(3):1709–15.

Suzuki YJ, Mizuno M, Tritschler HJ, Packer L. Redox regulation of NF-kappa B DNA binding activity by dihydrolipoate. *Biochemistry and Molecular Biology International* 1995;36(2):241–46.

Suzuki YJ, Tsuchiya M, Packer L. Lipoate prevents glucose-induced protein modifications. *Free Radical Research Communications* 1992;17(3):211–17.

Tan WF, Lin LP, Li MH, Zhang YX, Tong YG, Xiao D, Ding J. Quercetin, a dietary-derived flavonoid, possesses antiangiogenic potential. *European Journal of Pharmacology* 2003;459(2–3):255–62.

Tanaka K, Koga T, Konishi F, Nakamura M, Mitsuyama M, Himeno K, Nomoto K. Augmentation of host defense by unicellular green alga, *Chlorella vulgaris*, to *Escherichia coli* infection. *Infection and Immunity* 1986;53:267–71.

Tanaka K, Yamada A, Noda K, Hasegawa T, Okuda M, Shoyama Y, Nomoto K. A novel glycoprotein obtained from *Chlorella vulgaris* strain CK22 shows antimetastatic immunopotentiation. *Cancer Immunology, Immunotherapy* 1998;45:313–20.

Tanaka K, Yamada A, Noda K, Shoyama Y, Kubo C, Nomoto K. Oral administration of a unicellular green algae, *Chlorella vulgaris*, prevents stress-induced ulcer. *Planta Medica* 1997;63:465–66.

Te C, Gentile JM, Baguley BC, et al. In vivo effects of chlorophyllin on the antitumour agent cyclophosphamide. *International Journal of Cancer* 1997;70:84–9.

Teikari JM, Rautalahti M, Haukka J, Jarvinen P, Hartman AM, Virtamo J, Albanes D, Heinonen O. Incidence of cataract operations in Finnish male smokers unaffected by alpha tocopherol or beta carotene supplements. *Journal of Epidemiology and Community Health* 1998;52:468–72.

Terman A. Garbage catastrophe theory of aging: imperfect removal of oxidative damage? *Redox Report* 2001;6(1):15–26. Review.

Thies F, Garry JM, Yaqoob P, Rerkasem K, Williams J, Shearman CP, Gallagher PJ, Calder PC, Grimble RF. Association of n-3 polyunsaturated fatty acids with stability of atherosclerotic plaques: a randomised controlled trial. *Lancet* 2003;361 (9356):477–85.

Tijburg LBM, Mattern T, Folts JD, Weisgerber UM, Katan MB. Tea flavonoids and cardiovascular diseases: a review. *Critical Reviews in Food Science and Nutrition* 1997;37: 771–85.

Todoric J, Loffler M, Huber J, Bilban M, Reimers M, Kadl A, Zeyda M, Waldhausl W, Stulnig TM. Adipose tissue inflammation induced by high-fat diet in obese diabetic mice is prevented by n-3 polyunsaturated fatty acids. *Diabetologia* 2006;49(9):2109–19. [Epub ahead of print]

Toniolo P, Van Kappel AL, Akhmedkhanov A, Ferrari P, Kato I, Shore RE, Riboli E. Serum carotenoids and breast cancer. *American Journal of Epidemiology* 2001;153 (12):1142–47.

Torres-Duran PV, Miranda-Zamora R, Paredes-Carbajal MC, Mascher D, Diaz-Zagoya JC, Juarez-Oropeza MA. *Spirulina maxima* prevents induction of fatty liver by carbon tetrachloride in the rat. *Biochemistry and Molecular Biology International* 1998; 44:787–93.

Torstensen BE, Bell JG, Rosenlund G, Henderson RJ, Graff IE, Tocher DR, Lie O, Sargent JR. Tailoring of Atlantic salmon (Salmo salar L.) flesh lipid composition and sensory quality by replacing fish oil with a vegetable oil blend. *Journal of Agricultural and Food Chemistry.* 2005;53(26):10166–78.

Toyokuni S. Reactive oxygen species-induced molecular damage and its application in pathology. *Pathology International* 1999;49(2):91–102. Review.

Trent LK, Thieding-Cancel D. Effects of chromium picolinate on body composition. *Journal of Sports Medicine and Physical Fitness* 1995;35(4):273–80.

Tucker KL, Qiao N, Scott T, Rosenberg I, Spiro A 3rd. High homocysteine and low B vitamins predict cognitive decline in aging men: the Veterans Affairs Normative Aging Study. *American Journal of Clinical Nutrition* 2005;82(3):627–35.

Tudek B, Peryt B, Miloszewska J, Szymczyk T, Przybyszewska M, Janik P, et al. The effect of wheat sprout extract on benzo(a)pyrene and 7,2-dimethylbenz(a) anthracene activity. *Neoplasma* 1998;35:515–23.

Turujman SA, Wamer WG, Wei RR, Albert RH. Rapid liquid chromatographic method to distinguish wild salmon from aquacultured salmon fed synthetic astaxanthin. *Journal of AOAC International* 1997;80(3):622–32.

Vadiraja BB, Gaikwad NW, Madyastha KM. Hepatoprotective effect of C-phycocyanin: protection for carbon tetrachloride and R-(+)-pulegone-mediated hepatotoxicity in rats. *Biochemical and Biophysical Research Communications* 1998;249:428–31.

van Doorn HE, van der Kruk GC, van Holst GJ. Large scale determination of glucosinolates in brussels sprouts samples after degradation of endogenous glucose. *Journal of Agricultural and Food Chemistry* 1999;47(3):1029–34.

Vancheri C, Mastruzzo C, Sortino MA, Crimi N. The lung as a privileged site for the beneficial actions of PGE2. *Trends in Immunology* 2004;25:40–6.

Vena JE, Graham S, Freudenheim J, Marshall J, Zielezny M, Swanson M, Sufrin G. Diet in the epidemiology of bladder cancer in western New York. *Nutrition and Cancer* 1992;18:255–64.

Vendemiale G, Grattagliano I, Altomare E. An update on the role of free radicals and antioxidant defense in human disease. *International Journal of Clinical & Laboratory Research* 1999;29(2):49–55.

Vincent JB. The potential value and toxicity of chromium picolinate as a nutritional supplement, weight loss agent and muscle development agent. *Sports Medicine* 2003;33(3):213–30. Review.

Vinson JA, Teufel K, Wu N. Red wine, de-alcoholised red wine, and especially grape juice, inhibit atherosclerosis in a hamster model. *Atherosclerosis* 2001;156(1): 67–72.

Viola G, Salvador A, Vedaldi D, Fortunato E, Disaro S, Basso G, Queiroz MJ. Induction of apoptosis by photoexcited tetracyclic compound derivatives of benzo[b]thiophenes and pyridines. *Journal of Photochemistry and Photobiology B, Biology* 2006;82(2):105–16.

Vitale S, West S, Hallfrisch J, Alston C, Wang E, Moorman C, Muller D, Singh V, Taylor HR. Plasma antioxidants and risk of cortical and nuclear cataract. *Epidemiology* 1993;4:195–203.

Vlad M, Bordas E, Caseanu E, Uza G, Creteanu E, Polinicenco C. Effect of cuprofilin on experimental atherosclerosis. *Biological Trace Element Research* 1995;48(1): 99–109.

Volpe SL, Huang HW, Larpadisorn K, Lesser II. Effect of chromium supplementation and exercise on body composition, resting metabolic rate and selected biochemical parameters in moderately obese women following an exercise program. *Journal of the American College of Nutrition* 2001;20(4):293–306.

Voutilainen S, Nurmi T, Mursu J, Rissanen TH. Carotenoids and cardiovascular health. *American Journal of Clinical Nutrition* 2006;83(6):1265–71. Review.

Waladkhani AR, Clemens MR. Effect of dietary phytochemicals on cancer development (review). *International Journal of Molecular Medicine* 1998;1(4):747–53. Review.

Walker LS, Bemben MG, Bemben DA, Knehans AW. Chromium picolinate effects on body composition and muscular performance in wrestlers. *Medical Science and Sports Exercise.* 1998;30(12):1730–37.

Wang H, Cao G, Prior RL. Total antioxidant capacity of fruits. *Journal of Agricultural and Food Chemistry* 1996;44(3):701–5.

Wang S, Chen B, Sun C. [Regulation effect of curcumin on blood lipids and antioxidation in hyperlipidemia rats]. *Wei Sheng Yan Jiu* 2000;29(4):240–42. Chinese.

Wei YH, Lu CY, Lee HC, Pang CY, Ma YS. Oxidative damage and mutation to mitochondrial DNA and age-dependent decline of mitochondrial respiratory function. *Annals of the New York Academy of Science* 1998;854:155–70. Review.

Weisburger JH. Chemopreventive effects of cocoa polyphenols on chronic diseases. *Experimental Biology and Medicine (Maywood).* 2001;226(10):891–97. Review.

Wilhelm J. Metabolic aspects of membrane lipid peroxidation. *Acta Universitatis Carollinae Medica Monographia* 1990;137:1–53. Review.

Willerson JT, Ridker PM. Inflammation as a cardiovascular risk factor. *Circulation* 2004;109(21 suppl 1):II2–10. Review.

Wright TI, Spencer JM, Flowers FP. Chemoprevention of nonmelanoma skin cancer. *Journal of the American Academy of Dermatology* 2006;54(6):933–46; quiz, 947–50. Review.

Xu Y, He L, Xu L, Liu Y. [Advances in immunopharmacological study of *Lycium barbarum* L.]. *Zhong Yao Cai* 2000;23(5):295–98. Review. Chinese.

Yamagishi M, Natsume M, Osakabe N, Nakamura H, Furukawa F, Imazawa T, Nishikawa A, Hirose M. Effects of cacao liquor proanthocyanidins on PhIP-induced mutagenesis in vitro, and in vivo mammary and pancreatic tumorigenesis in female Sprague-Dawley rats. *Cancer Letters* 2002;185(2):123–30.

Yamagishi M, Natsume M, Osakabe N, Okazaki K, Furukawa F, Imazawa T, Nishikawa A, Hirose M. Chemoprevention of lung carcinogenesis by cacao liquor proanthocyanidins in a male rat multi-organ carcinogenesis model. *Cancer Letters* 2003;191(1):49–57.

Yang HN, Lee EH, Kim HM. *Spirulina platensis* inhibits anaphylactic reaction. *Life Sciences* 1997;61:1237–44.

Ye X, Krohn RL, Liu W, Joshi SS, Kuszynski CA, McGinn TR, Bagchi M, Preuss HG, Stohs SJ, Bagchi D. The cytotoxic effects of a novel IH636 grape seed proanthocyanidin extract on cultured human cancer cells. *Molecular and Cellular Biochemistry* 1999;196(1–2):99–108.

Yim MB, Yim HS, Lee C, Kang SO, Chock PB. Protein glycation: creation of catalytic sites for free radical generation. *Annals of the New York Academy of Science* 2001;928:48–53.

Yin J, Tezuka Y, Kouda K, Tran QL, Miyahara T, Chen Y, Kadota S. Antiosteoporotic activity of the water extract of *Dioscorea spongiosa*. *Biological & Pharmaceutical Bulletin* 2004;27(4):583–86.

Young RW, Beregi JS Jr. Use of chlorophyllin in the care of geriatric patients. *Journal of the American Geriatrics Society* 1980;28:46–7.

Zampelas A, Panagiotakos DB, Pitsavos C, Das UN, Chrysohoou C, Skoumas Y, Stefanadis C. Fish consumption among healthy adults is associated with decreased levels of inflammatory markers related to cardiovascular disease. The ATTICA Study. *Journal of the American College of Cardiology* 2005;46(1):120–24.

Zebrack JS, Muhlestein JB, Horne BD, Anderson JL; Intermountain Heart Collaboration Study Group. C-reactive protein and angiographic coronary artery disease: independent and additive predictors of risk in subjects with angina. *Journal of the American College of Cardiology* 2002;39(4):632–37.

Zern TL, Fernandez ML. Cardioprotective effects of dietary polyphenols. *Journal of Nutrition* 2005;135(10):2291–94. Review.

Zhang LX, Cooney RV, Bertram JS. Carotenoids enhance gap junctional communication and inhibit lipid peroxidation in C3H/10T1/2 cells: relationship to their cancer chemopreventive action. *Carcinogenesis* 1991;12:2109–14.

Zhao G, Etherton TD, Martin KR, West SG, Gillies PJ, Kris-Etherton PM. Dietary alpha-linolenic acid reduces inflammatory and lipid cardiovascular risk factors in hypercholesterolemic men and women. *Journal of Nutrition* 2004;134:2991–97.

Zheng W, Sellers TA, Doyle TJ, et al. Retinol, antioxidant vitamins, and cancer of the upper digestive tract in a prospective cohort study of postmenopausal women. *American Journal of Epidemiology* 1995;142:955–60.

Zhi F, Zheng W, Chen P, He M. [Study on the extraction process of polysaccharide from *Lycium barbarum*]. *Zhong Yao Cai* 2004;27(12):948–50. Chinese.

Ziegler D, Hanefeld M, Ruhnau KJ, Meissner HP, Lobisch M, Schutte K, Gries FA. Treatment of symptomatic diabetic peripheral neuropathy with the anti-oxidant alpha-lipoic acid. A 3-week multicentre randomized controlled trial (ALADIN Study). *Diabetologia* 1995;38(12):1425–33.

Ziegler D, Reljanovic M, Mehnert H, Gries FA. Alpha-lipoic acid in the treatment of diabetic polyneuropathy in Germany: current evidence from clinical trials. *Experimental and Clinical Endocrinology & Diabetes* 1999;107(7):421–30. Review.

Ziegler RG. Vegetables, fruits, and carotenoids and the risk of cancer. *American Journal of Clinical Nutrition* 1991;53(suppl 1):251S–59S. Review.

Zs-Nagy I. The membrane hypothesis of aging: its relevance to recent progress in genetic research. *Journal of Molecular Medicine* 1997;75(10):703–14. Review.

Zs-Nagy I. The role of membrane structure and function in cellular aging: a review. *Mechanisms of Ageing and Development* 1979;9(3–4):237–46. Review.

Zs-Nagy I, Semsei I. Centrophenoxine increases the rates of total and mRNA synthesis in the brain cortex of old rats: an explanation of its action in terms of the membrane hypothesis of aging. *Experimental Gerontology* 1984;19(3):171–78.

CHAPTER 2

Belury MA et al. The conjugated linoleic acid (CLA) isomer, t10c12-CLA, is inversely associated with changes in body weight and serum leptin in subjects with type 2 diabetes mellitus. *Journal of Nutrition* 2003;133(1):257S–60S.

Benito P, Nelson GJ, Kelley DS, Bartolini G, Schmidt PC, Simon V. The effect of conjugated linoleic acid on plasma lipoproteins and tissue fatty acid composition in humans. *Lipids* 2001;36(3):229–36. Erratum in: *Lipids* 2001;36(8):857.

Blankson H, Stakkestad JA, Fagertun H, Thom E, Wadstein J, Gudmundsen O. Conjugated linoleic acid reduces body fat mass in overweight and obese humans. *Journal of Nutrition* 2000;130(12):2943–48.

Curran JE, Jowett JB, Elliott KS, Gao Y, Gluschenko K, Wang J, Abel Azim DM, Cai G, Mahaney MC, Comuzzie AG, Dyer TD, Walder KR, Zimmet P, MacCluer JW, Collier GR, Kissebah AH, Blangero J. Genetic variation in selenoprotein S influences inflammatory response. *Nature Genetics* 2005;37(11):1234–41. Epub 2005 Oct 9.

Gao Y, Hannan NR, Wanyonyi S, Konstantopolous N, Pagnon J, Feng HC, Jowett JB, Kim KH, Walder K, Collier GR. Activation of the selenoprotein SEPS1 gene expression by pro-inflammatory cytokines in HepG2 cells. *Cytokine* 2006;33(5):246–51. Epub 2006 Mar 30.

Gaullier JM, Halse J, Hoye K, Kristiansen K, Fagertun H, Vik H, Gudmundsen O. Supplementation with conjugated linoleic acid for 24 months is well tolerated by and reduces body fat mass in healthy, overweight humans. *Journal of Nutrition* 2005;135(4):778–84.

Gevrey JC, Malapel M, Philippe J, Mithieux G, Chayvialle JA, Abello J, Cordier-Bussat M. Protein hydrolysates stimulate proglucagon gene transcription in intestinal endocrine cells via two elements related to cyclic AMP response element. *Diabetologia* 2004;47(5):926–36. Epub 2004 Apr 14.

Haugen M, Alexander J. [Can linoleic acids in conjugated CLA products reduce overweight problems?] *Tidsskrift for den Norske Laegeforening* 2004;124(23):3051–54. Norwegian.

Kamphuis MM, Lejeune MP, Saris WH, Westerterp-Plantenga MS. Effect of conjugated linoleic acid supplementation after weight loss on appetite and food intake in overweight subjects. *European Journal of Clinical Nutrition* 2003;57(10): 1268–74.

Kamphuis MM, Lejeune MP, Saris WH, Westerterp-Plantenga MS. The effect of conjugated linoleic acid supplementation after weight loss on body weight regain, body composition, and resting metabolic rate in overweight subjects. *International Journal of Obesity and Related Metabolic Disorders* 2003;27(7):840–47.

Khan B, Arayne MS, Naz S, Mukhtar N. Hypoglycemic activity of aqueous extract of some indigenous plants. *Pakistan Journal of Pharmaceutical Sciences* 2005;18(1):62–4.

Kurpad AV, Raj R, Amarnath L. Use of *Caralluma fimbriata* extract to reduce weight. *Official South African Journal of Clinical Nutrition* 2005, 18(suppl. 1).

Lawrence RM, Choudary S. *Caralluma fimbriata* in the treatment of obesity. Western Geriatric Research Institute, Los Angeles, CA. 12th Annual World Congress of Anti-Aging Medicines, December 2004.

Malpuech-Brugere C, Verboeket-van de Venne WP, Mensink RP, Arnal MA, Morio B, Brandolini M, Saebo A, Lassel TS, Chardigny JM, Sebedio JL, Beaufrere B. Effects of two conjugated linoleic acid isomers on body fat mass in overweight humans. *Obesity Research* 2004;12(4):591–98.

McMillan-Price J, Petocz P, Atkinson F, O'Neill K, Samman S, Steinbeck K, Caterson I, Brand-Miller J. Comparison of 4 diets of varying glycemic load on weight loss and cardiovascular risk reduction in overweight and obese young adults: a randomized controlled trial. *Archives of Internal Medicine* 2006;166(14):1466–75.

Mithieux G, Misery P, Magnan C, Pillot B, Gautier-Stein A, Bernard C, Rajas F, Zitoun C. Portal sensing of intestinal gluconeogenesis is a mechanistic link in the diminution of food intake induced by diet protein. *Cell Metabolism* 2005;2(5): 321–29.

Moloney F, Yeow TP, Mullen A, Nolan JJ, Roche HM. Conjugated linoleic acid supplementation, insulin sensitivity, and lipoprotein metabolism in patients with type 2 diabetes mellitus. *American Journal of Clinical Nutrition* 2004;80(4):887–95.

Nagao K, Inoue N, Wang YM, Hirata J, Shimada Y, Nagao T, Matsui T, Yanagita I. The 10trans,12cis isomer of conjugated linoleic acid suppresses the development of hypertension in Otsuka Long-Evans Tokushima fatty rats. *Biochemical and Biophysical Research Communications* 2003;306;1:134–38.

Noakes M, Keogh JB, Foster PR, Clifton PM. Effect of an energy-restricted, high-protein, low-fat diet relative to a conventional high-carbohydrate, low-fat diet on weight loss, body composition, nutritional status, and markers of cardio-vascular health in obese women. *American Journal of Clinical Nutrition* 2005;81(6): 1298–306.

Nordmann AJ, Nordmann A, Briel M, Keller U, Yancy WS Jr, Brehm BJ, Bucher HC. Effects of low-carbohydrate vs low-fat diets on weight loss and cardiovascular risk factors: a meta-analysis of randomized controlled trials. *Archives of Internal Medicine* 2006;166(3):285–93. Erratum in: *Archives of Internal Medicine* 2006;166(8): 932.

Phillips KM, Ruggio DM, Ashraf-Khorassani M. Phytosterol composition of nuts and seeds commonly consumed in the United States. *Journal of Agricultural and Food Chemistry* 2005;53(24):9436–45.

Riserus U, Berglund L, Vessby B. Conjugated linoleic acid (CLA) reduced abdominal adipose tissue in obese middle-aged men with signs of the metabolic syndrome: a randomised controlled trial. *International Journal of Obesity and Related Metabolic Disorders* 2001;25(8):1129–35.

Riserus U, Vessby B, Arnlov J, Basu S. Effects of cis-9,trans-11 conjugated linoleic acid supplementation on insulin sensitivity, lipid peroxidation, and proinflammatory markers in obese men. *American Journal of Clinical Nutrition* 2004;80(2): 279–83.

Smedman A, Vessby B. Conjugated linoleic acid supplementation in humans—metabolic effects. *Lipids* 2001;36;8:773–81.

Thom E, Wadstein J, Gudmundsen O. Conjugated linoleic acid reduces body fat in healthy exercising humans. *Journal of International Medical Research* 2001;29;5: 392–96.

Whigham LD, O'Shea M, Mohede IC, Walaski HP, Atkinson RL. Safety profile of conjugated linoleic acid in a 12-month trial in obese humans. *Food and Chemical Toxicology* 2004;42(10):1701–9.

Yancy WS Jr, Olsen MK, Guyton JR, Bakst RP, Westman EC. A low-carbohydrate, ketogenic diet versus a low-fat diet to treat obesity and hyperlipidemia: a randomized, controlled trial. *Annals of Internal Medicine* 2004;140(10):769–77.

Zambell KL, Keim NL, Van Loan MD, Gale B, Benito P, Kelley DS, Nelson GJ. Conjugated linoleic acid supplementation in humans: effects on body composition and energy expenditure. *Lipids* 2000;35(7):777–82.

CHAPTER 3

Barel A, Calomme M, Timchenko A, De Paepe K, Demeester N, Rogiers V, Clarys P, Vanden Berghe D. Effect of oral intake of choline-stabilized orthosilicic acid on skin, nails, and hair in women with photodamaged skin. *Archives of Dermatological Research* 2005;297(4):147–53. Erratum in: *Archives of Dermatological Research* 2006;297(8):381.

Black DM, Cummings SR, Karpf DB, Cauley JA, Thompson DE, Nevitt MC, Bauer DC, Genant HK, Haskell WL, Marcus R, Ott SM, Torner JC, Quandt SA, Reiss TF, Ensrud KE. Randomized trial of effect of alendronate on the risk of fracture in women with existing vertebral fractures. *Lancet* 1996;348:1535–41.

Boivin M, Flourie B, Rizza RA, Go VL, DiMagno EP. Gastrointestinal and metabolic effects of amylase inhibition in diabetics. *Gastroenterology* 1988;94:387–94.

Boivin M, Zinsmeister AR, Go VL, DiMagno EP. Effect of a purified amylase inhibitor on carbohydrate metabolism after a mixed meal in healthy humans. *Mayo Clinic Proceedings* 1987;62:249–55.

Bo-Linn GW, Santa Ana CA, Morawski SG, Fordtran JS. Starch blockers—their effect on calorie absorption from a high-starch meal. *New England Journal of Medicine* 1982;307:1413–16.

Bone health and osteoporosis: a report of the Surgeon General (2004). U.S. Department of Health and Human Services, Washington, DC, 2004. Accessed June 8, 2005, at http://www.surgeongeneral.gov/library/bonehealth/content.html.

Brugge WR, Rosenfeld MS. Impairment of starch absorption by a potent amylase inhibitor. *American Journal of Gastroenterology* 1987;82:718–22.

Calomme M, Geusens P, Demeester N, Behets GJ, D'Haese P, Sindambiwe JB, Van Hoof V, Vanden Berghe D. Partial prevention of long-term femoral bone loss in aged ovariectomized rats supplemented with choline-stabilized orthosilicic acid. *Calcified Tissue International* 2006;78(4):227–32.

Carlson GL, Li BU, Bass P, Olsen WA. A bean alpha-amylase inhibitor formulation (starch blocker) is ineffective in man. *Science* 1983;219:393–95.

Cederholm T, Hedstrom M. Nutritional treatment of bone fracture. *Current Opinion in Clinical Nutrition and Metabolic Care* 2005;8(4):377–81.

Chapuy MC, Arlot ME, Duboeuf F, Brun J, Crouzet B, Arnaud S, Delmas PD, Meunier PJ. Vitamin D₃ and calcium to prevent hip fractures in elderly women. *New England Journal of Medicine* 1992;327:1637–42.

Cummings SR, Melton LJ 3rd. Epidemiology and outcomes of osteoporotic fractures. *Lancet* 2002;359(9319):1761–67.

Dawson-Hughes B, Dallal GE, Krall EA, Harris S, Sokoll LJ, Falconer G. Effect of vitamin D supplementation on wintertime and overall bone loss in healthy postmenopausal women. *Annals of Internal Medicine* 1991;115(7):505–12.

Dawson-Hughes B, Harris SS, Krall EA, Dallal GE. Effect of calcium and vitamin D supplementation on bone density in men and women 65 years of age or older. *New England Journal of Medicine* 1997;337(10):670–6.

Dawson-Hughes B, Harris SS, Krall EA, Dallal GE. Effect of withdrawal of calcium and vitamin D supplements on bone mass in elderly men and women. *American Journal of Clinical Nutrition* 2000;72(3):745–50.

Dawson-Hughes B, Harris SS, Krall EA, Dallal GE, Falconer G, Green CL. Rates of bone loss in postmenopausal women randomly assigned to one of two dosages of vitamin D. *American Journal of Clinical Nutrition* 1995;61(5):1140–45.

Di Daniele N, Carbonelli MG, Candeloro N, Iacopino L, De Lorenzo A, Andreoli A. Effect of supplementation of calcium and vitamin D on bone mineral density and bone mineral content in peri- and post-menopause women; a double-blind, randomized, controlled trial. *Pharmacological Research* 2004;50(6):637–41.

Elliott WJ. Clinical features in the management of selected hypertensive emergencies. *Progress in Cardiovascular Diseases* 2006;48(5):316–25. Review.

Englyst HN, Veenstra J, Hudson GJ. Measurement of rapidly available glucose (RAG) in plant foods: a potential in vitro predictor of the glycaemic response. *British Journal of Nutrition* 1996;75(3):327–37.

Ettinger B, Black DM, Mitlak BH, Knickerbocker RK, Nickelsen T, Genant HK, Christiansen C, Delmas PD, Zanchetta JR, Stakkestad J, Gluer CC, Krueger K, Cohen FJ, Eckert S, Ensrud KE, Avioli LV, Lips P, Cummings SR. Reduction of vertebral fracture risk in postmenopausal women with osteoporosis treated with raloxifene: results from a 3-year randomized clinical trial. *JAMA* 1999;282:637–45.

Garrow JS, Scott PF, Heels S, Nair KS, Halliday D. A study of 'starch blockers' in man using 13C-enriched starch as a tracer. *Human Nutrition Clinical Nutrition* 1983;37:301–5.

Gillespie WJ, Avenell A, Henry DA, O'Connell DL, Robertson J. Vitamin D and vitamin D analogues for preventing fractures associated with involutional and post-menopausal osteoporosis. *Cochrane Database of Systematic Reviews* 2001;(1): CD000227. Review.

Glerup H, Mikkelsen K, Poulsen L, Hass E, Overbeck S, Thomsen J, Charles P, Eriksen EF. Commonly recommended daily intake of vitamin D is not sufficient if sunlight exposure is limited. *Journal of Internal Medicine* 2000;247(2):260–68.

Gordon-Larsen P, McMurray RG, Popkin BM. Adolescent physical activity and inactivity vary by ethnicity: The National Longitudinal Study of Adolescent Health. *Journal of Pediatrics* 1999;135(3):301–6.

Granfeldt Y, Drews A, Bjorck I. Arepas made from high amylose corn flour produce favorably low glucose and insulin responses in healthy humans. *Journal of Nutrition* 1995;125(3):459–65.

Grant AM, Avenell A, Campbell MK, McDonald AM, MacLennan GS, McPherson GC, Anderson FH, Cooper C, Francis RM, Donaldson C, Gillespie WJ, Robinson CM, Torgerson DJ, Wallace WA; RECORD Trial Group. Oral vitamin D₃ and calcium for secondary prevention of low-trauma fractures in elderly people (Randomised Evaluation of Calcium Or vitamin D, RECORD): a randomised placebo-controlled trial. *Lancet* 2005;365:1621–28. Published online April 28, 2005 1001ID.1016/S0140-6736(05)63013-9.

Green KH, Wong SC, Weiler HA. The effect of dietary n-3 long-chain polyunsaturated fatty acids on femur mineral density and biomarkers of bone metabolism in healthy, diabetic and dietary-restricted growing rats. *Prostaglandins, Leukotrienes, and Essential Fatty Acids* 2004;71(2):121–30.

Guerrero-Romero F, Rodriguez-Moran M. Hypomagnesemia, oxidative stress, inflammation, and metabolic syndrome. *Diabetes Metab Res Rev.* 2006 Apr 5; [Epub ahead of print]

Harrington JT, Broy SB, Derosa AM, Licata AA, Shewmon DA. Hip fracture patients are not treated for osteoporosis: a call to action. *Arthritis and Rheumatism* 2002; 47(6):651–54.

Harris ST, Watts NB, Genant HR, McKeever CD, Hangartner T, Keller M, Chesnut CH 3rd, Brown J, Eriksen FF, Hoseyni MS, Axelrod DW, Miller PD. Effects of risedronate treatment on vertebral and nonvertebral fractures in women with postmenopausal osteoporosis: a randomized controlled trial. *JAMA* 1999;282: 1344–52.

Heaney RP. Nutritional factors in osteoporosis. *Annual Review of Nutrition* 1993;13: 287–316.

Heaney RP. Thinking straight about calcium. *New England Journal of Medicine* 1993;328: 503–5.

Higgins JA. Resistant starch: metabolic effects and potential health benefits. *Journal of AOAC International* 2004;87(3):761–68. Review.

Higgins JA, Higbee DR, Donahoo WT, Brown IL, Bell ML, Bessesen DH. Resistant starch consumption promotes lipid oxidation. *Nutrition & Metabolism* (London). 2004;1(1):8.

Hollenbeck CB, Coulston AM, Quan R, Becker TR, Vreman HJ, Stevenson DK, Reaven GM. Effects of a commercial starch blocker preparation on carbohydrate digestion and absorption: in vivo and in vitro studies. *American Journal of Clinical Nutrition* 1983;38:498–503.

Hollis BW, Wagner CL. Assessment of dietary vitamin D requirements during pregnancy and lactation. *American Journal of Clinical Nutrition* 2004;79(5):717–26. Review.

Holt PR, Thea D, Yang MY, Kotler DP. Intestinal and metabolic responses to an alpha-glucosidase inhibitor in normal volunteers. *Metabolism* 1988;37:1163–70.

Hunter D, Major P, Arden N, Swaminathan R, Andrew T, MacGregor AJ, Keen R, Snieder H, Spector TD. A randomized controlled trial of vitamin D supplementation on preventing postmenopausal bone loss and modifying bone metabolism using identical twin pairs. *Journal of Bone and Mineral Research* 2000;15: 2276–83.

Imada Y, Yoshioka S, Ueda T, Katayama S, Kuno Y, Kawahara R. Relationships between serum magnesium levels and clinical background factors in patients with mood disorders. *Psychiatry and Clinical Neurosciences* 2002;56(5):509–14.

Kendall CW, Emam A, Augustin LS, Jenkins DJ. Resistant starches and health. *Journal of AOAC International* 2004;87(3):769–74. Review.

Konishi M. [Cell membrane transport of magnesium]. *Clinical Calcium* 2005;15(2): 233–38. 8. Review. Japanese.

Korotkova M, Ohlsson C, Hanson LA, Strandvik B. Dietary n-6:n-3 fatty acid ratio in the perinatal period affects bone parameters in adult female rats. *British Journal of Nutrition* 2004;92(4):643–38.

Krall EA, Sahyoun N, Tannenbaum S, Dallal GE, Dawson-Hughes B. Effect of vitamin D intake on seasonal variations in parathyroid hormone secretion in postmenopausal women. *New England Journal of Medicine* 1989;321(26):1777–83.

Lankisch M, Layer P, Rizza RA, DiMagno EP. Acute postprandial gastrointestinal and metabolic effects of wheat amylase inhibitor (WAI) in normal, obese, and diabetic humans. *Pancreas* 1998;17(2):176–81.

LeBoff MS, Kohlmeier L, Hurwitz S, Franklin J, Wright J, Glowacki J. Occult vitamin D deficiency in postmenopausal US women with acute hip fracture. *JAMA* 1999;281(16):1505–11.

Leibson CL, Tosteson AN, Gabriel SE, Ransom JE, Melton LJ. Mortality, disability, and nursing home use for persons with and without hip fracture: a population-based study. *Journal of the American Geriatrics Society* 2002;50(10):1644–50.

Lindsay R, Meunier PJ. Osteoporosis: review of the evidence for prevention, diagnosis, and treatment and cost-effectiveness analysis. *Osteoporosis International* 1998;8(suppl 14):S1–S588.

Lips P, Graafmans WC, Ooms ME, et al. Vitamin D supplementation and fracture incidence in elderly persons. A randomized, placebo-controlled clinical trial. *Annals of Internal Medicine* 1996;124:400–6.

Mazur A, Maier JA, Rock E, Gueux E, Nowacki W, Rayssiguier Y. Magnesium and the inflammatory response: Potential physiopathological implications. *Archives of Biochemistry and Biophysics* 2006 Apr 19; [Epub ahead of print]

McKenna MJ, Freaney R. Secondary hyperparathyroidism in the elderly: means to defining hypovitaminosis D. *Osteoporosis International* 1998;8(suppl 2):S3–S6.

Meier C, Woitge HW, Witte K, Lemmer B, Seibel MJ. Supplementation with oral vitamin D₃ and calcium during winter prevents seasonal bone loss: a randomized controlled open-label prospective trial. *Journal of Bone and Mineral Research* 2004; 19(8):1221–30. Epub.

Melin AL, Wilske J, Ringertz H, Saaf M. Vitamin D status, parathyroid function and femoral bone density in an elderly Swedish population living at home. *Aging (Milan, Italy)* 1999;11(3):200–7.

Mihara M, Inoue D, Matsumoto T. [Vitamin D and its derivatives as anti-osteoporotic drugs]. *Clinical Calcium* 2005;15(4):597–604. Japanese.

Mitrou PN, Albanes D, Pietinen P, et al. Intakes of calcium, dairy products, and prostate cancer risk in the ATBC Study Abstract #3688, Panagiota Mitrou, National Cancer Institute, Bethesda, MD. Poster Session B, 5:15 p.m., Tuesday, Nov. 1, 2005. Accessed online November 19, 2005, at http://researchfestival. nih.gov/search.taf?_function=detail&t_Posters_uid1=805.

Murck H. Magnesium and affective disorders. *Nutritional Neuroscience* 2002;5(6): 375–89. Review.

Nair RR, Nair P. Alteration of myocardial mechanics in marginal magnesium deficiency. *Magnesium Research* 2002;15(3–4):287–306. Review.

National Osteoporosis Foundation. America's bone health: the state of osteoporosis and low bone mass in our nation. National Osteoporosis Foundation, Washington, DC, 2002.

National Osteoporosis Foundation. Pocket guide to the prevention and treatment of osteoporosis. National Osteoporosis Foundation, Washington, DC, 1998, p. 8.

Nieves JW. Osteoporosis: the role of micronutrients. *American Journal of Clinical Nutrition* 2005;81(5):1232S–9S.

Reginster JY. The high prevalence of inadequate serum vitamin D levels and implications for bone health. *Current Medical Research and Opinion* 2005;21(4):579–86.

Reid IR, Ames RW, Evans MC, Gamble GD, Sharpe SJ. Effect of calcium supplementation on bone loss in postmenopausal women. *New England Journal of Medicine* 1993;328:460–64.

Reid IR, Ames RW, Evans MC, Gamble GD, Sharpe SJ. Long-term effects of calcium supplementation on bone loss and fractures in postmenopausal women: a randomized controlled trial. *American Journal of Medicine* 1995;98:331–35.

Report of the Surgeon General's workshop on osteoporosis and bone health; Dec. 12–13, 2002. U.S. Department of Health and Human Services, Washington, DC, 2003. Available from http://www.surgeongeneral.gov/topics/bonehealth/.

Richmond J, Aharonoff GB, Zuckerman JD, Koval KJ. Mortality risk after hip fracture. *Journal of Orthopaedic Trauma* 2003;17(suppl 8):S2–5.

Riggs BL, Melton LJ 3rd. The worldwide problem of osteoporosis: insights afforded by epidemiology. *Bone* 1995;17(suppl 5):505S–11S.

Riis B, Thomsen K, Christiansen C. Does calcium supplementation prevent postmenopausal bone loss? A double-blind, controlled clinical study. *New England Journal of Medicine* 1987;316:173–77.

Robertson MD, Currie JM, Morgan LM, Jewell DP, Frayn KN. Prior short-term consumption of resistant starch enhances postprandial insulin sensitivity in healthy subjects. *Diabetologia* 2003;46(5):659–65.

Rosanoff A. [Magnesium and hypertension]. *Clinical Calcium.* 2005;15(2):255–60. Review. Japanese.

Salkeld G, Cameron ID, Cumming RG, Easter S, Seymour J, Kurrle SE, Quine S. Quality of life related to fear of falling and hip fracture in older women: a time trade off study. *BMJ* 2000;320(7231):341–46.

Sato Y, Asoh T, Kondo I, Satoh K. Vitamin D deficiency and risk of hip fractures among disabled elderly stroke patients. *Stroke.* 2001;32:1673–77.

Schiller JS, Coriaty-Nelson Z, Barnes P. Early release of selected estimates based on data from the 2003 National Health Interview Survey. National Center for Health Statistics, Hyattsville, MD, 2004. Available from http://www.cdc.gov/nchs/about/major/nhis/released200406.htm.

Schindler C, Dobrev D, Grossmann M, Francke K, Pittrow D, Kirch W. Mechanisms of beta-adrenergic receptor-mediated venodilation in humans. *Clinical Pharmacology and Therapeutics* 2004;75(1):49–59.

Shimosawa T, Fujita T. [Magnesium and N-type calcium channel]. *Clinical Calcium* 2005;15(2):239–44. Japanese.

Sontia B, Touyz RM. Role of magnesium in hypertension. *Archives of Biochemistry and Biophysics.* 2006 May 24; [Epub ahead of print]

Steingrimsdottir L, Gunnarsson O, Indridason OS, Franzson L, Sigurdsson G. Relationship between serum parathyroid hormone levels, vitamin D sufficiency, and calcium intake. *JAMA* 2005;294(18):2336–41.

Sun L, Tamaki H, Ishimaru T, Teruya T, Ohta Y, Katsuyama N, Chinen I. Inhibition of osteoporosis due to restricted food intake by the fish oils DHA and EPA and perilla oil in the rat. *Bioscience, Biotechnology, and Biochemistry* 2004;68(12):2613–15.

Thomas MK, Lloyd-Jones DM, Thadhani R, Shaw AC, Deraska DJ, Kitch BT, Vamvakas E, Dick IM, Prince RL, Finkelstein JS. Hypovitaminosis D in medical inpatients. *New England Journal of Medicine* 1998;338(12):777–83.

Tilyard MW, Spears GFS, Thomson J, Dovey S. Treatment of postmenopausal osteoporosis with calcitriol or calcium. *New England Journal of Medicine* 1992;326: 357–62.

Udani J, Hardy M, Madsen DC. Blocking carbohydrate absorption and weight loss: a clinical trial using phase 2 brand proprietary fractionated white bean extract. *Alternative Medicine Review* 2004;9(1):63–9.

Watkins BA, Li Y, Seifert MF. Dietary ratio of n-6/n-3 PUFAs and docosahexaenoic acid: actions on bone mineral and serum biomarkers in ovariectomized rats. *Journal of Nutritional Biochemistry* 2006;17(4):282–89.

Webb AR, Pilbeam C, Hanafin N, Holick MF. An evaluation of the relative contributions of exposure to sunlight and of diet to the circulating concentrations of 25-hydroxyvitamin D in an elderly nursing home population in Boston. *American Journal of Clinical Nutrition* 1990;51(6):1075–81.

Weiss LA, Barrett-Connor E, von Muhlen D. Ratio of n-6 to n-3 fatty acids and bone mineral density in older adults: the Rancho Bernardo Study. *American Journal of Clinical Nutrition* 2005;81(4):934–38.

Wortsman J, Matsuoka LY, Chen TC, Lu Z, Holick MF. Decreased bioavailability of vitamin D in obesity. *American Journal of Clinical Nutrition*. 2000;72(3):690–93. Erratum in: *American Journal of Clinical Nutrition* 2003;77(5):1342.

Wright JD, Wang CY, Kennedy-Stevenson J, Ervin RB. Dietary intakes of ten key nutrients for public health, United States: 1999–2000. *Advance Data* 2003;(334):104.

Zingmond DS, Melton LJ 3rd, Silverman SL. Increasing hip fracture incidence in California Hispanics, 1983 to 2000. *Osteoporosis International* 2004;15(8):603–10.

CHAPTER 4

Aggarwal BB, Kumar A, Bharti AC. Anticancer potential of curcumin: preclinical and clinical studies. *Anticancer Research* 2003;23(1A):363–98.

Aggarwal BB, Shishodia S. Suppression of the nuclear factor-kappaB activation pathway by spice-derived phytochemicals: reasoning for seasoning. *Annals of the New York Academy of Science* 2004;1030:434–41.

Aggarwal S, Ichikawa H, Takada Y, Sandur SK, Shishodia S, Aggarwal BB. Curcumin (diferuloylmethane) down-regulates expression of cell proliferation and anti-apoptotic and metastatic gene products through suppression of IkappaBalpha kinase and Akt activation. *Molecular Pharmacology* 2006;69(1):195–206.

Alkadhi KA. Endplate channel actions of a hemicholinium-3 analog, DMAE. *Naunyn-Schmiedeberg's Archives of Pharmacology* 1986;332(3):230–35.

Alvaro D, Cantafora A, Gandin C, Masella R, Santini MT, Angelico M. Selective hepatic enrichment of polyunsaturated phosphatidylcholines after intravenous administration of dimethylethanolamine in the rat. *Biochimica et Biophysica Acta* 1989;1006(1):116–20.

Anderson RA, Broadhurst CL, Polansky MM, Schmidt WF, Khan A, Flanagan VP, Schoene NW, Graves DJ. Isolation and characterization of polyphenol type-A polymers from cinnamon with insulin-like biological activity. *Journal of Agricultural and Food Chemistry* 2004;52(1):65–70.

Arafa HM. Curcumin attenuates diet-induced hypercholesterolemia. *Medical Science Monitor* 2005;11(7):BR228–34.

Arion VY, Zimina IV, Lopuchin YM. Contemporary views on the nature and clinical application of thymus preparations. *Russian Journal of Immunology* 1997;2(3–4): 157–66.

Association of Early Childhood Educators, Ontario, Canada. The importance of touch for children. Posted August 1997 at http://collections.ic.gc.ca/child/docs/00000949.htm.

Balasubramaniam A. Clinical potentials of neuropeptide Y family of hormones. *American Journal of Surgery* 2002;183(4):430–34.

Ben-Efraim S, Keisari Y, Ophir R, Pecht M, Trainin N, Burstein Y. Immunopotentiating and immunotherapeutic effects of thymic hormones and factors with special emphasis on thymic humoral factor THF-gamma2. *Critical Reviews in Immunology* 1999;19(4):261–84.

Berczi I, Chalmers IM, Nagy E, Warrington RJ. The immune effects of neuropeptides. *Baillière's Clinical Rheumatology* 1996;10(2):227–57.

Bharti AC, Donato N, Singh S, Aggarwal BB. Curcumin (diferuloylmethane) downregulates the constitutive activation of nuclear factor-kappa B and IkappaBalpha kinase in human multiple myeloma cells, leading to suppression of proliferation and induction of apoptosis. *Blood* 2003;101(3):1053–62.

Bierhaus A, Chevion S, Chevion M, Hofmann M, Quehenberger P, Illmer T, Luther T, Berentshtein E, Tritschler H, Muller M, Wahl P, Ziegler R, Nawroth PP. Advanced glycation end product-induced activation of NF-kappaB is suppressed by alpha-lipoic acid in cultured endothelial cells. *Diabetes* 1997;46(9):1481–90.

Bissett DL, Chatterjee R, Hannon DP. Photoprotective effect of superoxide-scavenging antioxidants against ultraviolet radiation-induced chronic skin damage in the hairless mouse. *Photodermatology, Photoimmunology & Photomedicine* 1990;7(2):56–62.

Black PH. Stress and the inflammatory response: a review of neurogenic inflammation. *Brain, Behavior, and Immunity* 2002;16(6):622–53.

Bodey B. Thymic hormones in cancer diagnostics and treatment. *Expert Opinion on Biological Therapy* 2001;1(1):93–107.

Bodey B, Bodey B Jr, Siegel SE, Kaiser HE. Review of thymic hormones in cancer diagnosis and treatment. *International Journal of Immunopharmacology* 2000;22(4): 261–73.

Bozin B, Mimica-Dukic N, Simin N, Anackov G. Characterization of the volatile composition of essential oils of some lamiaceae spices and the antimicrobial and antioxidant activities of the entire oils. *Journal of Agricultural and Food Chemistry* 2006;54(5):1822–28.

Broadhurst CL, Polansky MM, Anderson RA. Insulin-like biological activity of culinary and medicinal plant aqueous extracts in vitro. *Journal of Agricultural and Food Chemistry* 2000;48(3):849–52.

Brouet I, Ohshima H. Curcumin, an anti-tumour promoter and anti-inflammatory agent, inhibits induction of nitric oxide synthase in activated macrophages. *Biochemical and Biophysical Research Communications* 1995;206(2):533–40.

Cakatay U, Telci A, Kayali R, Sivas A, Akcay T. Effect of alpha-lipoic acid supplementation on oxidative protein damage in the streptozotocin-diabetic rat. *Research in Experimental Medicine (Berlin).* 2000;199(4):243–51.

Calabrese V, Scapagnini G, Colombrita C, Ravagna A, Pennisi G, Giuffrida Stella AM, Galli F, Butterfield DA. Redox regulation of heat shock protein expression in aging and neurodegenerative disorders associated with oxidative stress: a nutritional approach. *Amino Acids* 2003;25(3–4):437–44.

Chainani-Wu N. Safety and anti-inflammatory activity of curcumin: a component of turmeric (*Curcuma longa*). *Journal of Alternative and Complementary Medicine* 2003; 9(1):161–68.

Chan MM, Huang HI, Fenton MR, Fong D. In vivo inhibition of nitric oxide synthase gene expression by curcumin, a cancer preventive natural product with anti-inflammatory properties. *Biochemical Pharmacology.* 1998;55(12):1955–62.

Chan MM. Inhibition of tumor necrosis factor by curcumin, a phytochemical. *Biochemical Pharmacology* 1995;49(11):1551–56.

Chauhan DP. Chemotherapeutic potential of curcumin for colorectal cancer. *Current Pharmaceutical Design.* 2002;8(19):1695–706. Review.

Cole AC, Gisoldi EM, Grossman RM. Clinical and consumer evaluations of improved facial appearance after 1 month use of topical dimethylaminoethanol. Poster presentation, American Academy of Dermatology, Feb. 22–26, 2002, New Orleans.

Colven RM, Pinnell SR. Topical vitamin C in aging. *Clinical Dermatology* 1996;14(2): 227–34.

Conceicao de Oliveira M, Sichieri R, Sanchez Moura A. Weight loss associated with a daily intake of three apples or three pears among overweight women. *Nutrition* 2003;19(3):253–56.

Conney AH, Lysz T, Ferraro T, Abidi TF, Manchand PS, Laskin JD, Huang MT. Inhibitory effect of curcumin and some related dietary compounds on tumor promotion and arachidonic acid metabolism in mouse skin. *Advances in Enzyme Regulation* 1991;31:385–96. Review.

Datar P, Srivastava S, Coutinho E, Govil G. Substance P: structure, function, and therapeutics. *Current Topics in Medicinal Chemistry* 2004;4(1):75–103. Review.

Davis TP, Konings PN. Peptidases in the CNS: formation of biologically active, receptor-specific peptide fragments. *Critical Reviews in Neurobiology* 1993;7(3–4):163–74.

Deodhar, SD, Preliminary studies on anti-rheumatic activity of curcumin. *Indian Journal of Medical Research* 1980;71:632–34.

Ding M, Lu Y, Bowman L, Huang C, Leonard S, Wang L, Vallyathan V, Castranova V, Shi X. Inhibition of AP-1 and neoplastic transformation by fresh apple peel extract. *Journal of Biological Chemistry* 2004 12;279(11):10670–76.

Dorai T, Cao YC, Dorai B, Buttyan R, Katz AE. Therapeutic potential of curcumin in human prostate cancer. III. Curcumin inhibits proliferation, induces apoptosis, and inhibits angiogenesis of LNCaP prostate cancer cells in vivo. *Prostate* 2001; 47(4):293–303.

Duvoix A, Blasius R, Delhalle S, Schnekenburger M, Morceau F, Henry E, Dicato M, Diederich M. Chemopreventive and therapeutic effects of curcumin. *Cancer Letters* 2005;223(2):181–90.

Duvoix A, Morceau F, Delhalle S, Schmitz M, Schnekenburger M, Galteau MM, Dicato M, Diederich M. Induction of apoptosis by curcumin: mediation by glutathione S-transferase P1-1 inhibition. *Biochemical Pharmacology* 2003;66(8): 1475–83.

Eberlein-Konig B, Placzek M, Przybilla B. Phototoxic lysis of erythrocytes from humans is reduced after oral intake of ascorbic acid and D-alpha-tocopherol. *Photodermatology, Photoimmunology & Photomedicine* 1997;13(5–6):173–77.

Eberlein-Konig B, Placzek M, Przybilla B. Protective effect against sunburn of combined systemic ascorbic acid (vitamin C) and D-alpha-tocopherol (vitamin E). *Journal of the American Academy of Dermatology* 1998;38(1):45–8.

Evans JL, Goldfine ID. Alpha-lipoic acid: a multifunctional antioxidant that improves insulin sensitivity in patients with type 2 diabetes. *Diabetes Technology & Therapeutics*. 2000 Autumn;2(3):401–13. Review.

Friedman MJ. What might the psychobiology of posttraumatic stress disorder teach us about future approaches to pharmacotherapy? *Journal of Clinical Psychiatry* 2000;61(suppl 7):44–51.

Frucht-Pery J, Feldman ST, Brown SI. The use of capsaicin in herpes zoster ophthalmicus neuralgia. *Acta Ophthalmologica Scandinavica* 1997;75(3):311–13.

Fuchs J, Kern H. Modulation of UV-light-induced skin inflammation by D-alpha-tocopherol and L-ascorbic acid: a clinical study using solar simulated radiation. *Free Radical Biology & Medicine* 1998;25(9):1006–12.

Fuchs J, Milbradt R. Antioxidant inhibition of skin inflammation induced by reactive oxidants: evaluation of the redox couple dihydrolipoate/lipoate. *Skin Pharmacology and Medicine* 1994;7(5):278–84.

Galli L, de Martino M, Azzari C, Bernardini R, Cozza G, de Marco A, Lucarini D, Sabatini C, Vierucci A. [Preventive effect of thymomodulin in recurrent respiratory infections in children]. *La Pediatria Medica e Chirurgica* 1990;12(3):229–32. Italian.

Gambert SR, Garthwaite TL, Pontzer CH, Cook EE, Tristani FE, Duthie EH, Martinson DR, Hagen TC, McCarty DJ. Running elevates plasma beta-endorphin immunoreactivity and ACTH in untrained human subjects. *Proceedings of the Society for Experimental Biology and Medicine* 1981;168(1):1–4.

Geenen V, Kecha O, Brilot F, Hansenne I, Renard C, Martens H. Thymic T-cell tolerance of neuroendocrine functions: physiology and pathophysiology. *Cellular and Molecular Biology (Noisy-le-Grand, France)* 2001;47(1):179–88.

Geesin JC, Gordon JS, Berg RA. Regulation of collagen synthesis in human dermal fibroblasts by the sodium and magnesium salts of ascorbyl-2-phosphate. *Skin Pharmacology and Medicine* 1993;6(1):65–71.

Gianoulakis C. Implications of endogenous opioids and dopamine in alcoholism: human and basic science studies. *Alcohol and Alcoholism Supplement* 1996;1:33–42.

Goldberg DJ, Russell BA. Combination blue (415 nm) and red (633 nm) LED phototherapy in the treatment of mild to severe acne vulgaris. *Journal of Cosmetic and Laser Therapy* 2006;8(2):71–5.

Goldstein AL, Badamchian M. Thymosins: chemistry and biological properties in health and disease. *Expert Opinion on Biological Therapy* 2004;4(4):559–73.

Goldstein AL, Schulof RS, Naylor PH, Hall NR. Thymosins and anti-thymosins: properties and clinical applications. *Medical Oncology and Tumor Pharmacotherapy* 1986; 3(3–4):211–21.

Goya RG, Console GM, Herenu CB, Brown OA, Rimoldi OJ. Thymus and aging: potential of gene therapy for restoration of endocrine thymic function in thymus-deficient animal models. *Gerontology* 2002;48(5):325–28.

Grossman RM, Gisoldi EM, Cole AC. Long term safety and efficacy evaluation of a new skin firming technology: dimethylaminoethanol. Poster presentation, American Academy of Dermatology, Feb. 22–26, 2002, New Orleans.

Gutzwiller JP, Degen L, Matzinger D, Prestin S, Beglinger C. Interaction between GLP-1 and CCK33 in inhibiting food intake and appetite in men. *American Journal of Physiology Regulatory, Integrative and Comparative Physiology.* 2004;287(3): R562–67.

Hagen TM, Liu J, Lykkesfeldt J, Wehr CM, Ingersoll RT, Vinarsky V, Bartholomew JC, Ames BN. Feeding acetyl-L-carnitine and lipoic acid to old rats significantly improves metabolic function while decreasing oxidative stress. *Proceedings of the National Academy of the Sciences in the United States of America* 2002;99(4):1870–75. Erratum in: *Proceedings of the National Academy of the Sciences in the United States of America* 2002;99(10):7184.

Han D, Handelman G, Marcocci L, Sen CK, Roy S, Kobuchi H, Tritschler HJ, Flohe L, Packer L. Lipoic acid increases de novo synthesis of cellular glutathione by improving cystine utilization. *Biofactors* 1997;6(3):321–38.

Han SS, Keum YS, Seo HJ, Surh YJ. Curcumin suppresses activation of NF-kappaB and AP-1 induced by phorbol ester in cultured human promyelocytic leukemia cells. *Journal of Biochemistry and Molecular Biology* 2002;35(3):337–42.

Hill AJ, Peikin SR, Ryan CA, Blundell JE. Oral administration of proteinase inhibitor II from potatoes reduces energy intake in man. *Physiology & Behavior* 1990;48(2): 241–46.

Holmes A, Heilig M, Rupniak NM, Steckler T, Griebel G. Neuropeptide systems as novel therapeutic targets for depression and anxiety disorders. *Trends in Pharmacological Sciences* 2003;24(11):580–88.

Hughes J, Kosterlitz HW, Smith TW. The distribution of methionine-enkephalin and leucine-enkephalin in the brain and peripheral tissues. *British Journal of Pharmacology* 1977;120(suppl 4):428–36; discussion, 426–27.

Imparl-Radosevich J, Deas S, Polansky MM, Baedke DA, Ingebritsen TS, Anderson RA, Graves DJ. Regulation of PTP-1 and insulin receptor kinase by fractions from cinnamon: implications for cinnamon regulation of insulin signalling. *Hormone Research* 1998;50(3):177–82.

Jarvill-Taylor KJ, Anderson RA, Graves DJ. A hydroxychalcone derived from cinnamon functions as a mimetic for insulin in 3T3-L1 adipocytes. *Journal of the American College of Nutrition* 2001;20(4):327–36.

Jessop DS, Harbuz MS, Lightman SL. CRH in chronic inflammatory stress. *Peptides* 2001;22(5):803–7. Review.

Jobin C, Bradham CA, Russo MP, Juma B, Narula AS, Brenner DA, Sartor RB. Curcumin blocks cytokine-mediated NF-kappa B activation and proinflammatory gene expression by inhibiting inhibitory factor I-kappa B kinase activity. *Journal of Immunology* 1999;163(6):3474–83.

Kagan VE, Shvedova A, Serbinova E, Khan S, Swanson C, Powell R, Packer L. Dihydrolipoic acid—a universal antioxidant both in the membrane and in the aqueous phase. Reduction of peroxyl, ascorbyl and chromanoxyl radicals. *Biochemical Pharmacology* 1992;44(8):1637–49.

Kang G, Kong PJ, Yuh YJ, Lim SY, Yim SV, Chun W, Kim SS. Curcumin suppresses lipopolysaccharide-induced cyclooxygenase-2 expression by inhibiting activator protein 1 and nuclear factor kappaB bindings in BV2 microglial cells. *Journal of Pharmacological Sciences* 2004;94(3):325–28.

Karunagaran D, Rashmi R, Kumar TR. Induction of apoptosis by curcumin and its implications for cancer therapy. *Current Cancer Drug Targets* 2005;5(2):117–29.

Kastin AJ, Zadina JE, Olson RD, Banks WA. The history of neuropeptide research: version 5.a. *Annals of the New York Academy of Science* 1996;780:1–18. Review.

Katsuno M, Aihara M, Kojima M, Osuna H, Hosoi J, Nakamura M, Toyoda M, Matsuda H, Ikezawa Z. Neuropeptides concentrations in the skin of a murine (NC/Nga mice) model of atopic dermatitis. *Journal of Dermatological Science* 2003; 33(1):55–65.

Kempaiah RK, Srinivasan K. Beneficial influence of dietary curcumin, capsaicin and garlic on erythrocyte integrity in high-fat fed rats. *Journal of Nutritional Biochemistry* 2005 Oct 25; [Epub ahead of print]

Kempaiah RK, Srinivasan K. Influence of dietary spices on the fluidity of erythrocytes in hypercholesterolaemic rats. *British Journal of Nutrition* 2005;93(1):81–91.

Khan A, Safdar M, Ali Khan MM, Khattak KN, Anderson RA. Cinnamon improves glucose and lipids of people with type 2 diabetes. *Diabetes Care* 2003;26(12): 3215–18.

Khavinson VKh. Peptides and Ageing. *Neuro Endocrinology Letters* 2002;23(suppl 3): 11–14.

Khavinson VKh, Morozov VG. Peptides of pineal gland and thymus prolong human life. *Neuro Endocrinology Letters* 2003;24(3–4):233–40. Review.

Khor TO, Keum YS, Lin W, Kim JH, Hu R, Shen G, Xu C, Gopalakrishnan A, Reddy B, Zheng X, Conney AH, Kong AN. Combined inhibitory effects of curcumin and phenethyl isothiocyanate on the growth of human PC-3 prostate xenografts in immunodeficient mice. *Cancer Research* 2006;66(2):613–21.

Kocak G, Aktan F, Canbolat O, Ozogul C, Elbeg S, Yildizoglu-Ari N, Karasu C. Alpha-lipoic acid treatment ameliorates metabolic parameters, blood pressure, vascular reactivity and morphology of vessels already damaged by streptozotocin-diabetes. *Diabetes, Nutrition & Metabolism* 2000;13(6):308–18.

Komarcevic A. [The modern approach to wound treatment]. *Medicinski Pregled* 2000;53(7–8):363–68. Croatian. Review.

Kosterlitz HW, Corbett AD, Paterson SJ. Opioid receptors and ligands. *NIDA Research Monograph* 1989;95:159–66. Review.

Kouttab NM, Prada M, Cazzola P. Thymomodulin: biological properties and clinical applications. *Medical Oncology and Tumor Pharmacotherapy* 1989;6(1):5–9. Review.

Kramer MS, Winokur A, Kelsey J, Preskorn SH, Rothschild AJ, Snavely D, Ghosh K, Ball WA, Reines SA, Munjack D, Apter JT, Cunningham L, Kling M, Bari M, Getson A, Lee Y. Demonstration of the efficacy and safety of a novel substance P (NK1) receptor antagonist in major depression. *Neuropsychopharmacology* 2004; 29(2):385–92.

Krishnaswamy K, Polasa K. Diet, nutrition & cancer—the Indian scenario. *Indian Journal of Medical Research* 1995;102:200–9. Review.

Kumar AP, Garcia GE, Ghosh R, Rajnarayanan RV, Alworth WL, Slaga TJ. 4-Hydroxy-3-methoxybenzoic acid methyl ester: a curcumin derivative targets Akt/NF kappa B cell survival signaling pathway: potential for prostate cancer management. *Neoplasia* 2003;5(3):255–66.

Kunt T, Forst T, Wilhelm A, Tritschler H, Pfuetzner A, Harzer O, Engelbach M, Zschaebitz A, Stofft E, Beyer J. Alpha-lipoic acid reduces expression of vascular cell adhesion molecule-1 and endothelial adhesion of human monocytes after stimulation with advanced glycation end products. *Clinical Science* (London) 1999; 96(1):75–82.

Lambert JD, Hong J, Yang GY, Liao J, Yang CS. Inhibition of carcinogenesis by polyphenols: evidence from laboratory investigations. *American Journal of Clinical Nutrition* 2005;81(suppl 1):284S–91S. Review.

Leu TH, Maa MC. The molecular mechanisms for the antitumorigenic effect of curcumin. *Current Medicinal Chemistry Anti-cancer Agents* 2002;2(3):357–70. Review.

Li L, Aggarwal BB, Shishodia S, Abbruzzese J, Kurzrock R. Nuclear factor-kappaB and IkappaB kinase are constitutively active in human pancreatic cells, and their down-regulation by curcumin (diferuloylmethane) is associated with the suppression of proliferation and the induction of apoptosis. *Cancer* 2004;101 (10):2351–62.

Li L, Zhou JH, Xing ST, Chen ZR. [Effect of thymic factor D on lipid peroxide, glutathione, and membrane fluidity in liver of aged rats]. *Zhongguo Yao Li Xue Bao* 1993;14(4):382–84. Chinese.

Liacini A, Sylvester J, Li WQ, Huang W, Dehnade F, Ahmad M, Zafarullah M. Induction of matrix metalloproteinase-13 gene expression by TNF-alpha is mediated by MAP kinases, AP-1, and NF-kappaB transcription factors in articular chondrocytes. *Experimental Cell Research* 2003;288(1):208–17.

Lim GP, Chu T, Yang F, Beech W, Frautschy SA, Cole GM. The curry spice curcumin reduces oxidative damage and amyloid pathology in an Alzheimer transgenic mouse. *Journal of Neuroscience* 2001;21(21):8370–77.

Lin JK, Lin-Shiau SY. Mechanisms of cancer chemoprevention by curcumin. *Proceedings of the National Science Council, Republic of China. Part B, Life Science* 2001;25(2): 59–66.

Lin JK, Pan MH, Lin-Shiau SY. Recent studies on the biofunctions and biotransformations of curcumin. *Biofactors* 2000;13(1–4):153–58.

Linetsky M, James HL, Ortwerth BJ. Spontaneous generation of superoxide anion by human lens proteins and by calf lens proteins ascorbylated in vitro. *Experimental Eye Research* 1999;69(2):239–48.

Liu XY, Guo FL, Wu LM, Liu YC, Liu ZL. Remarkable enhancement of antioxidant activity of vitamin C in an artificial bilayer by making it lipo-soluble. *Chemistry and Physics of Lipids* 1996;83(1):39–43.

Low TL, Goldstein AL. Thymosins: structure, function and therapeutic applications. *Thymus* 1984;6(1–2):27–42. Review.

Maiorano V, Chianese R, Fumarulo R, Costantino E, Contini M, Carnimeo R, Cazzola P. Thymomodulin increases the depressed production of superoxide anion by alveolar macrophages in patients with chronic bronchitis. *International Journal of Tissue Reactions* 1989;11(1):21–5.

Mang B, Wolters M, Schmitt B, Kelb K, Lichtinghagen R, Stichtenoth DO, Hahn A. Effects of a cinnamon extract on plasma glucose, HbA, and serum lipids in diabetes mellitus type 2. *European Journal of Clinical Investigation* 2006;36(5): 340–44.

Martin-Du-Pan RC. [Thymic hormones. Neuroendocrine interactions and clinical use in congenital and acquired immune deficiencies]. *Annales d'endocrinologie* 1984;45(6):355–68. French.

Melhem MF, Craven PA, Derubertis FR. Effects of dietary supplementation of alpha-lipoic acid on early glomerular injury in diabetes mellitus. *Journal of the American Society of Nephrology* 2001;12(1):124–33.

Melhem MF, Craven PA, Liachenko J, DeRubertis FR. Alpha-lipoic acid attenuates hyperglycemia and prevents glomerular mesangial matrix expansion in diabetes. *Journal of the American Society of Nephrology* 2002;13(1):108–16.

Meyer M, Pahl HL, Baeuerle PA. Regulation of the transcription factors NF-kappa B and AP-1 by redox changes. *Chemico-biological Interactions* 1994;91(2–3):91–100.

Meyer M, Schreck R, Baeuerle PA. H_2O_2 and antioxidants have opposite effects on activation of NF-kappa B and AP-1 in intact cells: AP-1 as secondary antioxidant-responsive factor. *EMBO Journal* 1993;12(5):2005–15.

Midaoui AE, Elimadi A, Wu L, Haddad PS, de Champlain J. Lipoic acid prevents hypertension, hyperglycemia, and the increase in heart mitochondrial superoxide production. *American Journal of Hypertension* 2003;16(3):173–79.

Mohandas KM, Desai DC. Epidemiology of digestive tract cancers in India. V. Large and small bowel. *Indian Journal of Gastroenterology* 1999;18(3):118–21.

Mohandas KM, Jagannath P. Epidemiology of digestive tract cancers in India. VI. Projected burden in the new millennium and the need for primary prevention. *Indian Journal of Gastroenterology* 2000;19(2):74–8.

Morgan CA 3rd, Wang S, Southwick SM, Rasmusson A, Hazlett G, Hauger RL, Charney DS. Plasma neuropeptide-Y concentrations in humans exposed to military survival training. *Biological Psychiatry* 2000;47(10):902–9.

Nagy I, Floyd RA. Electron spin resonance spectroscopic demonstration of the hydroxyl free radical scavenger properties of dimethylaminoethanol in spin trapping experiments confirming the molecular basis for the biological effects of centrophenoxine. *Archives of Gerontology and Geriatrics* 1984;3(4):297–310.

Nagy I, Nagy K. On the role of cross-linking of cellular proteins in aging. *Mechanisms of Ageing and Development* 1980;14(1–2):245–51.

Narayan S. Curcumin, a multi-functional chemopreventive agent, blocks growth of colon cancer cells by targeting beta-catenin-mediated transactivation and cell-cell adhesion pathways. *Journal of Molecular Histology* 2004;35(3):301–7. Review.

Nayama S, Takehana M, Kanke M, Itoh S, Ogata E, Kobayashi S. Protective effects of sodium-L-ascorbyl-2 phosphate on the development of UVB-induced damage in cultured mouse skin. *Biological & Pharmaceutical Bulletin* 1999;22(12):1301–5.

Newman N, Lee DVM. Use of a calcium ascorbate supplement in therapy of obstructive pulmonary disease. *Pharmacokinetics–AAEP Proceedings* 1997;43.

Obrenovich ME, Monnier VM. Vitamin B_1 blocks damage caused by hyperglycemia. *Science of Aging Knowledge Environment* 2003;2003(10):PE6.

Onoda M, Inano H. Effect of curcumin on the production of nitric oxide by cultured rat mammary gland. *Nitric Oxide* 2000;4(5):505–15.

Ookawara T, Kawamura N, Kitagawa Y, Taniguchi N. Site-specific and random fragmentation of Cu,Zn-superoxide dismutase by glycation reaction. Implication of reactive oxygen species. *Journal of Biological Chemistry* 1992;267(26):18505–10.

Pacher P, Kecskemeti V. Trends in the development of new antidepressants. Is there a light at the end of the tunnel? *Current Medicinal Chemistry* 2004;11(7):925–43.

Pacher P, Kohegyi E, Kecskemeti V, Furst S. Current trends in the development of new antidepressants. *Current Medicinal Chemistry* 2001;8(2):89–100. Review.

Packer L, Kraemer K, Rimbach G. Molecular aspects of lipoic acid in the prevention of diabetes complications. *Nutrition* 2001;17(10):888–95. Review.

Packer L, Roy S, Sen CK. Alpha-lipoic acid: a metabolic antioxidant and potential redox modulator of transcription. *Advances in Pharmacology* 1996;38:79–101.

Packer L, Witt EH, Tritschler HJ. Alpha-lipoic acid as a biological antioxidant. *Free Radical Biology & Medicine* 1995;19(2):227–50. Review.

Paez X, Hernandez L, Baptista T. [Advances in the molecular treatment of depression]. *Revista de neurologia* 2003;37(5):459–70. Spanish. Review.

Pan MH, Lin-Shiau SY, Lin JK. Comparative studies on the suppression of nitric oxide synthase by curcumin and its hydrogenated metabolites through down-regulation of IkappaB kinase and NFkappaB activation in macrophages. *Biochemical Pharmacology* 2000;60(11):1665–76.

Pani G, Colavitti R, Bedogni B, Fusco S, Ferraro D, Borrello S, Galeotti T. Mitochondrial superoxide dismutase: a promising target for new anticancer therapies. *Current Medicinal Chemistry* 2004;11(10):1299–308.

Park JM, Adam RM, Peters CA, Guthrie PD, Sun Z, Klagsbrun M, Freeman MR. AP-1 mediates stretch-induced expression of HB-EGF in bladder smooth muscle cells. *American Journal of Physiology* 1999;277(2 Pt 1):C294–301.

Parker J. Do It Now Foundation. http://www.doitnow.org/.

Perricone NV. Photoprotective and anti-inflammatory effects of topical ascorbyl palmitate. *Journal of Geriatric Dermatology* 1993;1(1):5–10.

Perricone NV. Skin whiteners containing hydroxytetronic acid: United States Patent 6417226. Skin whitening compositions contain alpha-hydroxytetronic acid or an alpha-hydroxy tetronic derivative, and, in some cases, hydroquinone, an alpha-hydroxy acid such as glycolic acid, and a fatty acid ester of ascorbic acid such as ascorbyl palmitate.

Perricone NV. Topical 5% alpha lipoic acid cream in the treatment of cutaneous rhytids. *Dermatologic Surgery* 2000;20(3).

Perricone NV. Topical vitamin C ester (ascorbyl palmitate). Adapted from the first annual symposium on aging skin, San Diego, CA, February 21–23, 1997. *Journal of Geriatric Dermatology* 1997;5(4):162–70.

Perricone NV. Treatment of psoriasis with topical ascorbyl palmitate. *Clinical Research* 1991;39:535A.

Perricone N, Nagy K, Horvath F, Dajko G, Uray I, Zs-Nagy I. The hydroxyl free radical reactions of ascorbyl palmitate as measured in various in vitro models. *Biochemical and Biophysical Research Communications* 1999;262(3):661–65.

Perricone N, Nagy K, Horvath F, Dajko G, Uray I, Zs-Nagy I. Alpha lipoic acid (ALA) protects proteins against the hydroxyl free radical-induced alterations: rationale for its geriatric application. *Archives of Gerontology and Geriatrics* 1999;29(1):45–56.

Pert CB, Pasternak G, Snyder SH. Opiate agonists and antagonists discriminated by receptor binding in brain. *Science* 1973;182(119):1359–61.

Phan TT, See P, Lee ST, Chan SY. Protective effects of curcumin against oxidative damage on skin cells in vitro: its implication for wound healing. *Journal of Trauma* 2001;51(5):927–31.

Plummer SM, Holloway KA, Manson MM, Munks RJ, Kaptein A, Farrow S, Howells L. Inhibition of cyclo-oxygenase 2 expression in colon cells by the chemopreventive agent curcumin involves inhibition of NF-kappaB activation via the NIK/IKK signalling complex. *Oncogene* 1999;18(44):6013–20.

Podda M, Rallis M, Traber MG, Packer L, Maibach HI. Kinetic study of cutaneous and subcutaneous distribution following topical application of [7,8-14C]rac-alpha-lipoic acid onto hairless mice. *Biochemical Pharmacology* 1996;52(4): 627–33.

Podda M, Tritschler HJ, Ulrich H, Packer L. Alpha-lipoic acid supplementation prevents symptoms of vitamin E deficiency. *Biochemical and Biophysical Research Communications* 1994;204(1):98–104.

Podda M, Zollner TM, Grundmann-Kollmann M, Thiele JJ, Packer L, Kaufmann R. Activity of alpha-lipoic acid in the protection against oxidative stress in skin. *Current Problems in Dermatology* 2001;29:43–51.

Preuss HG, Echard B, Enig M, Brook I, Elliott TB. Minimum inhibitory concentrations of herbal essential oils and monolaurin for gram-positive and gram-negative bacteria. *Molecular and Cellular Biochemistry* 2005;272(1–2):29–34.

Qin B, Nagasaki M, Ren M, Bajotto G, Oshida Y, Sato Y. Cinnamon extract prevents the insulin resistance induced by a high-fructose diet. *Hormone and Metabolic Research* 2004;36(2):119–25.

Qin B, Nagasaki M, Ren M, Bajotto G, Oshida Y, Sato Y. Cinnamon extract (traditional herb) potentiates in vivo insulin-regulated glucose utilization via enhancing insulin signaling in rats. *Diabetes Research and Clinical Practice* 2003;62(3):139–48.

Rains C, Bryson HM. Topical capsaicin. A review of its pharmacological properties and therapeutic potential in post-herpetic neuralgia, diabetic neuropathy and osteoarthritis. *Drugs & Aging* 1995;7(4):317–28. Review.

Ramirez-Tortosa MC, Mesa MD, Aguilera MC, Quiles JL, Baro L, Ramirez-Tortosa CL, Martinez-Victoria E, Gil A. Oral administration of a turmeric extract inhibits LDL oxidation and has hypocholesterolemic effects in rabbits with experimental atherosclerosis. *Atherosclerosis* 1999;147(2):371–78.

Rao CV, et al. Antioxidant activity of curcumin and related compounds. Lipid peroxide formation in experimental inflammation. *Cancer Research* 1993;55:259.

Rasmusson AM, Hauger RL, Morgan CA, Bremner JD, Charney DS, Southwick SM. Low baseline and yohimbine-stimulated plasma neuropeptide Y (NPY) levels in combat-related PTSD. *Biological Psychiatry* 2000;47(6):526–39.

Reber F, Geffarth R, Kasper M, Reichenbach A, Schleicher ED, Siegner A, Funk RH. Graded sensitiveness of the various retinal neuron populations on the glyoxal-mediated formation of advanced glycation end products and ways of protection. *Graefe's Archive for Clinical and Experimental Ophthalmology* 2003;241(3): 213–25. Epub 2003 Feb 07.

Ritenbaugh C. Diet and prevention of colorectal cancer. *Current Oncology Reports* 2000;2(3):225–33. Review.

Rosenblat G, Perelman N, Katzir E, Gal-Or S, Jonas A, Nimni ME, Sorgente N, Neeman I. Acylated ascorbate stimulates collagen synthesis in cultured human foreskin fibroblasts at lower doses than does ascorbic acid. *Connective Tissue Research* 1998;37(3–4):303–11.

Ross D, Mendiratta S, Qu ZC, Cobb CE, May JM. Ascorbate 6-palmitate protects human erythrocytes from oxidative damage. *Free Radical Biology & Medicine* 1999;26(1–2):81–9.

Roy S, Sen CK, Tritschler HJ, Packer L. Modulation of cellular reducing equivalent homeostasis by alpha-lipoic acid. Mechanisms and implications for diabetes and ischemic injury. *Biochemical Pharmacology* 1997;53(3):393–99.

Rukkumani R, Aruna K, Varma PS, Rajasekaran KN, Menon VP. Comparative effects of curcumin and its analog on alcohol- and polyunsaturated fatty acid-induced alterations in circulatory lipid profiles. *Journal of Medicinal Food* 2005;8(2):256–60.

Saliou C, Kitazawa M, McLaughlin L, Yang JP, Lodge JK, Tetsuka T, Iwasaki K, Cillard J, Okamoto T, Packer L. Antioxidants modulate acute solar ultraviolet radiation-induced NF-kappa-B activation in a human keratinocyte cell line. *Free Radical Biology & Medicine* 1999;26(1–2):174–83.

Satoskar RR, Shah SJ, Shenoy SG. Evaluation of anti-inflammatory property of curcumin (diferuloyl methane) in patients with postoperative inflammation. *International Journal of Clinical Pharmacology, Therapy, and Toxicology* 1986;24(12):651–54.

Schulof RS. Thymic peptide hormones: basic properties and clinical applications in cancer. *Critical Reviews in Oncology/Hematology* 1985;3(4):309–76. Review.

Semsei I, Zs-Nagy I. Superoxide radical scavenging ability of centrophenoxine and its salt dependence in vitro. *Free Radical Biology & Medicine* 1985;1(5–6):403–8.

Sen CK, Packer L. Antioxidant and redox regulation of gene transcription. *FASEB Journal* 1996;10:709–20.

Shah BH, Nawaz Z, Pertani SA, Roomi A, Mahmood H, Saeed SA, Gilani AH. Inhibitory effect of curcumin, a food spice from turmeric, on platelet-activating factor–and arachidonic acid–mediated platelet aggregation through inhibition of thromboxane formation and Ca2+ signaling. *Biochemical Pharmacology* 1999;58(7):1167–72.

Shan B, Cai YZ, Sun M, Corke H. Antioxidant capacity of 26 spice extracts and characterization of their phenolic constituents. *Journal of Agricultural and Food Chemistry* 2005;53(20):7749–59.

Sharma RA, Gescher AJ, Steward WP. Curcumin: the story so far. *European Journal of Cancer* 2005;41(13):1955–68. Review.

Sharma SC, Mukhtar H, Sharma SK, Krishna Murt CR. Lipid peroxide formation in experimental inflammation. *Biochemical Pharmacology* 1972;21:1210.

Shindo Y, Witt E, Packer L. Antioxidant defense mechanisms in murine epidermis and dermis and their responses to ultraviolet light. *Journal of Investigative Dermatology* 1993;100(3):260–65.

Silva AP, Cavadas C, Grouzmann E. Neuropeptide Y and its receptors as potential therapeutic drug targets. *Clinica Chimica Acta* 2002;326(1–2):3–25. Review.

Singh S, Aggarwal BB. Activation of transcription factor NF-kappa B is suppressed by curcumin (diferuloylmethane). *Journal of Biological Chemistry* 1995;270(42): 24995–5000. Erratum in: *Journal of Biological Chemistry* 1995;270(50):30235.

Sinha R, Anderson DE, McDonald SS, Greenwald P. Cancer risk and diet in India. *Journal of Postgraduate Medicine* 2003;49(3):222–28. Review.

Siwak DR, Shishodia S, Aggarwal BB, Kurzrock R. Curcumin-induced antiproliferative and proapoptotic effects in melanoma cells are associated with suppression of IkappaB kinase and nuclear factor kappaB activity and are independent of the B-Raf/mitogen-activated/extracellular signal-regulated protein kinase pathway and the Akt pathway. *Cancer* 2005;104(4):879–90.

Smart RC, Crawford CL. Effect of ascorbic acid and its synthetic lipophilic derivative ascorbyl palmitate on phorbol ester-induced skin-tumor promotion in mice. *American Journal of Clinical Nutrition* 1991;54(suppl 6):1266S–73S.

Soliman KF, Mazzio EA. In vitro attenuation of nitric oxide production in C6 astrocyte cell culture by various dietary compounds. *Proceedings of the Society for Experimental Biology and Medicine* 1998;218(4):390–97.

Soni KB, Kuttan R. Effect of oral curcumin administration on serum peroxides and cholesterol levels in human volunteers. *Indian Journal of Physiology and Pharmacology* 1992;(36):273, 293.

Sreekanth KS, Sabu MC, Varghese L, Manesh C, Kuttan G, Kuttan R. Antioxidant activity of Smoke Shield in-vitro and in-vivo. *Journal of Pharmacy and Pharmacology* 2003;55(6):847–53.

Srimal R, Dhawan B. Pharmacology of diferuloyl methane (curcumin), a nonsteroidal anti-inflammatory agent. *Journal of Pharmacy and Pharmacology* 1973;(25) 447–52.

Srinivas L, Shalini VK, Shylaja M. Turmerin: a water-soluble antioxidant peptide from turmeric [*Curcuma longa*]. *Archives of Biochemistry and Biophysics* 1992;292(2): 617–23.

Srivasta R, Srimal RC. Modification of certain inflammation-induced biochemical changes by curcumin. *Indian Journal of Medical Research* 1985;(81):215–23.

Surh YJ. Anti-tumor promoting potential of selected spice ingredients with antioxidative and anti-inflammatory activities: a short review. *Food and Chemical Toxicology* 2002;40(8):1091–97.

Surh YJ, Chun KS, Cha HH, Han SS, Keum YS, Park KK, Lee SS. Molecular mechanisms underlying chemopreventive activities of anti-inflammatory phytochemicals: down-regulation of COX-2 and iNOS through suppression of NF-kappa B activation. *Mutation Research* 2001;480–81:243–68. Review.

Surh YJ, Han SS, Keum YS, Seo HJ, Lee SS. Inhibitory effects of curcumin and capsaicin on phorbol ester-induced activation of eukaryotic transcription factors, NF-kappaB and AP-1. *Biofactors* 2000;12(1–4):107–12.

Susan M, Rao MNA. Induction of glutathione S-transferase activity by curcumin in mice. *Arzneimittel-Forschung* 1992;42:962.

Suzuki YJ, Aggarwal BB, Packer L. Alpha-lipoic acid is a potent inhibitor of NF-kappa B activation in human T cells. *Biochemical and Biophysical Research Communications* 1992;189(3):1709–15.

Suzuki YJ, Mizuno M, Tritschler HJ, Packer L. Redox regulation of NF-kappa B DNA binding activity by dihydrolipoate. *Biochemistry and Molecular Biology International* 1995;36(2):241–46.

Suzuki YJ, Tsuchiya M, Packer L. Lipoate prevents glucose-induced protein modifications. *Free Radical Research Communications* 1992;17(3):211–17.

Tada H, Nakashima A, Awaya A, Fujisaki A, Inoue K, Kawamura K, Itoh K, Masuda H, Suzuki T. Effects of thymic hormone on reactive oxygen species-scavengers and renal function in tacrolimus-induced nephrotoxicity. *Life Sciences* 2002; 70(10):1213–23.

Tebbe B, Wu S, Geilen CC, Eberle J, Kodelja V, Orfanos CE. L-ascorbic acid inhibits UVA-induced lipid peroxidation and secretion of IL-1alpha and IL-6 in cultured human keratinocytes in vitro. *Journal of Investigative Dermatology* 1997; 108(3):302–6.

Toyoda M, Morohashi M. New aspects in acne inflammation. *Dermatology* 2003; 206(1):17–23.

Toyoda M, Nakamura M, Makino T, Hino T, Kagoura M, Morohashi M. Nerve growth factor and substance P are useful plasma markers of disease activity in atopic dermatitis. *British Journal of Dermatology* 2002;147(1):71–9.

Toyoda M, Nakamura M, Morohashi M. Neuropeptides and sebaceous glands. *European Journal of Dermatology* 2002;12(5):422–27. Review.

Tremblay JF, Sire DJ, Lowe NJ, Moy RL. Light-emitting diode 415 nm in the treatment of inflammatory acne: an open-label, multicentric, pilot investigation. *Journal of Cosmetic and Laser Therapy* 2006;8(1):31–3.

University of Texas MD Anderson Cancer Center. Herbal/plant therapies: turmeric (*Curcuma longa* Linn.) and curcumin. 2002, updated May, 2004. Accessed Feb. 18, 2006, at http://www.mdanderson.org/departments/cimer/display.cfm?id= fa324b1c-b0ca-4e93-903082f85808558f&method=displayfull&pn=6eb86a59-ebd9-11d4-810100508b603a14.

Wang S, Chen B, Sun C. [Regulation effect of curcumin on blood lipids and antioxidation in hyperlipidemia rats]. *Wei Sheng Yan Jiu* 2000;29(4):240–42. Chinese.

Yu MJ, McCowan JR, Thrasher KJ, Keith PT, Luttman CA, Ho PP, Towner RD, Bertsch B, Horng JS, Um SL, et al. Phenothiazines as lipid peroxidation inhibitors and cytoprotective agents. *Journal of Medicinal Chemistry* 1992;35(4):716–24.

Ziegler D, Reljanovic M, Mehnert H, Gries FA. Alpha-lipoic acid in the treatment of diabetic polyneuropathy in Germany: current evidence from clinical trials. *Experimental and Clinical Endocrinology & Diabetes* 1999;107(7):421–30. Review.

Zs-Nagy I. On the role of intracellular physicochemistry in quantitative gene expression during aging and the effect of centrophenoxine. A review. *Archives of Gerontology and Geriatrics* 1989;9(3):215–29.

Zs-Nagy I, Semsei I. Centrophenoxine increases the rates of total and mRNA synthesis in the brain cortex of old rats: an explanation of its action in terms of the membrane hypothesis of aging. *Experimental Gerontology* 1984;19(3):171–78.

CHAPTER 5

Adimoelja A. Phytochemicals and the breakthrough of traditional herbs in the management of sexual dysfunctions. *International Journal of Andrology* 2000;(suppl 3)2:82–4.

Ang HH, Cheang HS. Effects of *Eurycoma longifolia* jack on laevator ani muscle in both uncastrated and testosterone-stimulated castrated intact male rats. *Archives of Pharmacal Research* 2001;24(5):437–40.

Ang HH, Ikeda S, Gan EK. Evaluation of the potency activity of aphrodisiac in *Eurycoma longifolia* Jack. *Phytotherapy Research* 2001;15(5):435–36.

Ang HH, Lee KL. Effect of *Eurycoma longifolia* Jack on libido in middle-aged male rats. *Journal of Basic and Clinical Physiology and Pharmacology* 2002;13(3):249–54.

Ang HH, Lee KL. Effect of *Eurycoma longifolia* Jack on orientation activities in middle-aged male rats. *Fundamental & Clinical Pharmacology* 2002;16(6):479–83.

Ang HH, Lee KL, Kiyoshi M. *Eurycoma longifolia* Jack enhances sexual motivation in middle-aged male mice. *Journal of Basic and Clinical Physiology and Pharmacology* 2003;14(3):301–38.

Ang HH, Lee KL, Kiyoshi M. Sexual arousal in sexually sluggish old male rats after oral administration of *Eurycoma longifolia* Jack. *Journal of Basic and Clinical Physiology and Pharmacology* 2004;15(3–4):303–9.

Ang HH, Ngai TH. Aphrodisiac evaluation in non-copulator male rats after chronic administration of *Eurycoma longifolia* Jack. *Fundamental & Clinical Pharmacology* 2001;15(4):265–68.

Ang HH, Ngai TH, Tan TH. Effects of *Eurycoma longifolia* Jack on sexual qualities in middle aged male rats. *Phytomedicine* 2003;10(6–7):590–93.

Ang HH, Sim MK. *Eurycoma longifolia* increases sexual motivation in sexually naive male rats. *Archives of Pharmacal Research* 1998;21(6):779–81.

Ang HH, Sim MK. *Eurycoma longifolia* Jack and orientation activities in sexually experienced male rats. *Biological & Pharmaceutical Bulletin* 1998;21(2):153–55.

Ang HH, Sim MK. *Eurycoma longifolia* Jack enhances libido in sexually experienced male rats. *Experimental Animals* 1997;46(4):287–90.

Balick MJ, Lee R. Maca: From traditional crop to energy and libido stimulant. *Alternative Therapies in Health and Medicine* 2002;8(3):96–8.

Baranov VB. Experimental trials of herbal adaptogen effect on the quality of operation activity, mental and professional work capacity. Contract 93-11-615, stage

2, phase I. Moscow, Russia, Russian Federation Ministry of Health Institute of Medical and Biological Problems, 1994.

Brown RP, Gerbarg PL, Muskin PR. Alternative therapies in psychiatry. In Tasman A, Lieberman J, Kay J (ed.): *Psychiatry*, 2nd ed. West Sussex, England: Wiley & Sons, 2002.

Brown RP, Gerbarg PL, Ramazanov Z. *Rhodiola rosea*: a phytomedicinal overview. *Herbalgram* 2002;56:40–52.

Cicero AF, Bandieri E, Arletti R. *Lepidium meyenii* Walp. improves sexual behaviour in male rats independently from its action on spontaneous locomotor activity. *Journal of Ethnopharmacology* 2001;75(2–3):225–29.

Cyranoski D. Malaysian researchers bet big on home-grown Viagra. *Nature Medicine* 2005;11(9):912.

Darbinyan V, Kteyan A, Panossian A, Gabrielian E, Wikman G, Wagner H. *Rhodiola rosea* in stress induced fatigue—a double blind cross-over study of a standardized extract SHR-5 with a repeated low-dose regimen on the mental performance of healthy physicians during night duty. *Phytomedicine* 2000;7(5):365–71.

Ebrahim S, May M, Ben Shlomo Y, McCarron P, Frankel S, Yarnell J, Davey Smith G. Sexual intercourse and risk of ischaemic stroke and coronary heart disease: the Caerphilly study. *Journal of Epidemiology and Community Health* 2002;56(2):99–102.

Ebrahim SH, McKenna MT, Marks JS. Sexual behaviour: related adverse health burden in the United States. *Sexually Transmitted Infections* 2005;81(1):38–40.

Gerasimova HD. Effect of *Rhodiola rosea* extract on ovarian functional activity. In: *Proceedings of the Scientific Conference on Endocrinology and Gynecology*. Sverdlovsk, Russia. 1970 Sept. 15–16. Siberian Branch of the Russian Academy of Sciences. pp. 46–48.

Gonzales GF, Cordova A, Vega K, Chung A, Villena A, Gonez C, Castillo S. Effect of *Lepidium meyenii* (MACA) on sexual desire and its absent relationship with serum testosterone levels in adult healthy men. *Andrologia* 2002;34(6):367–72.

Gonzales GF, Ruiz A, Gonzales C, Villegas L, Cordova A. Effect of *Lepidium meyenii* (maca) roots on spermatogenesis of male rats. *Asian Journal of Andrology* 2001;3(3):231–33.

Katharine Dexter McCormick Library/Planned Parenthood Federation of America. The Health Benefits of Sexual Expression. Published in cooperation with the Society for the Scientific Study of Sexuality. Accessed Feb. 12, 2006, at http://www.plannedparenthood.org/pp2/portal/files/portal/medicalinfo/sexualhealth/white-030401-sexual-expression.pdf.

Kimoto H, Haga S, Sato K, Touhara K. Sex-specific peptides from exocrine glands stimulate mouse vomeronasal sensory neurons. *Nature* 2005;437(7060):898–901.

Komar VV, Kit SM, Sischuk LV, Sischuk VM. Effect of *Rhodiola rosea* on the human mental activity. *Pharmaceutical Journal* 1981;36(4):62–64.

Kurkin VA, Zapesochnaya GG. Chemical composition and pharmacological characteristics of *Rhodiola rosea* [review]. *Journal of Medicinal Plants* 1985;1231–445.

Lazarova MB, Petkov VD, Markovska VL, Petkov VV, Mosharrof A. Effects of meclofenoxate and extr. *Rhodiolae rosea* L. on electroconvulsive shock-impaired learning and memory in rats. *Methods and Findings in Experimental and Clinical Pharmacology* 1986;8(9):547–52.

Lupien SJ, de Leon M, de Santi S, Convit A, Tarshish C, Nair NP, Thakur M, McEwen BS, Hauger RL, Meaney MJ. Cortisol levels during human aging predict hippocampal atrophy and memory deficits. *Nature Neuroscience* 1998;1(1):69–73.

Marina TF. Effect of *Rhodiola rosea* extract on bioelectrical activity of the cerebral cortex isolated to a different extent from the brain. In Saratikov AS(ed.): *Stimulants of the Central Nervous System.* Tomsk, Russia: Tomsk State University Press; 1968, pp. 27–31.

Marina TF, Alekseeva LP. Effect of *Rhodiola rosea* extract on electroencephalograms in rabbit. In Saratikov AS (ed.): *Stimulants of the Central Nervous System.* Tomsk, Russia: Tomsk State University Press, 1968, pp. 22–26.

McKay D. Nutrients and botanicals for erectile dysfunction: examining the evidence. *Alternative Medicine Review* 2004;9(1):4–16.

Olson R, Dulac C, Bjorkman PJ. MHC homologs in the nervous system—they haven't lost their groove. *Current Opinion in Neurobiology* 2006;16(3):351–57. Epub 2006 May 15.

Petkov VD, Yonkov D, Mosharoff A, Kambourova T, Alova L, Petkov VV, Todorov I. Effects of alcohol aqueous extract from *Rhodiola rosea* L. roots on learning and memory. *Acta Physiologica et Pharmacologica Bulgarica* 1986;12(1):3–16.

Petridou E, Giokas G, Kuper H, Mucci LA, Trichopoulos D. Endocrine correlates of male breast cancer risk: a case-control study in Athens, Greece. *British Journal of Cancer* 2000;83(9):1234–37.

Russian Federation Ministry of Health and Medical Industry. *Russian National Pharmacopoeia.* Pharmacopoeia article: PA 42-2126-83, liquid extract of *Rhodiola rosea* root and rhizome. Moscow, Russia, Russian Federation Ministry of Health and Medical Industry, 1983.

Saratikov A, Marina TF, Fisanova LL. Effect of golden root extract on processes of serotonin synthesis in CNS. *Journal of Biological Sciences* 1978;6:142.

Saratikov AS, Krasnov EA. Clinical studies of *Rhodiola.* In Saratikov AS, Krasnov EA (eds.): *Rhodiola Rosea Is a Valuable Medicinal Plant (Golden Root).* Tomsk, Russia: Tomsk State University Press, 1987, pp. 216–27.

Saratikov AS, Krasnov EA. The influence of *Rhodiola* on endocrine glands and the liver. In Saratikov AS, Krasnov EA (eds.): *Rhodiola Rosea Is a Valuable Medicinal Plant (Golden Root).* Tomsk, Russia: Tomsk State University Press, 1987, pp. 180–93.

Saratikov AS, Krasnov EA, Khnikina LA, Duvidson LM. Isolation and chemical analysis of individual biologically active constituents of *Rhodiola rosea. Proceedings of the Siberian Academy of Sciences. Biology* 1967;1:54–60.

Spasov AA, Mandrikov VB, Mironova IA. The effect of the preparation rhodiosin on the psychophysiological and physical adaptation of students to an academic load. *Eksperimental'naia i klinicheskaia farmakologiia* 2000;63(1):76–78.

Spasov AA, Wikman GK, Mandrikov VB, Mironova IA, Neumoin VV. A double-blind, placebo-controlled pilot study of the stimulating and adaptogenic effect of *Rhodiola rosea* SHR-5 extract on the fatigue of students caused by stress during an examination period with a repeated low-dose regimen. *Phytomedicine* 2000; 7(2):85–89.

Stancheva SL, Mosharrof A. Effect of the extract of *Rhodiola rosea* L. on the content of the brain biogenic monoamines. *Medecine Physiologie Comptes Rendus de l'Académie Bulgare des Sciences* 1987;40(6):85–87.

Wedekind C, Penn D. MHC genes, body odours, and odour preferences. *Nephrology, Dialysis, Transplantation* 2000;15(9):1269–71. Review.

Weeks D, James J. *Secrets of the Superyoung.* New York: Berkley Books, 1998.

Weeks DJ. Sex for the mature adult: health, self-esteem and countering ageist stereotypes. *Sexual and Relationship Therapy* 2002;17(3),231–40.

Zheng BL, He K, Kim CH, Rogers L, Shao Y, Huang ZY, Lu Y, Yan SJ, Qien LC, Zheng QY. Effect of a lipidic extract from lepidium meyenii on sexual behavior in mice and rats. *Urology* 2000;55(4):598–602.

CHAPTER 6

Albert M, Jones K, Savage C, Berkman L, Seeman T, Blazer D, Rowe J. Predictors of cognitive change in older persons: MacArthur Studies of Successful Aging. *Psychology and Aging* 1995;10;578–89.

Barnes DE, Yaffe K, Satariano WA, Tager IB. A longitudinal study of cardiorespiratory fitness and cognitive function in healthy older adults. *Journal of the American Geriatrics Society* 2003;51:459–65.

Carmelli D, Swan GE, LaRue A, Eslinger PJ. Correlates of change in cognitive function in survivors from the Western Collaborative Group Study. *Neuroepidemiology* 1997;16:285–95.

Colcombe S, Kramer AF. Fitness effects on the cognitive function of older adults: a meta-analytic study. *Psychological Science* 2003;14:125–30.

Colcombe SJ, Erickson KI, Raz N, Webb AG, Cohen NJ, McAuley E, Kramer AF. Aerobic fitness reduces brain tissue loss in aging humans. *Journals of Gerontology. Series A, Biological Sciences and Medical Sciences* 2003;58:176–80.

Colcombe SJ, Kramer AF, Erickson KI, Scalf P, McAuley E, Cohen NJ, Webb A, Jerome GJ, Marquez DX, Elavsky S. Cardiovascular fitness, cortical plasticity, and aging. *Proceedings of the National Academy of the Sciences of the United States of America* 2004; 101:3316–21.

Friedland RP, Fritsch T, Smith KA, Koss E, Lerner AJ, Chen CH, Petot GJ, Debanne SM. Patients with Alzheimer's disease have reduced activities in midlife compared with healthy control-group members. *Proceedings of the National Academy of the Sciences of the United States of America* 2001;98:3440–45.

Han A, Robinson V, Judd M, Taixiang W, Wells G, Tugwell P. Tai chi for treating rheumatoid arthritis. *Cochrane Database System Review* 2004;(3):CD004849. Review.

Kramer AF, Colcombe SJ, McAuley E, Eriksen KI, Scalf P, Jerome GJ, Marquez DX, Elavsky S, Webb AG. Enhancing brain and cognitive function of older adults through fitness training. *Journal of Molecular Neuroscience* 2003;213–21.

Laurin D, Verreault R, Lindsay J, MacPherson K, Rockwood K. Physical activity and risk of cognitive impairment and dementia in elderly persons. *Archives of Neurology* 2001;58:498–504.

Li F, Fisher KJ, Harmer P, McAuley E. Delineating the impact of tai chi training on physical function among the elderly. *American Journal of Preventive Medicine* 2002; 23(suppl 2):92–97.

National Institutes of Health. Cognitive and Emotional Health Project Physical Activity and Cardiorespiratory Fitness. Accessed Aug. 11, 2006, at http://trans.nih.gov/CEHP/index.htm.

Réquéna Y. *Chi Kung: The Chinese Art of Mastering Energy.* Rochester, VT: Healing Arts Press, 1997.

Song R, Lee EO, Lam P, Bae SC. Effects of tai chi exercise on pain, balance, muscle strength, and perceived difficulties in physical functioning in older women with osteoarthritis: a randomized clinical trial. *Journal of Rheumatology* 2003;30(9): 2039–44.

Taylor-Piliae RE, Froelicher ES. Effectiveness of tai chi exercise in improving aerobic capacity: a meta-analysis. *Journal of Cardiovascular Nursing* 2004;19(1):48–57.

Taylor-Piliae RE, Haskell WL, Stotts NA, Froelicher ES. Improvement in balance, strength, and flexibility after 12 weeks of tai chi exercise in ethnic Chinese adults with cardiovascular disease risk factors. *Alternative Therapies in Health and Medicine* 2006;12(2):50–8.

Verghese J, Lipton RB, Katz MJ, Hall CB, Derby CA, Kuslansky G, Ambrose AF, Sliwinski M, Buschke H. Leisure activities and the risk of dementia in the elderly. *New England Journal of Medicine* 2003;348:2508–16.

Wang C, Collet JP, Lau J. The effect of tai chi on health outcomes in patients with chronic conditions: a systematic review. *Archives of Internal Medicine* 2004;164(5): 493–501. Review.

Wayne PM, Krebs DE, Wolf SL, Gill-Body KM, Scarborough DM, McGibbon CA, Kaptchuk TJ, Parker SW. Can tai chi improve vestibulopathic postural control? *Archives of Physical Medicine and Rehabilitation* 2004;85(1):142–52. Review.

Yaffe K, Barnes D, Nevitt M, Lui LY, Covinsky K. A prospective study of physical activity and cognitive decline in elderly women: women who walk. *Archives of Internal Medicine* 2001;161:1703–8.

CHAPTER 7

AAP 2000 Red Book: Report of the Committee on Infectious Diseases, 25th ed. Elk Grove Village, IL: American Academy of Pediatrics, 2000.

Adlercreutz CH, Goldin BR, Gorbach SL, Hockerstedt KA, Watanabe S, Hamalainen EK, Markkanen MH, Makela TH, Wahala KT, Adlercreutz T. Soybean phytoestrogen intake and cancer risk. *Journal of Nutrition* 1995;125:757S–70S.

Anderson J, Johnstone BM, Cook-Newell ME. Meta-analysis of the effects of soy protein intake on serum lipiods. *New England Journal of Medicine* 1995;333;276–82.

Afzal M, Al-Hadidi D, Menon M, Pesek J, Dhami MS. Ginger: an ethnomedical, chemical and pharmacological review. *Drug Metabolism and Drug Interactions* 2001; 18(3–4):159–90. Review.

Agerholm-Larsen L, Raben A, Haulrik N, Hansen AS, Manders M, Astrup A. Effect of 8 week intake of probiotic milk products on risk factors for cardiovascular diseases. *European Journal of Clinical Nutrition* 2000;54(4):288–97.

Aggarwal BB, Kumar A, Bharti AC. Anticancer potential of curcumin: preclinical and clinical studies. *Anticancer Research* 2003;23(1A):363–98. Review.

Ahmed RS, Seth V, Banerjee BD. Influence of dietary ginger (*Zingiber officinales* Rosc) on antioxidant defense system in rat: comparison with ascorbic acid. *Indian Journal of Experimental Biology* 2000;38(6):604–6.

Altman RD, Marcussen KC. Effects of a ginger extract on knee pain in patients with osteoarthritis. *Arthritis and Rheumatism* 2001;44:2531–38.

Anderson JW, Deakins DA, Floore TL, Smith BM, Whitis SE. Dietary fiber and coronary heart disease. *Critical Reviews in Food Science and Nutrition* 1990;29:95–147.

Anderson JW, Gustafson NJ. Hypocholesterolemic effect of oat and bean products. *American Journal of Clinical Nutrition* 1988;48:749–53.

Anderson JW, Gustafson NJ, Spencer DB, Tietyen J, Bryant CA. Serum lipid response of hypercholesterolemic men to single and divided doses of canned beans. *American Journal of Clinical Nutrition* 1990;51:1013–19.

Anderston JW, Johnstone BM, Cook-Newell ME. 1995. Meta-analysis of the effects of soy protein intake on serum lipids. *New England Journal of Medicine* 333:276–82.

Antonio MA, Hawes SE, Hillier SL. The identification of vaginal *Lactobacillus* species and the demographic and microbiologic characteristics of women colonized by these species. *Journal of Infectious Diseases* 1999;180(6):1950–56.

Bazzano LA, He J, Ogden LG, Loria C, Vupputuri S, Myers L, Whelton PK. Legume consumption and risk of coronary heart disease in US men and women. *Archives of Internal Medicine* 2001;161:2573–78.

Bengmark S. Colonic food: pre- and probiotics. *American Journal of Gastroenterology* 2000;95(suppl 1):S5–7.

Bomba A, Nemcova R, Gancarcikova S, Herich R, Pistl J, Revajova V, Jonecova Z, Bugarsky A, Levkut M, Kastel R, Baran M, Lazar G, Hluchy M, Marsalkova S, Posivak J. The influence of omega-3 polyunsaturated fatty acids (omega-3 pufa) on lactobacilli adhesion to the intestinal mucosa and on immunity in gnotobiotic piglets. *Berliner und Munchener tierarztliche Wochenschrift* 2003;116(7–8):312–16.

Borchers AT, Keen CL, Gershwin ME. The influence of yogurt/*Lactobacillus* on the innate and acquired immune response. *Clinical Reviews in Allergy & Immunology* 2002;22(3):207–30. Review.

Bordia A, Verma SK, Srivastava KC. Effect of ginger (*Zingiber officinale Rosc.*) and fenugreek (*Trigonella foenumgraecum* L.) on blood lipids, blood sugar and platelet aggregation in patients with coronary artery disease. *Prostaglandins, Leukotrienes, and Essential Fatty Acids* 1997;56:379–84.

Bressani R, Elías LG. The nutritional role of polyphenols in beans. In JH Hulse (ed.): *Polyphenols in Cereals and Legumes* (IDRC-145e). Ottawa, Ontario, Canada, International Development Research Centre, 1979.

Bressani R, Elías LG, Braham JE. Reduction of digestibility of legume protein by tannins. In: *Workshop on Physiological Effects of Legumes in the Laymen Diet*, XII International Congress of Nutrition, San Diego, CA, August 1981.

Brouet I, Ohshima H. Curcumin, an anti-tumour promoter and anti-inflammatory agent, inhibits induction of nitric oxide synthase in activated macrophages. *Biochemical and Biophysical Research Communications* 199517;206(2):533–40.

Burros M. Is there an extra ingredient in nonstick pans? *New York Times*, July 27, 2005. Accessed June 21, 2006 at http://www.nytimes.com/2005/07/27/dining/27well.html?ex=1151294400&en=7fe344b845338ff9&ei=5070.

Calabrese V, Scapagnini G, Colombrita C, Ravagna A, Pennisi G, Giuffrida Stella AM, Galli F, Butterfield DA. Redox regulation of heat shock protein expression in aging and neurodegenerative disorders associated with oxidative stress: a nutritional approach. *Amino Acids* 2003;25(3–4):437–44.

Caragay AB. Cancer-preventative foods and ingredients. *Food Technology* 1992;46(4):65–68.

Carroll KK. Review of clinical studies on cholesterol lowering response to soy protein. *Journal of the American Dietetic Association* 1991;91:820–27.

Cav GH, Sofic E, Prior RL. Antioxidant capacity of tea and common vegetables. *Journal of Agricultural and Food Chemistry* 1996;44:(11)3426–31.

Cesarone MR, Belcaro G, Incandela L, Geroulakos G, Griffin M, Lennox A, DeSanctis MT, Acerbi G. Flight microangiopathy in medium-to-long distance flights: prevention of edema and microcirculation alterations with HR (Paroven, Venoruton; 0-(beta-hydroxyethyl)-rutosides): a prospective, randomized, controlled trial. *Journal of Cardiovascular Pharmacology and Therapeutics* 2002;7(suppl 1):S17–20.

Cesarone MR, Incandela L, DeSanctis MT, Belcaro G, Griffin M, Ippolito E, Acerbi G. Treatment of edema and increased capillary filtration in venous hypertension with HR (Paroven, Venoruton; 0-(beta-hydroxyethyl)-rutosides): a clinical, prospective, placebo-controlled, randomized, dose-ranging trial. *Journal of Cardiovascular Pharmacology and Therapeutics* 2002;7(suppl 1):S21–4.

Chainani-Wu N. Safety and anti-inflammatory activity of curcumin: a component of turmeric (*Curcuma longa*). *Journal of Alternative and Complementary Medicine* 2003;9(1):161–68. Review.

Chan MM. Inhibition of tumor necrosis factor by curcumin, a phytochemical. *Biochemical Pharmacology* 1995;49(11):1551–56.

Chan MM, Huang HI, Fenton MR, Fong D. In vivo inhibition of nitric oxide synthase gene expression by curcumin, a cancer preventive natural product with anti-inflammatory properties. *Biochemical Pharmacology* 1998;15;55(12):1955–62.

Chauhan DP. Chemotherapeutic potential of curcumin for colorectal cancer. *Current Pharmaceutical Design* 2002;8(19):1695–706. Review.

Chung WY, Yow CM, Benzie IF. Assessment of membrane protection by traditional Chinese medicines using a flow cytometric technique: preliminary findings. *Redox Report* 2003;8(1):31–3.

Cohen H, Ziv Y, Cardon M, Kaplan Z, Matar MA, Gidron Y, Schwartz M, Kipnis J. Maladaptation to mental stress mitigated by the adaptive immune system via depletion of naturally occurring regulatory CD4+CD25+ cells. *Journal of Neurobiology* 2006;66(6):552–63.

Conney AH, Lysz T, Ferraro T, Abidi TF, Manchand PS, Laskin JD, Huang MT. Inhibitory effect of curcumin and some related dietary compounds on tumor promotion and arachidonic acid metabolism in mouse skin. *Advances in Enzyme Regulation* 1991;31:385–96. Review.

Consumer Reports. Cookware: Top picks in pans. December 2005. Accessed June 21, 2006, at http://www.consumerreports.org/cro/home-garden/cooking-cleaning/cookware-1205/overview/index.htm.

Cyong JA. A pharmacological study of the antiinflammatory activity of Chinese herbs—a review. *International Journal of Acupuncture Electro-Therapy Research* 1982;(7): 173–202.

D'Souza AL, Rajkumar C, Cooke J, Bulpitt CJ. Probiotics in prevention of antibiotic associated diarrhoea: meta-analysis. *BMJ* 2002;324(7350):1361.

Danielsson G, Jungbeck C, Peterson K, Norgren L. A randomised controlled trial of micronised purified flavonoid fraction vs placebo in patients with chronic venous disease. *European Journal of Vascular and Endovascular Surgery* 2002;23(1):73–6.

Delzenne N, Cherbut C, Neyrinck A. Prebiotics: actual and potential effects in inflammatory and malignant colonic diseases. *Current Opinion in Clinical Nutrition and Metabolic Care* 2003;6(5):581–86.

Deodhar SD, Sethi R, Srimal RC. Preliminary studies on antirheumatic activity of curcumin. *Indian Journal of Medical Research* 1980;71:632–34.

Dhuley JN. Anti-oxidant effects of cinnamon (*Cinnamomum verum*) bark and greater cardamom (*Amomum subulatum*) seeds in rats fed high fat diet. *Indian Journal of Experimental Biology* 1999;37(3):238–42.

Dickerson C. Neuropeptide regulation of proinflammatory cytokine responses. *Journal of Leukocyte Biology* 1998;63(5):602–5.

Dorai T, Cao YC, Dorai B, Buttyan R, Katz AE. Therapeutic potential of curcumin in human prostate cancer. III. Curcumin inhibits proliferation, induces apoptosis, and inhibits angiogenesis of LNCaP prostate cancer cells in vivo. *Prostate* 2001;47(4):293–303.

Duenas M, Sun B, Hernandez T, Estrella I, Spranger MI. Proanthocyanidin composition in the seed coat of lentils (*Lens culinaris* L.) *Journal of Agricultural and Food Chemistry* 2003;51(27):7999–8004.

Dumitrescu AL. Influence of periodontal disease on cardiovascular diseases. *Romanian Journal of Internal Medicine* 2005;43(1–2):9–21.

Duvoix A, Morceau F, Delhalle S, Schmitz M, Schnekenburger M, Galteau MM, Dicato M, Diederich M. Induction of apoptosis by curcumin: mediation by glutathione S-transferase P1-1 inhibition. *Biochemical Pharmacology* 2003;66(8): 1475–83.

Elmer GW. Probiotics: "living drugs." *American Journal of Health-System Pharmacy* 2001; 58(12):1101–9.

Environmental Working Group. Canaries in the kitchen. Accessed June 21, 2006, at http://www.ewg.org/reports/toxicteflon/cookwaretips.php.

Epel ES, Blackburn EH, Lin J, Dhabhar FS, Adler NE, Morrow JD, Cawthon RM. Accelerated telomere shortening in response to life stress. *Proceedings of the National Academy of the Sciences in the United States of America* 2004;101(49):17312–15. Epub 2004 Dec. 1.

Epel ES, Lin J, Wilhelm FH, Wolkowitz OM, Cawthon R, Adler NE, Dolbier C, Mendes WB, Blackburn EH. Cell aging in relation to stress arousal and cardiovascular disease risk factors. *Psychoneuroendocrinology* 2006;31(3):277–87.

Fernandes G, Lawrence R, Sun D. Protective role of n-3 lipids and soy protein in osteoporosis. *Prostaglandins, Leukotrienes, and Essential Fatty Acids* 2003;68(6):361–72. Review.

Fernandez-Orozco R, Zielinski H, Piskula MK. Contribution of low-molecular-weight antioxidants to the antioxidant capacity of raw and processed lentil seeds. *Die Nahrung* 2003;47(5):291–99.

Floch MH, Hong-Curtiss J. Probiotics and functional foods in gastrointestinal disorders. *Current Gastroenterology Reports* 2001;3(4):343–50.

Food and Drug Administration HHS. Code of Federal Regulations. Office of the Federal Register National Archives and Records Administration. 1991. 21CFR, 131.200 (yogurt).

Friedrich MJ. A bit of culture for children: probiotics may improve health and fight disease. *JAMA* 2000;284(11):1365–66.

Fuhrman B, Rosenblat M, Hayek T, Coleman R, Aviram M. Ginger extract consumption reduces plasma cholesterol, inhibits LDL oxidation and attenuates development of atherosclerosis in atherosclerotic, apolipoprotein E-deficient mice. *Journal of Nutrition* 2000;130(5):1124–31.

Gaon D, Garcia H, Winter L, Rodriguez N, Quintas R, Gonzalez SN, Oliver G. Effect of *Lactobacillus* strains and *Saccharomyces boulardii* on persistent diarrhea in children. *Medicina (Buenos Aires)* 2003;63(4):293–98.

Gaon D, Garmendia C, Murrielo NO, de Cucco Games A, Cerchio A, Quintas R, Gonzalez SN, Oliver G. Effect of *Lactobacillus* strains (*L. casei* and *L. Acidophillus* strains cerela) on bacterial overgrowth-related chronic diarrhea. *Medicina (Buenos Aires)* 2002;62(2):159–63.

Geil PB, Anderson JW. Nutrition and health implications of dry beans: a review. *Journal of the American College of Nutrition* 1994;13(6):549–58. Review.

Ghosh S, Playford RJ. Bioactive natural compounds for the treatment of gastrointestinal disorders. *Clinical Science (London)* 2003;104(6):547–56. Review.

Grand RJ, et al. Lactose intolerance. UpToDate Electronic Database (Version 9.2) 2001.

Guardia T, Rotelli AE, Juarez AO, Pelzer LE. Anti-inflammatory properties of plant flavonoids. Effects of rutin, quercetin and hesperidin on adjuvant arthritis in rat. *Farmaco* 2001;56(9):683–87.

Han SS, Keum YS, Chun KS, Surh YJ. Suppression of phorbol ester-induced NF-kappaB activation by capsaicin in cultured human promyelocytic leukemia cells. *Archives of Pharmacal Research* 2002;25(4):475–79.

Han SS, Keum YS, Seo HJ, Chun KS, Lee SS, Surh YJ. Capsaicin suppresses phorbol ester-induced activation of NF-kappaB/Rel and AP-1 transcription factors in mouse epidermis. *Cancer Letters* 2001;164(2):119–26.

Han SS, Keum YS, Seo HJ, Surh YJ. Curcumin suppresses activation of NF-kappaB and AP-1 induced by phorbol ester in cultured human promyelocytic leukemia cells. *Journal of Biochemistry and Molecular Biology* 2002;35(3):337–42.

Health and nutritional properties of probiotics in food including powder milk with live lactic acid bacteria—joint expert consultation of the Food and Agriculture Organization of the United Nations and the World Health Organization. Cordoba, Argentina, 1–4 October 2001 (EN). Available at http://www.who.int/foodsafety/publications/fs_management/en/probiotics.pdf.

Ho C-T, Lee CY, Huang MT. *Phenolic Compounds in Food and Their Effects on Health. I: Analysis, Occurrence, and Chemistry.* American Chemical Society Symposium Series 506. American Chemical Society, Washington, DC, 1992.

Hughes VL, Hillier SL. Microbiologic characteristics of Lactobacillus products used for colonization of the vagina. *Obstetrics and Gynecology* 1990;75:244–48.

Ihme N, Kiesewetter H, Jung F, Hoffmann KH, Birk A, Muller A, Grutzner KI. Leg oedema protection from a buckwheat herb tea in patients with chronic venous insufficiency: a single-centre, randomised, double-blind, placebo-controlled clinical trial. *European Journal of Clinical Pharmacology* 1996;50(6):443–47.

Incandela L, Belcaro G, Renton S, DeSanctis MT, Cesarone MR, Bavera P, Ippolito E, Bucci M, Griffin M, Geroulakos G, Dugall M, Golden G, Acerbi G. HR (Paroven, Venoruton; 0-(beta-hydroxyethyl)-rutosides) in venous hypertensive microangiopathy: a prospective, placebo-controlled, randomized trial. *Journal of Cardiovascular Pharmacology and Therapeutics* 2002;7(suppl 1):S7–S10.

Incandela L, Cesarone MR, DeSanctis MT, Belcaro G, Dugall M, Acerbi G. Treatment of diabetic microangiopathy and edema with HR (Paroven, Venoruton; 0-(beta-hydroxyethyl)-rutosides): a prospective, placebo-controlled, randomized study. *Journal of Cardiovascular Pharmacology and Therapeutics* 2002;7(suppl 1):S11–5.

Isolauri E. Probiotics: from anecdotes to clinical demonstration. *Journal of Allergy and Clinical Immunology* 2001;108(6):1062.

Ito K, Nakazato T, Yamato K, Miyakawa Y, Yamada T, Hozumi N, Segawa K, Ikeda Y, Kizaki M. Induction of apoptosis in leukemic cells by homovanillic acid derivative, capsaicin, through oxidative stress: implication of phosphorylation of p53 at Ser-15 residue by reactive oxygen species. *Cancer Research* 2004;64(3): 1071–78.

Jambunathan R, Singh U. Studies on desi and kabuli chickpea (*Cicer arietinum* L.) cultivars. 3. Mineral and trace element composition. *Journal of Agricultural and Food Chemistry* 1981;29(5):1091–93.

Janssen PL, Meyboom S, van Staveren WA, Vegt F, Katan MB. Consumption of ginger (*Zingiber officinale* Roscoe) does not affect ex vivo platelet thromboxane production in humans. *European Journal of Clinical Nutrition* 1996;50:772–74.

Jobin C, Bradham CA, Russo MP, Juma B, Narula AS, Brenner DA, Sartor RB. Curcumin blocks cytokine-mediated NF-kappa B activation and proinflammatory gene expression by inhibiting inhibitory factor I-kappa B kinase activity. *Journal of Immunology* 1999;163(6):3474–83.

Joe B, Lokesh BR. Effect of curcumin and capsaicin on arachidonic acid metabolism and lysosomal enzyme secretion by rat peritoneal macrophages. *Lipids* 1997; 32(11):1173–80.

Joe B, Lokesh BR. Role of capsaicin, curcumin and dietary n-3 fatty acids in lowering the generation of reactive oxygen species in rat peritoneal macrophages. *Biochimica et Biophysica Acta* 1994;1224(2):255–63.

Kale AY, Paranjape SA, Briski KP. I.c.v. administration of the nonsteroidal glucocorticoid receptor antagonist, CP-472555, prevents exacerbated hypoglycemia during repeated insulin administration. *Neuroscience* 2006;140(2):555–65.

Kan H, Onda M, Tanaka N, Furukawa K. [Effect of green tea polyphenol fraction on 1,2-dimethylhydrazine (DMH)-induced colorectal carcinogenesis in the rat]. *Nippon Ika Daigaku Zasshi* 1996;63(2):106–16. Japanese.

Kang G, Kong PJ, Yuh YJ, Lim SY, Yim SV, Chun W, Kim SS. Curcumin suppresses lipopolysaccharide-induced cyclooxygenase-2 expression by inhibiting activator protein 1 and nuclear factor kappaB bindings in BV2 microglial cells. *Journal of Pharmacological Sciences* 2004;94(3):325–28.

Kaur IP, Chopra K, Saini A. Probiotics: potential pharmaceutical applications. *European Journal of Pharmaceutical Science* 2002;15:1–9.

Kawa JM, Taylor CG, Przybylski R. Buckwheat concentrate reduces serum glucose in streptozotocin-diabetic rats. *Journal of Agricultural and Food Chemistry* 2003;51(25): 7287–91.

Keating A, Chez RA. Ginger syrup as an antiemetic in early pregnancy. *Alternative Therapies in Health and Medicine* 2002;8:89–91.

Kennedy AR. The evidence for soybean products as cancer preventive agents. *Journal of Nutrition* 1995;125:733S–43S.

Kent HL. Epidemiology of vaginitis. *American Journal of Obstetrics and Gynecology* 1991; 165:1168–76.

Kiessling G, Schneider J, Jahreis G. Long-term consumption of fermented dairy products over 6 months increases HDL cholesterol. *European Journal of Clinical Nutrition* 2002;56(9):843–49.

Kihara N, de la Fuente SG, Fujino K, Takahashi T, Pappas TN, Mantyh CR. Vanilloid receptor-1 containing primary sensory neurones mediate dextran sulphate sodium induced colitis in rats. *Gut* 2003;52(5):713–19.

Kikuzaki H, Nakatani N. Antioxidant effects of some ginger constituents. *Journal of Food Science* 1993;58:1407.

Kiuchi F, Shibuya M, Sankawa U. Inhibitors of prostaglandin biosynthesis from ginger. *Chemical & Pharmaceutical Bulletin (Tokyo)* 1982;30(2):754–57.

Kolida S, Tuohy K, Gibson GR. Prebiotic effects of inulin and oligofructose. *British Journal of Nutrition* 2002;87(suppl)2:S193–97.

Kurzer MS, Xu X. Dietary phytoestrogens. *Annual Review of Nutrition* 1997;17:353–81.

Kwak JY. A capsaicin-receptor antagonist, capsazepine, reduces inflammation-induced hyperalgesic responses in the rat: evidence for an endogenous capsaicin-like substance. *Neuroscience* 1998;86(2):619–26.

Lee YB, et al. Antioxidant property in ginger rhizome and its application to meat products. *Journal of Food Science* 1986;51(1):20–3.

Leonard BE. The HPA and immune axes in stress: the involvement of the serotonergic system. *European Psychiatry* 2005;20(suppl)3:S302–6.

Li CH, Matsui T, Matsumoto K, Yamasaki R, Kawasaki T. Latent production of angiotensin I-converting enzyme inhibitors from buckwheat protein. *Journal of Peptide Science* 2002;8(6):267–74. Review.

Li SQ, Zhang QH. Advances in the development of functional foods from buckwheat. *Critical Reviews in Food Science and Nutrition* 2001;41(6):451–64.

Liacini A, Sylvester J, Li WQ, Huang W, Dehnade F, Ahmad M, Zafarullah M. Induction of matrix metalloproteinase-13 gene expression by TNF-alpha is mediated by MAP kinases, AP-1, and NF-kappaB transcription factors in articular chondrocytes. *Experimental Cell Research* 2003;288(1):208–17.

Lien HC, Sun WM, Chen YH, Kim H, Hasler W, Owyang C. Effects of ginger on motion sickness and gastric slow-wave dysrhythmias induced by circular vection. *American Journal of Gastrointestinal and Liver Physiology* 2003;284:G481–G89.

Liepke C, Adermann K, Raida M, Magert HJ, Forssmann WG, Zucht HD. Human milk provides peptides highly stimulating the growth of bifidobacteria. *European Journal of Biochemistry* 2002;269(2):712–18.

Lim GP, Chu T, Yang F, Beech W, Frautschy SA, Cole GM. The curry spice curcumin reduces oxidative damage and amyloid pathology in an Alzheimer transgenic mouse. *Journal of Neuroscience* 2001;21(21):8370–77.

Liu N, Huo G, Zhang L, Zhang X. [Effect of *Zingiber officinale* Rosc on lipid peroxidation in hyperlipidemia rats]. *Wei Sheng Yan Jiu* 2003;32(1):22–3. Chinese.

Lu P, Lai BS, Liang P, Chen ZT, Shun SQ. [Antioxidation activity and protective effection of ginger oil on DNA damage in vitro]. *Zhongguo Zhong Yao Za Zhi* 2003; 28(9):873–75. Chinese.

Lumb AB. Effect of dried ginger on human platelet function. *Journal of Thrombosis and Haemostasis* 1994;71:110–11.

Majamaa H. Probiotics: a novel approach in the management of food allergy. *Journal of Allergy and Clinical Immunology* 1997;99(2):179–85.

Majamaa H, Isolauri E. Probiotics: a novel approach in the management of food allergy. *Journal of Allergy and Clinical Immunology* 1997;99(2):179–85.

Menne E, Guggenbuhl N, Roberfroid M. Fn-type chicory inulin hydrolysate has a prebiotic effect in humans. *Journal of Nutrition* 2000;130(5):1197–99.

Messina M, Messina V. Increasing use of soy foods and their potential role in cancer prevention. *Journal of the American Dietetic Association* 1991;91:836–40.

Messina M, Messina V. *The Simple Soybean and Your Health.* Avery Publishing Group, Garden City, NY, 1994.

Messina MJ, Persky V, Setchell KD, Barnes S. Soy intake and cancer risk: a review of the in vitro and in vivo data. *Nutrition and Cancer* 1994;21(2):113–31.

Metchnikoff E. *The Prolongation of Life: Optimistic Studies.* New York: G. P. Putnam's Sons, 1908.

Miraglia del Giudice M Jr, De Luca MG, Capristo C. Probiotics and atopic dermatitis. A new strategy in atopic dermatitis. *Digestive and Liver Disease* 2002;34(suppl 2):S68–71.

Mitchell JA. Role of nitric oxide in the dilator actions of capsaicin-sensitive nerves in the rabbit coronary circulation. *Neuropeptides* 1997;31(4):333–38.

Murosaki S, Muroyama K, Yamamoto Y, Yoshikai Y. Antitumor effect of heat-killed Lactobacillus plantarum L-137 through restoration of impaired interleukin-12 production in tumor-bearing mice. *Cancer Immunology, Immunotherapy* 2000;49(3):157–64.

Nestel P, Cehun M, Pomeroy S, Abbey M, Duo L, Weldon G. Cholesterol-lowering effects of sterol esters and non-esterified sitostanol in margarine, butter and low-fat foods. *European Journal of Cardiovascular Nursing* 2001;55:1084–90.

Nyirjesy P, Weitz MV, Grody MH, Lorber B. Over-the-counter and alternative medicines in the treatment of chronic vaginal symptoms. *Obstetrics and Gynecology* 1997;90:50–53.

Oh GS, Pae HO, Seo WG, Kim NY, Pyun KH, Kim IK, Shin M, Chung HT. Capsazepine, a vanilloid receptor antagonist, inhibits the expression of inducible nitric oxide synthase gene in lipopolysaccharide-stimulated RAW264.7 macrophages through the inactivation of nuclear transcription factor-kappa B. *International Immunopharmacology* 2001;1(4):777–84.

Ohta T, Nakatsugi S, Watanabe K, Kawamori T, Ishikawa F, Morotomi M, Sugie S, Toda T, Sugimura T, Wakabayashi K. Inhibitory effects of Bifidobacterium-fermented soy milk on 2-amino-1-methyl-6-phenylimidazo[4,5-b]pyridine-induced rat mammary carcinogenesis, with a partial contribution of its component isoflavones. *Carcinogenesis* 2000;21(5):937–41.

Onoda M, Inano H. Effect of curcumin on the production of nitric oxide by cultured rat mammary gland. *Nitric Oxide* 2000;4(5):505–15.

Ostrakhovitch EA, Afanas'ev IB. Oxidative stress in rheumatoid arthritis leukocytes:

suppression by rutin and other antioxidants and chelators. *Biochemical Pharmacology* 2001;62(6):743–46.

Pan MH, Lin-Shiau SY, Lin JK. Comparative studies on the suppression of nitric oxide synthase by curcumin and its hydrogenated metabolites through down-regulation of IkappaB kinase and NFkappaB activation in macrophages. *Biochemical Pharmacology* 20001;60(11):1665–76.

Park JM, Adam RM, Peters CA, Guthrie PD, Sun Z, Klagsbrun M, Freeman MR. AP-1 mediates stretch-induced expression of HB-EGF in bladder smooth muscle cells. *American Journal of Physiology* 1999;277(2 Pt 1):C294–301.

Patel PS, Varney ML, Dave BJ, Singh RK. Regulation of constitutive and induced NF-kappaB activation in malignant melanoma cells by capsaicin modulates interleukin-8 production and cell proliferation. *Journal of Interferon & Cytokine Research* 2002;22(4):427–35.

Petruzzellis V, Troccoli T, Candiani C, Guarisco R, Lospalluti M, Belcaro G, Dugall M. Oxerutins (Venoruton): efficacy in chronic venous insufficiency—a double-blind, randomized, controlled study. *Angiology* 2002;53(3):257–63.

Phan TT, See P, Lee ST, Chan SY. Protective effects of curcumin against oxidative damage on skin cells in vitro: its implication for wound healing. *Journal of Trauma* 2001;51(5):927–31.

Plummer SM, Holloway KA, Manson MM, Munks RJ, Kaptein A, Farrow S, Howells L. Inhibition of cyclo-oxygenase 2 expression in colon cells by the chemopreventive agent curcumin involves inhibition of NF-kappaB activation via the NIK/IKK signalling complex. *Oncogene* 1999;18(44):6013–20.

Pongrojpaw D, Chiamchanya C. The efficacy of ginger in prevention of postoperative nausea and vomiting after outpatient gynecological laparoscopy. *Journal of the Medical Association of Thailand* 2003;86:244–50.

Potter SM. Overview of proposed mechanisms for the hypocholesterolemic effect of soy. *Journal of Nutrition* 1995;125:606S–11S.

Potter SM, Bakhit RM, Essex-Sorlie DL, Weingartner KE, Chapman KM, Nelson RA, Prabhudesai M, Savage WD, Nelson AI, Winter LW. Depression of plasma cholesterol in men by consumption of baked products containing soy protein. *American Journal of Clinical Nutrition* 1993;58:501–6.

Prasad NS, Raghavendra R, Lokesh BR, Naidu KA. Spice phenolics inhibit human PMNL 5-lipoxygenase. *Prostaglandins, Leukotrienes, and Essential Fatty Acids* 2004; 70(6):521–28.

Rafter JJ. Scientific basis of biomarkers and benefits of functional foods for reduction of disease risk: cancer. *British Journal of Nutrition* 2002;88(suppl 2): S219–24.

Ramirez-Tortosa MC, Mesa MD, Aguilera MC, Quiles JL, Baro L, Ramirez-Tortosa CL, Martinez-Victoria E, Gil A. Oral administration of a turmeric extract inhibits LDL oxidation and has hypocholesterolemic effects in rabbits with experimental atherosclerosis. *Atherosclerosis* 1999;147(2):371–78.

Rao BN. Bioactive phytochemicals in Indian foods and their potential in health promotion and disease prevention. *Asia Pacific Journal of Clinical Nutrition* 2003;12(1): 9–22.

Rao CV, et al. Antioxidant activity of curcumin and related compounds. Lipid peroxide formation in experimental inflammation. *Cancer Research* 1993;55:259.

Raubenheimer PJ, Young EA, Andrew R, Seckl JR. The role of corticosterone in human hypothalamic-pituitary-adrenal axis feedback. *Clinical Endocrinology* 2006;65(1):22–6.

Rautava S, Isolauri E. The development of gut immune responses and gut microbiota: effects of probiotics in prevention and treatment of allergic disease. *Current Issues in Intestinal Microbiology* 2002;3(1):15–22.

Reid G, Bocking A. The potential for probiotics to prevent bacterial vaginosis and preterm labor. *American Journal of Obstetrics and Gynecology* 2003;189(4):1202–8.

Reid G, Howard J, Gan BS. Can bacterial interference prevent infection? *Trends in Microbiology* 2001;9(9):424–28.

Reuter G. [Probiotics—possibilities and limitations of their application in food, animal feed, and in pharmaceutical preparations for men and animals]. *Berliner und Munchener tierarztliche Wochenschrift* 2001;114(11–12):410–19. German.

Rohleder N, Schommer NC, Hellhammer DH, Engel R, Kirschbaum C. Sex differences in glucocorticoid sensitivity of proinflammatory cytokine production after psychosocial stress. *Psychosomatic Medicine* 2001;63(6):966–72.

Rolfe RD. The role of probiotic cultures in the control of gastrointestinal health. *Journal of Nutrition* 2000;130(suppl 2):396S–402S. Review.

Roos K, Hakansson EG, Holm S. Effect of recolonisation with "interfering" streptococci on recurrences of acute and secretory otitis media in children: randomised placebo controlled trial. *BMJ* 2001;322:210.

Saavedra JM, Tschernia A. Human studies with probiotics and prebiotics: clinical implications. *British Journal of Nutrition* 2002;87(suppl 2):S241–46. Review.

Saito Y. The antioxidant effects of petroleum ether soluble and insoluble fractions from spices. *Journal of the Japanese Society of Nutrition and Food Science* 1976;29:505–10.

Satoskar RR, Shah SJ, Shenoy SG. Evaluation of anti-inflammatory property of curcumin (diferuloyl methane) in patients with postoperative inflammation. *International Journal of Clinical Pharmacology, Therapy, and Toxicology* 1986;24(12):651–54.

Schiffrin EJ, Blum S. Interactions between the microbiota and the intestinal mucosa. *European Journal of Clinical Nutrition* 2002;56(suppl 3):S60–4. Review.

Schultz M, Scholmerich J, Rath HC. Rationale for probiotic and antibiotic treatment strategies in inflammatory bowel diseases. *Digestive Diseases* 2003;21(2):105–28. Review.

Schulz KH, Gold S. Psychoneuroimmunology. The relationship between stress, immune system and health. *Bundesgesundheitsblatt, Gesundheitsforschung, Gesundheitsschutz* 2006;49(8):759–72. [Epub ahead of print]

Sephton SE, Kraemer HC, Neri E, Stites DP, Weissbecker I, Spiegel D. Improving methods of assessing natural killer cell cytotoxicity. *International Journal of Methods in Psychiatric Research* 2006;15(1):12–21.

Setchell KD, Lydeking-Olsen E. Dietary phytoestrogens and their effect on bone: evidence from in vitro and in vivo, human observational, and dietary intervention studies. *American Journal of Clinical Nutrition* 2003;78(suppl 3):593S–609S. Review.

Shah BH, Nawaz Z, Pertani SA, Roomi A, Mahmood H, Saeed SA, Gilani AH. Inhibitory effect of curcumin, a food spice from turmeric, on platelet-activating factor- and arachidonic acid-mediated platelet aggregation through inhibition of thromboxane formation and Ca2+ signaling. *Biochemical Pharmacology* 1999; 58(7):1167–72.

Shalev E, Battino S, Weiner E, Colodner R, Keness Y. Ingestion of yogurt containing *Lactobacillus acidophilus* compared with pasteurized yogurt as prophylaxis for recurrent candidal vaginitis and bacterial vaginosis. *Archives of Family Medicine* 1996;5(10):593–96.

Sharma SC, Mukhtar H, Sharma SK, Krishna Murt CR. Lipid peroxide formation in experimental inflammation. *Biochemical Pharmacology* 1972;21:1210.

Shutler SM, Bircher GM, Tredger JA, Morgan LM, Walker AF, Low AG. The effect of daily baked bean (Phaseolus vulgaris) consumption on the plasma lipid levels of young, normo-cholesterolaemic men. *British Journal of Nutrition* 1989;61: 257–65.

Simpson HCR, Lousley S, Geekie M, Simpson RW, Carter RD, Hockaday TDR, Mann JI. 1981. A high carbohydrate leguminous fibre diet improves all aspects of diabetic control. *Lancet* 1981;1(8210):1–5.

Singh S, Aggarwal BB. Activation of transcription factor NF-kappa B is suppressed by curcumin (diferuloylmethane). *Journal of Biological Chemistry* 1995;270(42): 24995–5000. Erratum in: *Journal of Biological Chemistry* 1995;270(50):30235.

Singh S, Natarajan K, Aggarwal BB. Capsaicin (8-methyl-N-vanillyl-6-nonenamide) is a potent inhibitor of nuclear transcription factor-kappa B activation by diverse agents. *Journal of Immunology* 1996;157(10):4412–20.

Smith BM, Whitis SE. 1990. Dietary fiber and coronary heart disease. *Critical Reviews in Food Science and Nutrition* 29:95–147.

Sobel JD. Overview of vaginitis. UpToDate Electronic Database (Version 9.2) 2001.

Soliman KF, Mazzio EA. In vitro attenuation of nitric oxide production in C6 astrocyte cell culture by various dietary compounds. *Proceedings of the Society for Experimental Biology and Medicine* 1998;218(4):390–97.

Soni KB, Kuttan R. Effect of oral curcumin administration on serum peroxides and cholesterol levels in human volunteers. *Indian Journal of Physiology and Pharmacology* 1992;(36):273, 293.

Sreekanth KS, Sabu MC, Varghese L, Manesh C, Kuttan G, Kuttan R. Antioxidant activity of Smoke Shield in-vitro and in-vivo. *Journal of Pharmacy and Pharmacology* 2003;55(6):847–53.

Srimal R, Dhawan B. Pharmacology of diferuloyl methane (curcumin), a nonsteroidal anti-inflammatory agent. *Journal of Pharmacy and Pharmacology* 1973;(25) 447–52.

Srinivas L, Shalini VK, Shylaja M. Turmerin: a water-soluble antioxidant peptide from turmeric [*Curcuma longa*]. *Archives of Biochemistry and Biophysics* 1992;292(2):617–23.

Srivasta R, Srimal RC. Modification of certain inflammation-induced biochemical changes by curcumin. *Indian Journal of Medical Research* 1985;(81):215–23.

Srivastava KC. Effect of onion and ginger consumption on platelet thromboxane production in humans. *Prostaglandins, Leukotrienes, and Essential Fatty Acids* 1989;35: 183–85.

Srivastava KC. Effects of aqueous extracts of onion, garlic and ginger on platelet aggregation and metabolism of arachidonic acid in the blood vascular system: in vitro study. *Prostaglandins, Leukotrienes, and Medicine* 1984;13:227–35.

Srivastava KC. Isolation and effects of some ginger components on platelet aggregation and eicosanoid biosynthesis. *Prostaglandins, Leukotrienes, and Medicine* 1986; 25:187–98.

Srivastava KC, Mustafa T. Ginger (*Zingiber officinale*) and rheumatic disorders. *Medical Hypotheses* 1989;29(1):25–8.

Stavric B. Antimutagens and anticarcinogens in foods. *Food and Chemical Toxicology* 1994;32(1):79–90.

Steele MG. The effect on serum cholesterol levels of substituting milk with a soya beverage. *Austrian Journal of Nutrition and Diet* 1992;49:24–28.

Steptoe A, Brydon L. Associations between acute lipid stress responses and fasting lipid levels 3 years later. *Health Psychology* 2005;24(6):601–7.

Suekawa M, Yuasa K, Isono M, Sone H, Ikeya Y, Sakakibara I, Aburada M, Hosoya E. [Pharmacological studies on ginger. IV. Effect of (6)-shogoal on the arachidonic cascade]. *Nippon Yakurigaku Zasshi* 1986;88(4):263–69. Japanese.

Surh YJ. Anti-tumor promoting potential of selected spice ingredients with antioxidative and anti-inflammatory activities: a short review. *Food and Chemical Toxicology* 2002;40(8):109–97.

Surh YJ, Chun KS, Cha HH, Han SS, Keum YS, Park KK, Lee SS. Molecular mechanisms underlying chemopreventive activities of anti-inflammatory phytochemicals: down-regulation of COX-2 and iNOS through suppression of NF-kappa B activation. *Mutation Research* 2001;480–81:243–68. Review.

Surh YJ, Han SS, Keum YS, Seo HJ, Lee SS. Inhibitory effects of curcumin and capsaicin on phorbol ester-induced activation of eukaryotic transcription factors, NF-kappaB and AP-1. *Biofactors* 2000;12(1–4):107–12.

Susan M, Rao MNA. Induction of glutathione S-transferase activity by curcumin in mice. *Arzneimittel-Forschung* 1992;42:962.

Tannock GW. *Normal Microflora*. New York: Chapman & Hall, 1995.

Tjendraputra E, Tran VH, Liu-Brennan D, Roufogalis BD, Duke CC. Effect of ginger constituents and synthetic analogues on cyclooxygenase-2 enzyme in intact cells. *Bioorganic Chemistry* 2001;29(3):156–63.

Tosevski DL, Milovancevic MP. Stressful life events and physical health. *Current Opinion in Psychiatry* 2006;19(2):184–89.

Turmeric for treating health ailments. Invented by Van Bich Nguyen, College Park, MD. No assignee. U.S. Patent 6,048,533. Issued April 11, 2000. This patent (and U.S. Patent 5,897,865, issued April 27, 1999) covers the therapeutic use of the common spice turmeric (*Curcuma longa*) for the treatment of skin disorders such as acne, blemishes, psoriasis, dandruff, dry skin, discoloration, irritation, and sun damage.

U.S. Department of Agriculture Nutrient Data Laboratory. Accessed Aug. 13, 2006, at http://www.ars.usda.gov/main/site_main.htm?modecode=12354500.

Udani J. *Lactobacillus acidophilus* to prevent traveler's diarrhea. *Alternative Medicine Alert* 1999;2:53–5.

Uhlig T, Kallus KW. The brain: a psychoneuroimmunological approach. *Current Opinion in Anaesthesiology* 2005;18(2):147–50.

Van Kessel K, Assefi N, Marrazzo J, Eckert L. Common complementary and alternative therapies for yeast vaginitis and bacterial vaginosis: a systematic review. *Obstetrical & Gynecological Survey* 2003;58(5):351–58. Review.

Vanderhoof VA. Probiotics: future directions. *American Journal of Clinical Nutrition* 2001; 73:1152S–55S.

Vitaliano PP, Persson R, Kiyak A, Saini H, Echeverria D. Caregiving and gingival symptom reports: psychophysiologic mediators. *Psychosomatic Medicine* 2005;67(6): 930–38.

Walling A. Therapeutic modulation of the psychoneuroimmune system by medical acupuncture creates enhanced feelings of well-being. *Journal of the American Academy of Nurse Practitioners* 2006;18(4):135–43. Review.

Wang CC, Chen LG, Lee LT, Yang LL. Effects of 6-gingerol, an antioxidant from ginger, on inducing apoptosis in human leukemic HL-60 cells. *In Vivo* 2003;17(6): 641–45.

Weisburger JH. Tea and health: the underlying mechanisms. *Proceedings of the Society for Experimental Biology and Medicine* 1999;220(4):271–75. Review.

Wood JR, et al. In vitro adherence of *Lactobacillus* species to vaginal epithelial cells. *American Journal of Obstetrics and Gynecology* 1985;153:740–43.

Zeneb MB, et al. Dairy (yogurt) augments fat loss and reduces central adiposity during energy restriction in obese subjects. *FASEB Journal* 2003;17(5):A1088.

Zhang J, Nagasaki M, Tanaka Y, Morikawa S. Capsaicin inhibits growth of adult T-cell leukemia cells. *Leukemia Research* 2003;27(3):275–83.

Index

About the Author

NICHOLAS PERRICONE, M.D., is the #1 *New York Times* best-selling author of *The Perricone Weight-Loss Diet, The Wrinkle Cure, The Perricone Prescription,* and *The Perricone Promise.* He is a board certified dermatologist, award-winning inventor, research scientist, and internationally renowned anti-aging expert. He is the focus of a series of award-winning PBS specials, and a popular guest on *Oprah, Today, 20/20, Good Morning America,* and *Larry King Live,* among other programs. He is currently adjunct professor of medicine at Michigan State University's College of Human Medicine. Visit the author's website at *www.nvperriconemd.com.*